Clinical Case Studies in Hematology

Clinical Case Studies in Hematology

Editor: Fiona Rogers

AMERICAN
MEDICAL PUBLISHERS
www.americanmedicalpublishers.com

AMERICAN
MEDICAL PUBLISHERS
www.americanmedicalpublishers.com

Cataloging-in-Publication Data

Clinical case studies in hematology / edited by Fiona Rogers.
p. cm.
Includes bibliographical references and index.
ISBN 979-8-88740-624-4
1. Hematology. 2. Blood--Diseases. 3. Internal medicine. I. Rogers, Fiona.
RC633 .H36 2023
616.15--dc23

American Medical Publishers,
41 Flatbush Avenue,
1st Floor, New York,
NY 11217, USA

ISBN 979-8-88740-624-4 (Hardback)

Contents

Preface

Over the recent decade, advancements and applications have progressed exponentially. This has led to the increased interest in this field and projects are being conducted to enhance knowledge. The main objective of this book is to present some of the critical challenges and provide insights into possible solutions. This book will answer the varied questions that arise in the field and also provide an increased scope for furthering studies.

Hematology is the study of blood and blood disorders. It encompasses a wide range of topics including the physiology of blood cells, the mechanisms of blood clotting, and the diagnosis and treatment of various blood diseases. Hematology plays a vital role in healthcare as it involves the evaluation and management of conditions such as anemia, leukemia, lymphoma and bleeding disorders. It uses a variety of diagnostic tools, including blood tests, bone marrow biopsies and imaging studies to diagnose and treat these conditions. Treatment options may include medications, blood transfusions, bone marrow transplants, or chemotherapy. This book is a compilation of chapters that discuss the most vital concepts and emerging trends in the field of hematology. It will serve as a reference to a broad spectrum of readers.

I hope that this book, with its visionary approach, will be a valuable addition and will promote interest among readers. Each of the authors has provided their extraordinary competence in their specific fields by providing different perspectives as they come from diverse nations and regions. I thank them for their contributions.

Editor

1

The First Case of E-Cigarette-Induced Polycythemia

Marika Okuni-Watanabe,[1] Keiji Kurata,[1,2] and Kimikazu Yakushijin[1,2]

[1]Department of Hematology, Kobe City Medical Center West Hospital, 2-4, Ichiban-cho, Nagata-ku, Kobe City, Hyogo 653-0013, Japan
[2]Department of Medical Oncology and Hematology, Kobe University Hospital, 7-5-2, Kusunoki-cho, Chuo-ku, Kobe City, Hyogo 650-0017, Japan

Correspondence should be addressed to Kimikazu Yakushijin; kyakushi@med.kobe-u.ac.jp

Academic Editor: Dennis Galanakis

A 71-year-old male smoker was referred to our hospital because of increased hemoglobin and hematocrit. At initial consultation, his hemoglobin and hematocrit levels were 21.8 g/dl and 64.8%, respectively. Other laboratory data and his cardiopulmonary functions were almost normal, and JAK2 V617F mutation was negative. He had smoked about 25 cigarettes per day for 50 years until the age of 70, when he switched from conventional smoking to electronic cigarettes (e-cigarettes). We requested that he quit e-cigarette use. Thereafter, his hemoglobin and hematocrit gradually decreased and normalized. Here, we report the first case of e-cigarette-induced polycythemia.

1. Introduction

Recently, the development of science and technology has been remarkable, with such innovations as the smartphone, tablet computer, electronic money, and virtual reality. These advances successfully enrich our lives; however, they might have unprecedented adverse effects, such as "computer vision syndrome," which causes users pain in their heads, necks, or shoulders and dry eye syndrome [1].

The electronic cigarette (e-cigarette) is one new invention developed with recent technology; it does not use fire, and is believed to be less hazardous than conventional tobacco. E-cigarettes are battery-operated devices that heat an e-liquid and produce aerosol that the users inhale, while conventional tobacco produces smoke by burning tobacco leaves [2]. E-cigarettes create the simulation of smoking, which can help users to reduce conventional tobacco consumption as they switch from conventional cigarettes to e-cigarettes [3]. It is also known that conventional tobacco may cause many kinds of diseases, one of which is polycythemia [4]; however, there have not yet been any reports on the relationship between e-cigarettes and polycythemia. Here, we report on the first case of e-cigarette-induced polycythemia.

2. Case Report

A 71-year-old male smoker was referred to our hospital because of increased hemoglobin and hematocrit. The laboratory data are shown in Table 1. At initial consultation, his hemoglobin and hematocrit levels were 21.8 g/dl and 64.8%, respectively. Eight years earlier, they had been 15.0 g/dl and 43%, respectively. Other laboratory data and his cardiopulmonary functions were approximately normal. Janus kinase 2 (JAK2 V617F) mutation was negative, and erythropoietin was not suppressed. A computed tomography scan revealed no malignancy in his entire body. He had smoked about 25 cigarettes per day for 50 years until he was 70 years old and switched from conventional smoking to e-cigarettes (electronic nonnicotine delivery system, approximately 40 puffs per day) one year before visiting our hospital.

Speculating about secondary polycythemia, we requested that he quit e-cigarette use. One month later, his hemoglobin and hematocrit had gradually decreased and normalized, as shown in Figure 1. He was diagnosed with e-cigarette-induced polycythemia. Written informed consent for this manuscript was obtained from this patient.

Table 1: Laboratory data.

WBC	5500	/μL
Neutrophils	44	%
Monocytes	7.5	%
Lymphocytes	46	%
Eosinophils	1.5	%
Basophils	0.5	%
Atypical lymphocytes	0.5	%
RBC	705×10^4	/μL
Hb	21.8	g/dL
Ht	64.8	%
Ret	12.9	‰
Plt	11.1×10^4	/μL
APTT	27.2	sec
PT-INR	1.06	
D-dimer	<1.0	mg/mL
TP	8.06	g/dL
Alb	4.96	g/dL
T-Bil	0.9	mg/dL
AST	39	U/L
ALT	27	U/L
LDH	224	U/L
γ-GTP	45	U/L
CK	65	U/L
BUN	12	mg/dL
Cre	0.67	mg/dL
eGFR	88.5	mL/min/1.73m^2
Na	143	mEq/L
K	4.1	mEq/L
Cl	102	mEq/L
CRP	0.12	mg/dL
Ferritin	233	ng/mL
CEA	3.9	ng/mL
AFP	1.5	ng/mL
CA19-9	5.7	U/mL
Erythropoietin	11.4	mIU/mL
IgG	1382	mg/dL
IgA	227	mg/dL
IgM	162	mg/dL
BNP	24.0	pg/mL
JAK2 V617F mutation	Negative	

3. Discussion

To the best of our knowledge, this is the first report of e-cigarette-induced polycythemia diagnosed by quitting e-cigarette. These days, e-cigarettes have been increasingly popular among smokers who want to stop smoking. As Hajek et al. reported that e-cigarettes could help smokers to quit or reduce tobacco better rather than nicotine replacement therapy [3], their use is likely to increase in the near future. There are hundreds of e-cigarette devices and thousands of e-liquids available globally today, and every e-liquid contains a variety of components and flavors. Therefore, we cannot easily compare various e-cigarettes and do not know much about their safety. However, based on this case, we have doubts about whether e-cigarette use is truly safe.

No research to date has indicated that e-cigarettes cause polycythemia. In this case, polycythemia was thought to be associated with e-cigarette smoking because the patient's hemoglobin and hematocrit levels decreased after quitting e-cigarette smoking. In conventional tobacco cases, carbon monoxide in cigarettes is known to combine with hemoglobin and inhibit hemoglobin from combining with oxygen, which leads to the secretion of erythropoietin and an increase in hemoglobin to compensate for hypoxia. However, it is unclear how e-cigarette use might cause polycythemia, and certain e-cigarettes might involve some carbon monoxide as in a conventional tobacco dose; we speculate that compounds that are only found in e-cigarettes might cause polycythemia because our patient had smoked for decades without polycythemia. It is known that e-cigarettes contain some metals, such as nickel, cadmium, and copper, to some degree [2]. Goldberg et al. suggest that cobalt chloride and nickel chloride seem to stimulate erythropoietin production through the heme protein, which is integrally involved in the oxygen-sensing mechanism using the human hepatoma cell line Hep3B, based on a report that rats with renal-injected nickel showed polycythemia, and nickel could be said to be associated with erythropoietin activity [5]. Thus, Goldberg and colleagues proposed the following hypothesis: cobalt and nickel could be substituted for ferrous iron in the porphyrin ring; however, cobalt hemoglobin binds oxygen with low affinity and nickel hemoglobin is unable to bind oxygen at all. Because of this, the substituted heme protein is locked in the deoxy conformation, mimicking stimulation of deoxygenated heme protein, which stimulates erythropoietin production [5]. Although we did not measure these metals in our patient, we speculate that some of them could be the cause of polycythemia in this case.

Polycythemia is a common disease in the hematology division. While polycythemia vera is known to be the cause of serious thrombosis, it is uncertain whether secondary polycythemia might increase the risk of thrombosis. However, as is it has been reported that secondary polycythemia might cause critical infarction or thrombosis [6–8], it is important to pay attention to e-cigarette smokers' polycythemia.

To date, there have been some reports of e-cigarette-related respiratory disorders, including eosinophilic pneumonitis [9], organizing pneumonia [10], hypersensitive pneumonitis [11], and acute respiratory distress syndrome [12]. Moreover, some researchers doubt the long-term safety of e-cigarettes. Recently, Layden et al. reported 53 cases with pulmonary illness related to e-cigarette use in two states in America [13]. They concluded that e-cigarettes should never be used by youths, young adults, pregnant women, or adults who do not currently use tobacco products although the pathophysiology and definitive causes have not yet been identified [13]. Moreover, Canistro et al. reported that e-cigarettes can raise the risk of cancer [14]. Thus, e-cigarettes might be more harmful than has been believed.

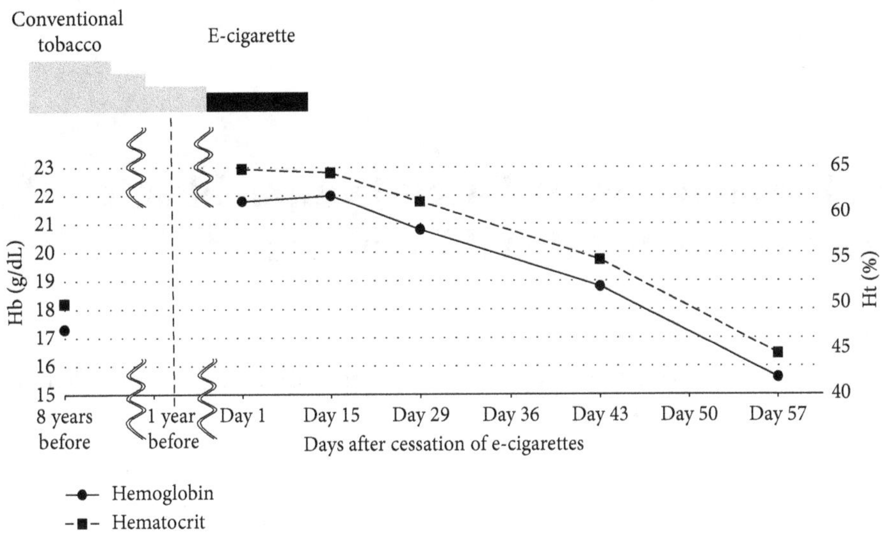

FIGURE 1: Clinical course. One month after quitting e-cigarette use, his hemoglobin and hematocrit gradually decreased and normalized on day 57.

In conclusion, we experienced the first case of "e-cigarette-induced polycythemia," which was directly clarified by complete hematological improvement after cessation of e-cigarette use. Although new products are generally convenient for human beings, we should reconsider what we are willing to accept from diversified viewpoints.

References

[1] S. Munshi, A. Varghese, and S. Dhar-Munshi, "Computer vision syndrome-a common cause of unexplained visual symptoms in the modern era," *International Journal of Clinical Practice*, vol. 71, no. 7, Article ID e12962, 2017.

[2] A. Bhatnagar, L. P. Whitsel, K. M. Ribisl et al., "Electronic cigarettes: a policy statement from the American Heart Association," *Circulation*, vol. 130, no. 16, pp. 1418–1436, 2014.

[3] P. Hajek, A. Phillips-Waller, D. Przulj et al., "A randomized trial of e-cigarettes versus nicotine-replacement therapy," *New England Journal of Medicine*, vol. 380, no. 7, pp. 629–637, 2019.

[4] J. R. Smith and S. A. Landaw, "Smokers' polycythemia," *New England Journal of Medicine*, vol. 298, no. 1, pp. 6–10, 1978.

[5] M. A. Goldberg, S. P. Dunning, and H. F. Bunn, "Regulation of the erythropoietin gene: evidence that the oxygen sensor is a heme protein," *Science*, vol. 242, no. 4884, pp. 1412-1415, 1988.

[6] P. Grant, P. Patel, and S. Singh, "Acute myocardial infarction secondary to polycythaemia in a case of cyanotic congenital heart disease," *International Journal of Cardiology*, vol. 9, no. 1, pp. 108–110, 1985.

[7] Y. Kobayashi, Y. Kobayashi, and A. Hirohata, "Left main coronary thrombotic occlusion due to secondary polycythemia in a normal sinus of valsalva," *The Journal of Invasive Cardiology*, vol. 25, no. 8, pp. 421-422, 2013.

[8] A. R. H. Sandoval, B. J. F. Robles, R. F. Andrus, and D. A. Y. Chon, "Transient ischaemic attack secondary to paraneoplastic erythrocytosis," *BMJ Case Reports*, vol. 2014, Article ID bcr2013202572, 2014.

[9] D. Thota and E. Latham, "Case report of electronic cigarettes possibly associated with eosinophilic pneumonitis in a previously healthy active-duty sailor," *The Journal of Emergency Medicine*, vol. 47, no. 1, pp. 15–17, 2014.

[10] M. S. Khan, F. Khateeb, J. Akhtar et al., "Organizing pneumonia related to electronic cigarette use: a case report and review of literature," *The Clinical Respiratory Journal*, vol. 12, no. 3, pp. 1295–1299, 2018.

[11] C. G. Sommerfeld, D. J. Weiner, A. Nowalk, and A. Larkin, "Hypersensitivity pneumonitis and acute respiratory distress syndrome from e-cigarette use," *Pediatrics*, vol. 141, no. 6, Article ID e20163927, 2018.

[12] Z. L. Arter, A. Wiggins, C. Hudspath, A. Kisling, D. C. Hostler, and J. M. Hostler, "Acute eosinophilic pneumonia following electronic cigarette use," *Respiratory Medicine Case Reports*, vol. 27, Article ID 100825, 2019.

[13] J. E. Layden, I. Ghinai, I. Pray et al., "Pulmonary illness related to e-cigarette use in Illinois and Wisconsin—preliminary report," *New England Journal of Medicine*, 2019.

[14] D. Canistro, F. Vivarelli, S. Cirillo et al., "E-cigarettes induce toxicological effects that can raise the cancer risk," *Scientific Reports*, vol. 7, no. 1, p. 2028, 2017.

An Unusual Presentation of T-Cell Lymphoblastic Lymphoma with Isolated Renal Involvement

Sultan Aydın Köker,[1] Alper Koker,[2] Adem Yasin Köksoy,[3] Yasemin Kayadibi,[4] Ülkü Gül Şiraz,[3] and Emine Tekin[3]

[1]*Department of Pediatric Hematology and Oncology, SBÜ Van Education and Research Hospital, Van, Turkey*
[2]*Department of Pediatric Intensive Care, Hatay State Hospital, Antakya, Hatay, Turkey*
[3]*Department of Pediatrics, SBÜ Van Education and Research Hospital, Van, Turkey*
[4]*Department of Radiology, SBÜ Van Education and Research Hospital, Van, Turkey*

Correspondence should be addressed to Alper Koker; kokeralper@gmail.com

Academic Editor: Vincent Ribrag

The clinical presentation of Non-Hodgkin lymphoma (NHL) is frequently associated with the involvement of the abdomen and mediastinal lymphadenopathies, but rarely the kidney, ovaries, and testicles. Here, we report a rare case of T-cell lymphoblastic lymphoma (T-LBL) presenting with bilateral nephromegaly without acute renal failure (ARF) as the first manifestation. A 30-month-old boy was admitted to the department of pediatric nephrology exhibiting abdominal distension. Physical examination revealed bilateral renal palpation up to the inguinal region. Elevated lactate dehydrogenase (LDH) levels were detected in his blood. Bilateral diffuse enlarged kidneys with increased hypoechogenicity were found on abdominal ultrasonography. In the next step, contrast-enhanced computed tomography showed diffusely enlarged kidneys, which were compressing the intestinal bowels and midline structures. Renal biopsy demonstrated precursor T-LBL. We wish to report our patient with renal T-LBL presenting with diffuse renal enlargement, which has rarely been reported in the literature.

1. Introduction

Non-Hodgkin lymphoma (NHL) is the fifth most common childhood malignancy in children under the age of 15 years, and it accounts for nearly 7% of childhood cancers in developed countries [1]. The median age at diagnosis is approximately ten years, and the incidence increases with age [1]. T-cell lymphoblastic lymphoma (T-LBL) comprises approximately 20% of NHL cases in childhood [2]. Clinically, 75% of patients with T-LBL present with an anterior mediastinal mass, and it may present with lymph node involvement [3]. Primary renal lymphoma (PRL) is described as an NHL involving the kidneys. PRL is very rare (1%) [4]. In the literature, about 70 cases of PRL have been defined, and the large B-cell type comprises the majority of cases [5].

Here, we report a rare case of precursor T-LBL presenting with bilaterally enlarged kidneys and isolated bilateral renal involvement without tumor lysis syndrome or acute renal failure (ARF).

2. Case Report

A 30-month-old, previously healthy male was admitted to the pediatric nephrology department presenting with abdominal distension. Upon physical examination, bilateral renal palpation up to the inguinal region was identified. The chest X-ray did not show a significantly enlarged mediastinum. Abdominal ultrasonography revealed diffuse bilateral renal enlargement. The echogenicity of the kidneys was also decreased and heterogeneous, while the normal bean-shape of the kidneys was preserved and there was no discrete mass formation. Hematological analysis revealed that the patient had a hemoglobin level of 14.7 g/dL, a white blood cell count of 8780 /mm^3, and a platelet count of 3.6×10^9/L. Serum levels of lactate dehydrogenase (LDH) and uric acid were

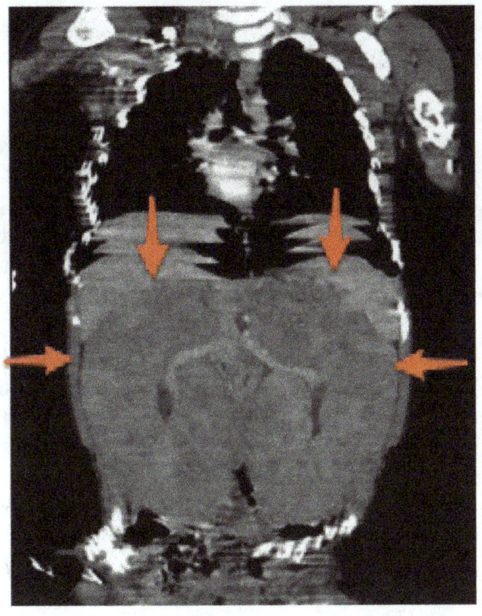

Figure 1: Coronal CT image shows bilaterally enlarged kidneys with decreased enhancement. Enhanced patchy parts are normal renal parenchyma; note the small size of normal parenchyma. Typical for diffuse lymphoma involvement, bilateral kidneys retain their normal bean-like shape.

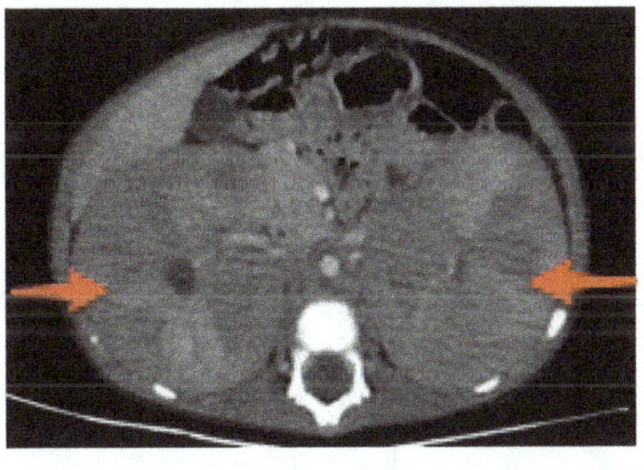

Figure 2: Axial CT image shows diffusely enlarged kidneys. Intestinal bowels and liver are compressed anteriorly.

increased to 1376 U/L and 6 mg/dL, respectively. Additional laboratory findings were normal. Contrast-enhanced computed tomography (CT) scanning showed normally shaped, but diffusely infiltrated kidneys with no normal renal parenchyma. The midline structures, liver, and spleen were also compressed (Figures 1 and 2). Bone marrow biopsy did not detect bone marrow involvement. Our patient was referred to another center for renal biopsy. A diagnostic renal biopsy was performed. The pathological results showed the presence of T-cell lymphoblastic lymphoma, with CD4−/CD8+ phenotype. Immunohistochemistry staining was positive for CD3, CD5, CD7, CD8, and CD1a and negative for CD20, CD79a, CD4, CD10, TdT, and CD99.

On the pediatric tumor committee, NHL-BFM 95 protocol is decided for the chemotherapy regimen [6]. Laboratory findings at the beginning of the treatment were potassium: 4.8 mEq/L, calcium: 9.2 mg/dL, and phosphorus: 3.3 mg/dL. Hyperuricemia, hyperkalemia, hyperphosphatemia, and hypocalcemia occurred on the fifth day of treatment. He had seizures three times, and arrhythmia appeared. After the hydration, urinary alkalinization, and allopurinol treatment started, rasburicase was added. Arrhythmia persisted. Because oliguria and renal failure developed, renal replacement therapy was begun. He died on the eighth day of chemotherapy due to sudden cardiac arrest and acute tumor lysis syndrome.

3. Discussion

Lymphomas, which account for approximately 60–70% of adult NHL, form less than 5% of the total childhood NHL. While approximately 55% of all cases with pediatric NHL have B-cell phenotype, 15–20% of them have T-LBL. The majority of children with T-LBL (50–70%) present with rapidly enlarging neck and mediastinal lymphadenopathy. Symptoms often include cough, wheezing, shortness of breath, and orthopnea, though swelling of the neck and face and superior vena cava syndrome can occur due to mediastinal involvement. However, patients can also present with extranodal involvement, including bone, testicles, skin, pancreas, and kidneys [2, 3]. The occurrence of primary renal lymphoma (PRL) is infrequent [7]. Most cases of PRL are of the B-cell type, and only a few cases were reported with the T-cell lineage [5]. Our patient had bilaterally enlarged kidneys. The most interesting aspect of our case is that primary renal involvement was the first presenting symptom of T-LBL. T-LBL occurs more commonly in males. Our patient was a male, in keeping with the literature. The incidence is stable across all pediatric age groups with a median age at diagnosis of 12 years [3]. Thus, our patient was very young according to the literature.

LDH can alter pyruvate to lactate. An increased LDH level suggests more severe tumor progression, tumor angiogenesis, and tumor burden in malignancy [8]. Serum LDH levels may be used in daily clinical practice. Elevated LDH may be a good indicator of cancer in cases like ours with diffuse renal infiltration and bilaterally enlarged kidneys.

For patients with suspected findings, CT is the most sensitive radiological modality, and it can be used for diagnosis, detection of extrarenal extension, staging, and follow-up. Renal lymphoid involvement can be seen as single or multiple masses, an extension of retroperitoneal disease, perirenal disease, or diffuse renal involvement. Preservation of renal shape in the infiltrative form could create challenges for the diagnosis [9]. Our patient had diffuse renal involvement.

The exploration of extranodal sites or excisional node biopsy is commonly performed for diagnosis. Immunohistochemical studies are also required to diagnose T-LBL. T-LBL is confirmed when lineage markers for B-cells (CD20) and NK cells (CD56) are negative and those for precursor T-cells (CD3 and CD5) are positive [10]. T-LBL was detected as a result of biopsy in our case because TdT and T-cell markers (CD3) were positive based on immunohistochemical analysis of tumor cells.

In a study of the German BFM group, the 5-year event-free survival was estimated at 90% among children who were given an ALL-type chemotherapy regimen [11]. Moreover, systemic chemotherapy can use a CHOP regimen for treatment. Median survival is usually <1 year [12], but the addition of rituximab to the combination chemotherapy has improved the survival rate [13]. Because patients with T-LBL have poorer outcomes despite this chemotherapy regimen and it is hard to fight tumor lysis syndrome and renal failure at the same time, our patient died on the eighth day of the NHL-BFM 95 protocol.

The clinical presentation of our patient with bilaterally enlarged kidneys, diffuse renal infiltration, and elevated LDH suggested a diagnosis of isolated renal involvement of lymphoma. Histopathological examination of the renal biopsy with immunohistochemical study determined the diagnosis of T-LBL. Biopsy and histopathology are essential for a definite diagnosis of lymphoma. We wished to report our case of T-LBL presenting with rare renal involvement.

Authors' Contributions

Sultan Aydın Köker formulated the research idea and study design; data acquisition was performed by Adem Yasin Köksoy; data analysis/interpretation was performed by Sultan Aydın Köker and Ülkü Gül Şiraz; statistical analysis was conducted by Yasemin Kayadibi and Emine Tekin; and Alper Koker was involved in supervision or mentorship.

References

[1] P. Kaatsch, "Epidemiology of childhood cancer," *Cancer Treatment Reviews*, vol. 36, no. 4, pp. 277–285, 2010.

[2] C. L. Percy, M. A. Smith, M. Linet et al., "Lymphomas and reticuloendothelial neoplasms," in *Cancer Incidence and Survival among Children and Adolescents: United States SEER Program 1975–1995*, L. A. G. Ries, M. A. Smith, J. G. Gurney et al., Eds., pp. 35–50, National Cancer Institute, Bethesda, MA, USA, 1999.

[3] S. Cortelazzo, M. Ponzoni, A. J. M. Ferreri, and D. Hoelzer, "Lymphoblastic lymphoma," *Critical Reviews in Oncology/Hematology*, vol. 79, no. 3, pp. 330–343, 2011.

[4] F. Barreto, M. F. Dall'Oglio, and M. Srougi, "Renal lymphoma: atypical presentation of a renal tumor," *International Brazilian Journal of Urology*, vol. 32, no. 2, pp. 190–192, 2006.

[5] R. Belbaraka, S. Boutayeb, M. Elyoubi, and H. Errihani, "Primary renal non-Hodgkin lymphoma: an unusual diagnosis for a renal mass," *Indian Journal of Cancer*, vol. 48, no. 2, pp. 255-256, 2011.

[6] W. Woessmann, K. Seidemann, G. Mann et al., "The impact of the methotrexate administration schedule and dose in the treatment of children and adolescents with B-cell neoplasms: a report of the BFM group study NHL-BFM95," *Blood*, vol. 105, no. 3, pp. 948–958, 2005.

[7] E. Paganelli, L. Arisi, M. E. Ferrari, G. Olivetti, and F. Tedeschi, "Primary non-Hodgkin's lymphoma of the kidney," *Haematologica*, vol. 74, pp. 301–304, 1989.

[8] Y. Kolev, H. Uetake, Y. Takagi, and K. Sugihara, "Lactate dehydrogenase-5 (LDH-5) expression in human gastric cancer: association with hypoxia-inducible factor (HIF-1α) pathway, angiogenic factors production and poor prognosis," *Annals of Surgical Oncology*, vol. 15, no. 8, pp. 2336–2344, 2008.

[9] B. A. Urban and E. K. Fishman, "Renal lymphoma: CT patterns with emphasis on helical CT," *Radiographics*, vol. 20, no. 1, pp. 197–212, 2000.

[10] S. H. Swerdlow, E. Campo, N. L. Harris et al., *World Health Organization Classification of Tumours of Haematopoietic and Lymphoid Tissues*, IARC Press, Lyon, France, 2008.

[11] A. Reiter, M. Schrappe, W. D. Ludwig et al., "Intensive ALL-type therapy without local radiotherapy provides a 90% event-free survival for children with T-cell lymphoblastic lymphoma: a BFM group report," *Blood*, vol. 95, no. 2, pp. 416–421, 2000.

[12] Y. Yasunaga, Y. Hoshida, M. Hashimoto, T. Miki, A. Okuyama, and K. Aozasa, "Malignant lymphoma of the kidney," *Journal of Surgical Oncology*, vol. 64, no. 3, pp. 207–211, 1997.

[13] L. Sellin, C. Friedl, G. Klein, R. Waldherr, L. C. Rump, and S. M. Weiner, "Acute renal failure due to a malignant lymphoma infiltration uncovered by renal biopsy," *Nephrology Dialysis Transplantation*, vol. 19, no. 10, pp. 2657–2660, 2004.

3

Bone Marrow Infiltration in Rosai–Dorfman Disease

Fatima Zahra Rahali[1,2] **Fatima Taher,**[2,3] **Houda Nassih**[2,3] **and Sanae Sayagh**[1,2]

[1]*Hematology Laboratory, University Hospital Centre Mohammed VI, Marrakesh, Morocco*
[2]*Faculty of Medicine and Pharmacy, Marrakesh, Morocco*
[3]*Department of Pediatrics, University Hospital Centre Mohammed VI, Marrakesh, Morocco*

Correspondence should be addressed to Fatima Zahra Rahali; fatimazahra.rahali@edu.uca.ac.ma

Academic Editor: Pier Paolo Piccaluga

Rosai–Dorfman disease (RDD) is a rare and benign nonLangerhans cell histiocytosis. RDD commonly affects children and young adults typically presenting with massive, painless, and bilateral cervical lymphadenopathy. Extranodal involvement is present in about 40% of cases, and bone marrow infiltration is rare and unusual. RDD prognosis is usually good, however, involvement of bone marrow is associated with poor prognosis. We report a case of RDD with bone marrow involvement occurring in a 5-year-old female. She was admitted for asthenia, gingival bleeding, and diffuse bone pain without fever. Physical examination showed pallor, petechiae over the abdomen, painless and bilateral cervical lymphadenopathy, and several bony nodules, without splenomegaly or hepatomegaly. Cell blood count revealed microcytic hypochromic anemia with thrombocytopenia. Bone marrow aspiration showed infiltration by large histiocytes with hypochromatic nuclei and abundant vacuolated cytoplasm without emperipolesis. Biopsies of bone marrow, lymph node, and bone revealed immunohistochemical features of RDD: the histiocytes were positive for CD68 and S100 protein, but negative for CD1a. The patient initially received symptomatic treatment. One week after admission, she died of septic shock before the final establishment of RDD diagnosis. This case report highlights that bone marrow involvement in RDD is rare and associated with poor prognosis. We also aim to emphasize the obligation of bone marrow exploration in patients with RDD and presenting cytopenias in order to make an early diagnosis of bone marrow infiltration.

1. Introduction

Rosai–Dorfman disease (RDD) is a rare and benign non-Langerhans cell histiocytosis [1–3]. The pathophysiology of this disorder is poorly understood [4]. According to the 2016 revised histiocytosis classification, RDD belongs to the "R Group" of histiocytosis which includes familial and sporadic RDD, while cutaneous RDD belongs to the "C Group" of histiocytosis [5]. RDD affects habitually children and young adults presenting with bilateral, painless cervical lymphadenopathy [4]. Extranodal involvement is present in about 40% of cases [4]. Bone marrow infiltration, as an extranodal manifestation, is rare and associated with poor prognosis [6, 7].

We report here a case of RDD with bone marrow involvement in a 5-year-old child. Through this case report, we aim to emphasize the importance of bone marrow exploration in patients with RDD and presenting cytopenias.

2. Case Presentation

A 5-year-old female from nonconsanguineous marriage, with a medical history of snoring without sleep apnea, had presented asthenia, gingival bleeding, and diffuse bone pain evolving for three months, without associated fever. Before admission to our hospital, the patient had visited a general practitioner who ordered blood tests. Initial cell blood count showed bicytopenia (microcytic hypochromic anemia at 10.1 g/dL and thrombocytopenia at 100 G/L) with low reticulocytes at $70250/mm^3$. The patient was referred to the hospital for further investigations. Physical examination showed pallor, gingival hypertrophy, and petechiae over the abdomen. Palpation revealed painless and bilateral cervical lymphadenopathy, without splenomegaly or hepatomegaly. The skeletal examination showed several bony nodules on the forehead, mandible, wrists, and knees.

Cell blood count revealed microcytic hypochromic anemia (hemoglobin = 10.4 g/dL; MCV = 77.4 fL; MCHC = 26.1 pg), thrombocytopenia (platelet count = 84 G/L), and normal white blood cell count at 4.56 G/L (neutrophils = 3.11 G/L; lymphocytes = 1.2 G/L). The erythrocyte sedimentation rate was elevated at 57 mm/hour. Biochemical parameters objectified hyperferritinemia at 241 ng/mL and a high level of lactate dehydrogenase at 688 U/L.

Peripheral blood smear showed anisopoikilocytosis with mild hypochromia, without platelet clumping. Bone marrow aspiration was normocellular with the absence of megakaryocytes. It was infiltrated by 31% of large histiocytes with hypochromatic nuclei and abundant vacuolated cytoplasm, without emperipolesis (Figure 1). An infiltration by mature histiocytic cells was also observed in bone marrow, lymph nodes, and bone biopsies (Figure 2). Immunohistochemically, the histiocytes were positive for CD68 and S100 protein but negative for CD1a (Figure 3). A diagnosis of RDD involving bone marrow and bones was made. No concurrent malignancy was detected. Lymph node tuberculosis was ruled out because there was no histological evidence. Antinuclear antibodies, anti-DNA antibodies, and rheumatoid factor were absent, which ruled out an associated autoimmune disease. Serological tests for hepatitis B and C, syphilis, and cytomegalovirus were negative.

Neck ultrasound confirmed the presence of bilateral cervical lymphadenopathies. Chest and neck CT scan revealed bilateral lytic bone lesion involving both scapulas and bilateral cervical lymphadenopathies.

The patient has first received analgesics as a symptomatic treatment. On day 6 of admission, the patient's clinical course was deteriorated. She presented signs of septic shock: fever at 40°, hypotension with increased C reactive protein at 47 mg/L. The patient was transferred to the pediatric intensive care unit for appropriate management. Empirical antibiotic therapy was initiated (imipenem + vancomycin). However, the blood culture was negative without any microbiological evidence. The patient died one week after admission to the hospital before the final establishment of RDD diagnosis.

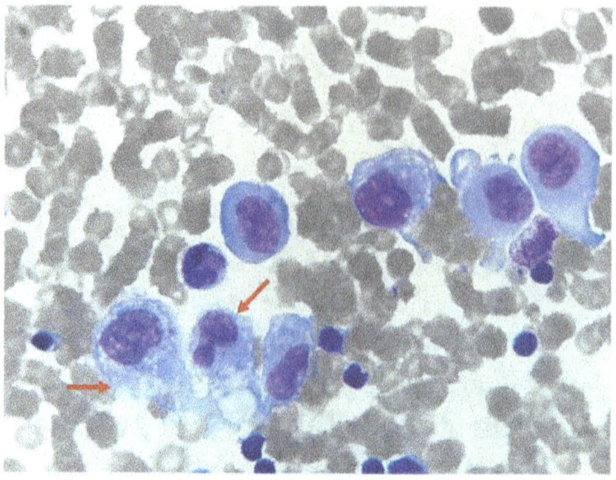

Figure 1: Bone marrow aspiration at high magnification ×100 showing bone marrow infiltration by histiocytic cells. Large histiocytes with hypochromatic nuclei and abundant vacuolated cytoplasm (arrow).

3. Discussion

Histiocytosis is a heterogeneous group of rare diseases distinguished by the accumulation of cells derived from macrophages or dendritic cells in diverse tissues and organs of children and adults [5, 8]. RDD is a rare and benign histiocytic disorder first described in 1965 by Destombes [1]. In 1969, Rosai and Dorfman described the same entity as "sinus histiocytosis with massive lymphadenopathy" [2]. In 1987, the Histiocyte Society classified RDD as a non-Langerhans cell histiocytosis [3]. Recently, according to the 2016 revised histiocytosis classification, RDD belongs to the "R Group" of histiocytosis which includes familial and sporadic RDD, while cutaneous RDD belongs to the "C Group" [5]. Sporadic RDD includes the classical nodal RDD, extranodal RDD, neoplasia-associated RDD, and immune disease-associated RDD [5]. RDD commonly affects children and young adults (mean age: 20.6 years) and frequently males of African descent [4–6, 9]. In our case, the patient was a 5-year-old female child, whereas the patients were male adults in Huang et al. and Zanelli et al. case reports [7, 10]. The pathophysiology of RDD is poorly understood [4]. It was considered as a reactive and non-neoplastic histiocytic disorder; however, recent studies described NRAS, KRAS, ARAF, and MAP2K1 mutations in nodal and extranodal RDD [4, 6]. Studies have supposed that herpes viruses, cytomegalovirus, Epstein-Barr virus, and HIV may be potential inciting agents, but no causative link has been demonstrated [4, 6]. In our patient, cytomegalovirus serology was negative. The other viral serologies were not performed.

Mutations in the SLC29A3 gene have been reported in familial cases of RDD [4, 6]. Sequencing studies to identify a germline predisposition to RDD were not pursued in our patient.

In classical sporadic RDD, the most frequent clinical presentation is bilateral painless massive lymphadenopathy with associated fever, night sweats, asthenia, and loss of weight [5]. Mediastinal and inguinal nodes may be associated [5, 9]. Extranodal manifestations are present in about 40% of cases, and the most frequent sites involved are skin, nasal cavity, bone, soft tissue, orbital tissue, and central nervous system [4, 5, 9]. The medical history of snoring in our patient suggests the possibility of Rosai–Dorfman disease with associated nasal cavity localisation. However, a CT scan of the nasal cavity and paranasal sinuses was not performed.

RDD diagnosis is confirmed by histology [5, 9]. Lymph node biopsy is characterized by the accumulation of large histiocytic cells with hypochromatic nuclei, abundant and pale cytoplasm, with emperipolesis which is a characteristic morphological feature of RDD [5, 8, 9]. However, emperipolesis is not specific and not required for RDD diagnosis [4]. In our patient, there was no observed emperipolesis. Biopsies of extranodal sites show the same histological features of histiocytes [9]. Immunohistochemically, the proliferative histiocytes are S100, CD68, and CD163 positive and are CD1a and CD207 negative [4, 5].

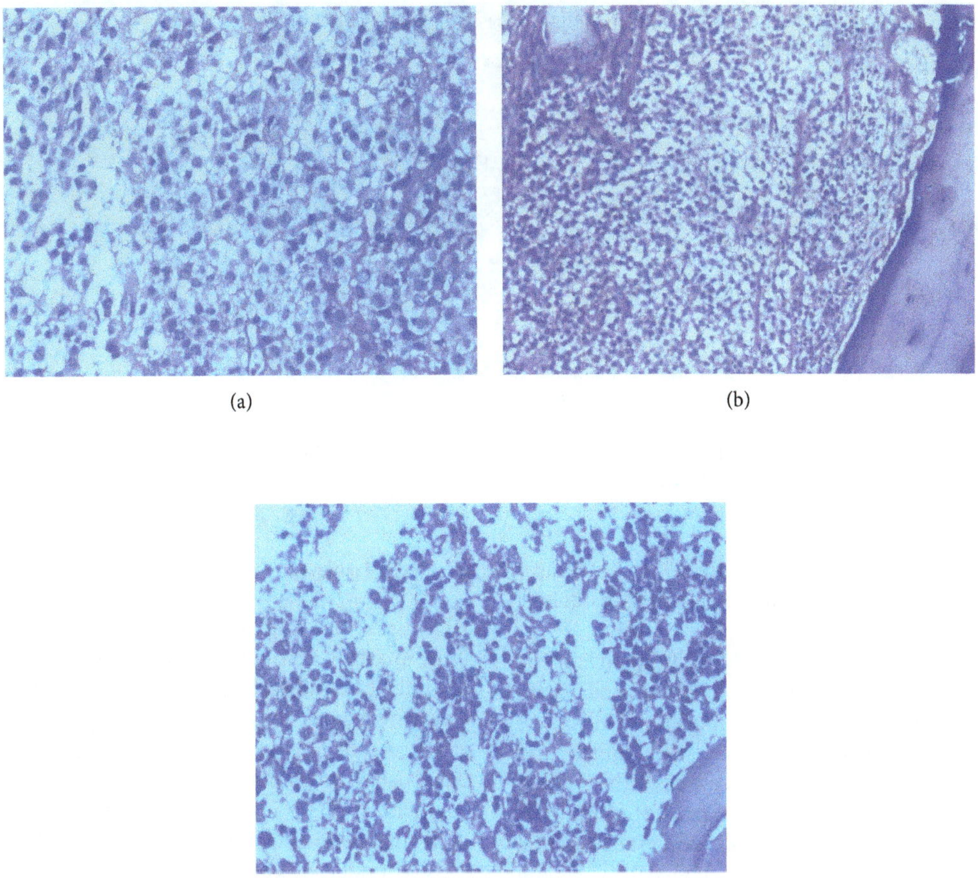

(a) (b) (c)

Figure 2: Biopsies showing infiltration by histiocytic cells. (a) Cervical lymph node biopsy, hematoxylin, and eosin, ×20. (b) Bone biopsy, hematoxylin, and eosin, ×10. (c) Bone marrow biopsy, hematoxylin, and eosin, ×10.

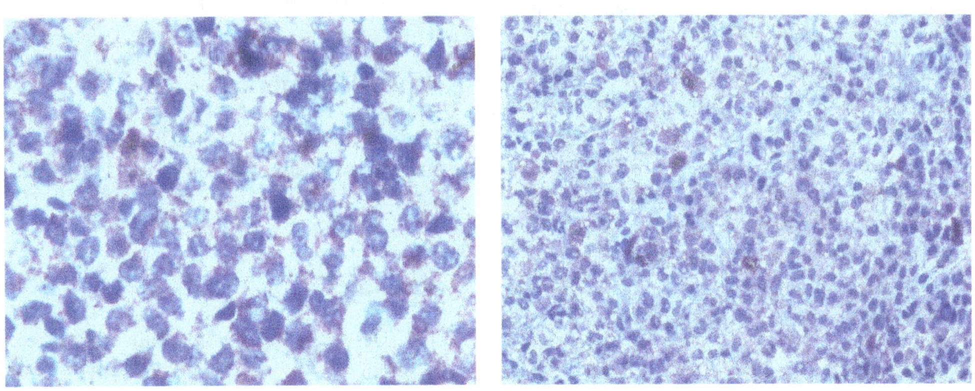

(a) (b)

Figure 3: Continued.

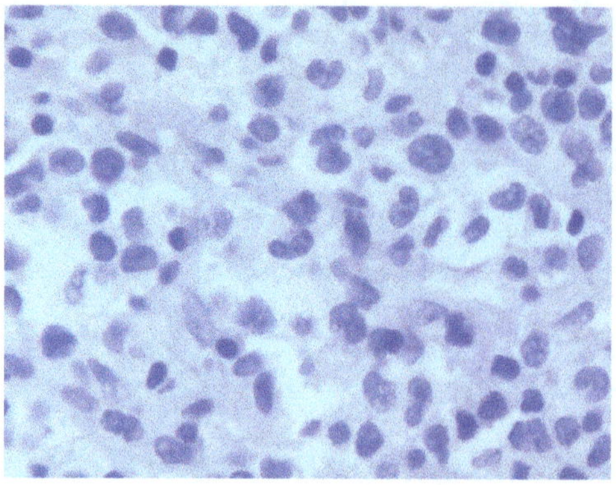

(c)

Figure 3: Immunohistochemical staining of lymph node biopsy. (a) CD68 expression by histiocytic cells. (b) S100 protein expression by histiocytic cells. (c) Histiocytic cells lack CD1a expression.

Bone involvement is reported in 5% to 10% of RDD cases [6]. Its common manifestation is bone pain with osteolytic bone lesions [5, 6].

Hematologic abnormalities in RDD include normocytic normochromic anemia (67% of cases), leukocytosis with neutrophilia (60% of cases), and thrombocytopenia [6]. As in Huang et al. case, our patient presented with anemia and thrombocytopenia, while in Zanelli et al. case, the patient had a mild pancytopenia [7, 10]. Bone marrow infiltration is rarely reported in the literature [6, 7, 10]. The first extranodal RDD involving the bone marrow was reported by Huang et al. in 2006 [7]. Bone marrow exploration was not performed in the past as a staging procedure, which explains the rare reported cases of bone marrow involvement in RDD [7, 10]. According to the consensus recommendations for the diagnosis and management of RDD by the American Society of Hematology, all patients with unexplained cytopenias or abnormal peripheral blood cells require bone marrow aspiration and biopsy [6].

Abnormal laboratory test results such as hyperferritinemia and high erythrocyte sedimentation rate are not specific and may be related to inflammation or infection [5]. It is recommended to carry out antinuclear antibodies and rheumatoid factor tests in order to screen for an associated immune disease [6]. These tests were negative in our patient, thus, there was no evidence of associated autoimmunity.

In our case, there was no malignancy detected, whereas Zanelli et al. reported a case of RDD involving bone marrow associated with acute myeloid leukemia [10].

RDD patients need a long-term follow-up searching for other possible tissues infiltration [11].

Many therapeutic strategies exist and depend on RDD manifestations, among these treatments: corticosteroids, chemotherapy, radiotherapy, immunomodulatory therapy, and surgery [6, 9].

Sporadic RDD has generally a good prognosis, especially nodal disease which is usually self-limited [4, 6]. Bony RDD prognosis is favorable in general [6]. Multifocal and extranodal RDD, including bone marrow involvement, have a poor prognosis [6, 7, 10].

4. Conclusion

RDD is a rare and benign histiocytic disorder. However, bone marrow involvement in RDD is associated with unfavorable prognosis. Hematologists and pathologists must be aware of the possible infiltration of bone marrow despite its rarity. According to the American Society of Hematology consensus recommendations for the diagnosis and management of RDD in 2018, it is required for RDD patients with unexplained cytopenias or abnormal peripheral blood cells to undergo bone marrow aspiration and biopsy.

Authors' Contributions

Rahali Fatima Zahra and Sayagh Sanae prepared and revised the manuscript. Taher Fatima and Nassih Houda participated in the manuscript preparation.

Acknowledgments

The authors thank Dr. Brahim Ben Hami for kindly providing the anatomopathology and immunohistochemistry images.

References

[1] P. Destombes, "Adenitis with lipid excess, in children or young adults, seen in the Antilles and in Mali.(4 cases)," *Bulletin de la Societe de pathologie exotique et de ses filiales*, vol. 58, no. 6, pp. 1169–1175, 1965.

[2] J. Rosai and R. F. Dorfman, "Sinus histiocytosis with massive lymphadenopathy. A newly recognized benign clinicopathological entity," *Archives of Pathology*, vol. 87, no. 1, pp. 63–70, 1969.

[3] T. Chu, G. J. D'Angio, B. Favara, S. Ladisch, M. Nesbit, and J. Pritchard, "Histiocytosis syndromes in children," *Lancet*, vol. 329, no. 8526, pp. 208-209, 1987.

[4] C. Bruce-Brand, J. W. Schneider, and P. Schubert, "Rosai-Dorfman disease: an overview," *Journal of Clinical Pathology*, vol. 73, no. 11, pp. 697–705, 2020.

[5] J. F. Emile, O. Abla, S. Fraitag et al., "Revised classification of histiocytoses and neoplasms of the macrophage-dendritic cell lineages," *Blood*, vol. 127, no. 22, pp. 2672–2681, 2016.
[6] O. Abla, E. Jacobsen, J. Picarsic et al., "Consensus recommendations for the diagnosis and clinical management of Rosai-Dorfman-Destombes disease," *Blood*, vol. 131, no. 26, pp. 2877–2890, 2018.
[7] Q. Huang, K. L. Chang, and L. M. Weiss, "Extranodal Rosai-Dorfman disease involving the bone marrow: a case report," *The American Journal of Surgical Pathology*, vol. 30, no. 9, pp. 1189–1192, 2006.
[8] J. F. Emile, F. Charlotte, C. Chassagne-Clement et al., "Histiocytoses: general classification and molecular criteria," *Presse Medicale*, vol. 46, no. 1, pp. 46–54, 2017.
[9] F. Cohen Aubart, J. Haroche, J.-F. Emile et al., "Rosai-Dorfman disease: diagnosis and therapeutic challenges," *La Revue de Medecine Interne*, vol. 39, no. 8, pp. 635–640, 2018.
[10] M. Zanelli, G. Goteri, M. C. Mengoli et al., "Rosai-dorfman disease involving bone marrow in association with acute myeloid leukemia," *International Journal of Surgical Pathology*, vol. 27, no. 4, pp. 396–398, 2019.
[11] B. Gramont, J. B. Gaultier, R. Duthel, S. Gouilloud, F. Forest, and P. Cathébras, "Two cases of histiocytoses in organs that were not expected," *La Revue de Medecine Interne*, vol. 37, pp. A141–A142, 2016.

4

A Single-Centre Experience of Post-COVID-19 Vaccine-Related Immune-Mediated Complications

David Palmer,[1] **Lauren Davis**,[1] **Helena Sivaloganathan**,[1] **and Timothy Chevassut**[1,2]

[1]*Royal Sussex County Hospitals, University Hospitals Sussex, Brighton BN2 5BE, UK*
[2]*Brighton and Sussex Medical School, University of Sussex, Brighton BN1 9PS, UK*

Correspondence should be addressed to David Palmer; david.palmer5@nhs.net

Academic Editor: Pier Paolo Piccaluga

The significant impact of the COVID-19 pandemic has resulted in a worldwide effort to develop effective vaccines. In the United Kingdom, the COVID-19 vaccine development and roll-out has been overwhelmingly successful in reducing infections and deaths. However, case reports have emerged of a rare syndrome of vaccine-induced immune thrombocytopenia and thrombosis (VITT), as well as cases of immune thrombocytopenia (ITP). This has necessitated a better understanding of these conditions. However, as both VITT and "vaccine-associated ITP" are emerging conditions, evidence on the clinical features, epidemiology, and management is still evolving. Subsequently, with the initiation of the COVID-19 vaccine booster program, it has become increasingly important to continue to collect accurate data on post-COVID-19 vaccine complications to aid with their prompt recognition and management. In this case series, we report on the presentations and management of seven cases of post-COVID-19 vaccine-related immune-mediated complications which occurred at our center between the months of March and July 2021.

1. Introduction

Vaccine-induced immune thrombocytopenia and thrombosis, or VITT, is a potentially severe condition featuring a combination of thrombocytopenia, high D-dimer levels, low fibrinogen, and thrombotic events, occurring 5–30 days following a dose of the COVID-19 vaccine [1]. These thrombotic events include cerebral venous sinus thrombosis, pulmonary embolus, splanchnic vein thrombosis, and arterial thromboses and can be life threatening [1, 2]. It was initially characterized after the AstraZeneca vaccine (ChAdOx1 nCoV-19) [1, 3] though there have also been reports after the Johnson & Johnson (AD26.COV2.S) and potentially the mRNA Pfizer-BioNTech (BNT162b2) and the Moderna (mRNA1273) vaccines [1, 4, 5]. It appears to mimic HIT (heparin-induced thrombocytopenia) with the production of anti-PF4 antibodies [3]. Further evidence suggests that these thrombotic events can be more severe than thromboses occurring in the absence of VITT [6], but the clinical presentation is highly variable and overlaps with other syndromes more reminiscent of immune thrombocytopenia [7].

2. Cases

2.1. Case 1. A 59-year-old woman with a past medical history of depression, hypertension, and hypothyroidism presented 19 days after her first dose of the AstraZeneca (ChAdOx1 nCoV-19) COVID-19 vaccine. Her initial symptoms were headaches, but she later developed severe pain and numbness in her left leg. On admission, she had a platelet count of 16×10^9/L, D-dimer of 36.00 ug/ml, and fibrinogen level of 2.6 g/L. An APTT and PT time were within normal range. She underwent a CT angiogram of the leg which showed an acute thrombus of the left common femoral artery (Figure 1). She was treated with two repeated doses of intravenous immunoglobulin, IVIg (1 g/kg), over two days, was started on an argatroban infusion, and was given four days of dexamethasone (40 mg once daily). Anti-PF4 antibodies were detected at 0.285 (OD units). By day six,

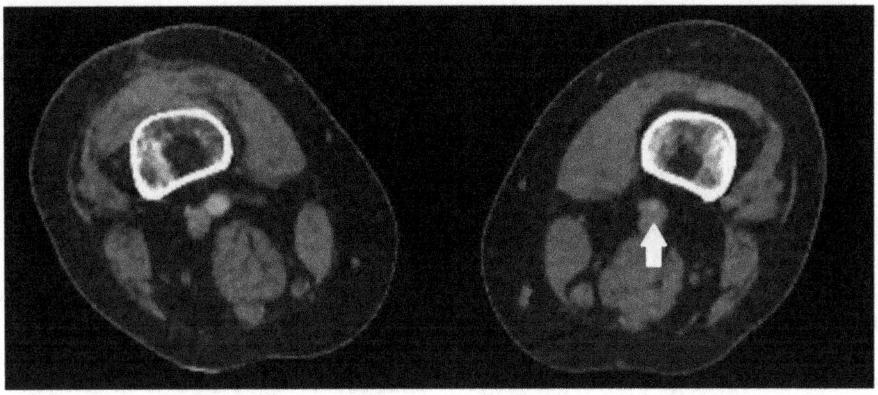

FIGURE 1: A CT angiogram demonstrates an occlusive thrombus (white arrow) of the left common femoral artery.

her platelet count had risen to 191×10^9/L. However, her leg had become increasingly ischaemic and was nonviable. Subsequently, she underwent a transfemoral above-knee amputation. Postoperatively, she was switched to fondaparinux and was later commenced on aspirin and rivaroxaban. Repeat anti-PF4 antibodies four weeks later were no longer elevated. She subsequently received a dose of the Pfizer (BNT162b2) vaccine without any complications.

2.2. Case 2. A 58-year-old man with a past medical history of depression and gastritis presented 11 days after his first dose of the AstraZeneca (ChAdOx1 nCoV-19) COVID-19 vaccine. He had a three-day history of headaches and generalized myalgia. On admission, he had a trough platelet count of 20×10^9/L, peak D-dimer of 54.30 ug/ml, and fibrinogen of 1.3 g/L. An APTT and PT time were within normal limits. He underwent a cerebral CT venogram and MR venogram which showed no evidence of a cerebral vein thrombus. An ultrasound scan of the abdomen showed no evidence of a splanchnic vein thrombus. Anti-PF4 antibodies were detected at 0.245 (OD units). He was given one dose of IVIg (1 mg/kg) and dexamethasone (40 mg once daily) for four days and started on the treatment dose of fondaparinux. By day seven, his platelet count had risen to 188×10^9/L, and by week five, his D-dimer and anti-PF4 antibodies were no longer elevated (<0.28 ug/ml and 0.141 OD units, respectively). He was switched to a six-month course of rivaroxaban and later went on to have a dose of the Pfizer (BNT162b2) vaccine without any complications.

2.3. Case 3. A 61-year-old woman with well-controlled rheumatoid arthritis on sulfasalazine presented 25 days after her first dose of the AstraZeneca (ChAdOx1 nCoV-19) COVID-19 vaccine. Her presenting symptoms were of bruising over the extremities, bleeding from the mouth, and a petechial rash over the legs. On admission, she had a platelet count of 5×10^9/L with an elevated D-dimer at 1.03 ug/ml. Anti-PF4 antibodies were detected at 0.247 (OD units). Her sulfasalazine was held. She initially had a poor response to IVIg (1 mg/kg) and four days of dexamethasone (40 mg once daily) which was switched at day six to 1 mg/kg of prednisolone when she received a further dose of IVIg. By day eight, her platelets had risen to over 50×10^9/L. For a further six weeks, her platelet count was maintained between 50 and 150×10^9/L and D-dimers were noted to fall to normal limits during this time. However, there was a subsequent fall in her platelet count shortly after this, associated again with rising D-dimer levels. She was subsequently commenced on eltrombopag and an improvement in her platelet count was sustained at over 50×10^9/L, associated with falling D-dimers. She later went on to have a dose of the Pfizer (BNT162b2) vaccine without any complications. She continues on eltrombopag and a low dose of prednisolone.

2.4. Case 4. A 66-year-old man with a history of benign prostatic hyperplasia presented 34 days following the first dose of his Pfizer (BNT162b2) COVID-19 vaccine, with epistaxis and bruising. On admission, his platelet count was 1×10^9/L and D-dimers were mildly elevated at 1.87 *u*g/ml. His anti-PF4 antibodies were positive at 0.285 OD units. He was given four days of dexamethasone (20 mg once daily) and IVIg (1 mg/kg). He had a good response to this treatment initially with platelets increasing to 108×10^9/L on day five. However, following this, his platelets dropped resulting in him being recommenced on both a weaning regime of prednisolone and eltrombopag. He had a good response to these agents, and the eltrombopag was discontinued after eight weeks with the platelet count remaining above 100×10^9/L. He was advised to get a second dose of either the AstraZeneca or Moderna COVID-19 vaccine.

2.5. Case 5. A 49-year-old woman with mild COPD presented 14 days after her first dose of the AstraZeneca (ChAdOx1 nCoV-19) COVID-19 vaccine. Her initial symptoms were bruising over the extremities and headaches. On admission, she had a platelet count of 26×10^9/L and normal D-dimers. A CT venogram followed by an MR venogram showed no evidence of cerebral vein thrombus. Anti-PF4 antibodies were strongly positive at 0.734 (OD units). She was given four days of dexamethasone (20 mg once daily) and IVIg (1 mg/kg). By day eight, her platelets had responded to 300×10^9/L. However, a week later they fell to less than 100×10^9/L. She was subsequently started on a weaning regime of prednisolone at (1 mg/kg) for which an ongoing response continues. She later went on to have a dose of the Pfizer (BNT162b2) vaccine without any complications.

2.6. Case 6. A 42-year-old man with no significant medical history presented 12 days after his first dose of the AstraZeneca (ChAdO × 1 nCoV-19) COVID-19 vaccine. His initial symptoms were a spreading petechial rash over both legs. On admission, his platelet count was 16×10^9/L and D-dimers were normal. Anti-PF4 antibodies were not elevated (0.0702 OD units). He was commenced on four days of dexamethasone (40 mg once daily) and given IVIg (1 mg/kg). By day seven, his platelet count had risen to 212×10^9/L and remains within normal limits since. He has not yet had a dose of an alternative COVID-19 vaccine.

2.7. Case 7. A 49-year-old woman with no medical history presented 21 days after her first dose of the AstraZeneca (ChAdO × 1 nCoV-19) COVID-19 vaccine. Her initial symptoms were bruising, blisters in the mouth, and a petechial rash. On admission, her platelet count was 1×10^9/L and D-dimers were normal. Anti-PF4 antibodies were not detected at elevated levels (0.172 OD units). She was given four days of dexamethasone (40 mg once daily) and IVIg (1 mg/kg). By day seven, there had been a limited response in her platelet count, remaining $<10 \times 10^9$/L; therefore, a repeat dose of IVIg (1 mg/kg) was given. By day 28, her platelet count had risen to 207×10^9/L and has remained within a normal range since. She has not yet had a second dose of an alternative COVID-19 vaccine.

3. Discussion

Presentations of VITT have been described as an autoimmune-prothrombotic disorder phenotypically comparable to "spontaneous HIT," but without any prior heparin exposure [8, 9]. In Case 1, based on the criteria set out by Pavord et al. [2], all five criteria had been met to satisfy a diagnosis of "definite VITT," whereas Case 2 only met the criteria for "probable VITT." Case 2 could be considered as "pre-VITT," previously described as the full syndrome in the absence of thrombosis [10]. Subsequently, a "subclinical" presentation based on the biochemical presence of thrombocytopenia, raised D-dimers, and anti-platelet factor 4 antibodies could precede any thrombotic events. Thus, VITT could exist on a spectrum, not always fulfilling the defined criteria, as has been suggested [11]. The timely implementation of anticoagulation, in this case, is likely to have averted thrombosis, most notably cerebral venous sinus thrombosis, which could have resulted in significant consequences for this patient, as has been reported [10, 12, 13]. Theoretically, repeat vaccine doses could further stimulate these "subclinical" anti-PF4 antibody levels, increasing the risk of VITT with second/booster doses, which has been suggested [14]. However, most cases to date have occurred following the first vaccine doses. Importantly, screening tests for VITT have not been recommended [15].

Perhaps receiving less initial attention than VITT, "vaccine-associated ITP" has been recognized as a complication of both the AstraZeneca (ChAdO × 1 nCoV-19) and Pfizer (BNT162b2) vaccines[7, 16–18]. In our center, we encountered patients who presented with suspected "vaccine-associated ITP" following both the AstraZeneca (ChAdO × 1 nCoV-19) and Pfizer (BNT162b2) vaccines (cases 3 to 7). Notably, the clinical presentation of each of these cases was similar to the sequelae seen in usual ITP, most commonly with a petechial rash and mucocutaneous bleeding. However, in each case, we report the variable levels of D-dimers measured and anti-PF4 antibodies detected. This could suggest an overlap between VITT and "vaccine-associated ITP," and whilst there remains a lack of understanding as to the different aetiological mechanisms, this heterogeneity of presentations might support the concept of a "spectrum" on which these conditions exist. The presentations, laboratory findings, management, and outcome have been summarised in Table 1.

3.1. The Role of Diagnostic Tests in VITT and "Vaccine-Associated ITP". As outlined by Pavord et al. [2], anti-PF4 antibodies form a key part of the diagnosis of VITT. In parallel to HIT, these antibodies are proposed to be an important mechanism in the pathophysiology of thrombocytopenia and thrombosis seen in VITT. Anti-PF4 antibodies from patients with VITT bind a similar site to heparin on PF4, creating immune complexes that activate platelets via Fcγ receptor IIa [19]. In HIT, this activation contributes to a hypercoagulable state, followed by platelet death [20]. In this case series, the same ELISA method was used to detect anti-PF4 antibodies, making their results comparable. For the most part, we have seen some correlation between anti-PF4 optical density and severity of disease supporting a causal role of these antibodies, as evidenced by the higher anti-PF4 antibody levels in Case 1, with arterial thrombosis, compared with Case 2, where no clinical thrombosis was demonstrated. The key exception to this in our cases was Case 5 where anti-PF4 antibody levels were strongly positive at 0.734 OD units. This raises a number of questions regarding the significance of these antibodies in this case, and further understanding is needed on anti-PF4 antibodies and their binding kinetics in relation to coagulation and thrombogenesis. Whilst it is possible that the anti-PF4 antibodies in Case 5 were nonpathogenic, possibly due to nonspecific binding, it does suggest that VITT and "vaccine-associated ITP" exist upon a spectrum of diseases.

In the diagnosis of HIT, the lower specificity of anti-PF4 immunoassays is an important consideration, necessitating the use of clinical judgment and a pre-test probability score [20]. The criteria set out by Pavord et al. [2] are a step toward the development of a clinical assessment tool, to further rationalize the use of antibody tests. Subsequent analysis is required to ensure the sensitivity and specificity of any scoring system, particularly if the disease processes of VITT and "vaccine-associated ITP" are intrinsically linked. It is clear that no

Table 1: A summary of the patients included in this case series.

Cases	Diagnosis	Presenting features	Laboratory findings	Management	Platelet recovery time	Outcome
Case 1	Definite VITT[2]	Headaches and critical limb ischemia	Platelet count: 16×10^9/L. D-dimer: 36.00 ug/ml. fibrinogen: 2.6 g/L. Anti-PF4 antibodies: 0.285	IVIg x2 Dexamethasone Argatroban IVI Surgical intervention Aspirin and rivaroxaban postoperatively	6 days	Transfemoral above-knee amputation. Anti-PF4 antibodies were not detected at 28 days
Case 2	Pre VITT/ Probable VITT[2]	Headaches and myalgia	Platelet count: 20×10^9/L. D-dimer: 54.30 ug/ml. fibrinogen: 1.3 g/L. Anti-PF4 antibodies: 0.245	IVIg Fondaparinux 6 months rivaroxaban	7 days	6 months rivaroxaban. Anti-PF4 antibodies were not detected at 35 days
Case 3	Vaccine-associated ITP	Mucocutaneous bleeding	Platelet count: 5×10^9/L. D-dimer: 1.03 ug/ml. Anti-PF4 antibodies: 0.247	IVIg Dexamethasone Prednisolone Eltrombopag	No full recovery of platelets when case series written	Continuous prednisolone and eltrombopag
Case 4	Vaccine-associated ITP	Mucocutaneous bleeding	Platelet count: 1×10^9/L. D-dimer: 1.87 ug/ml. Anti-PF4 antibodies: 0.285	IVIg Dexamethasone Prednisolone Eltrombopag	No full recovery of platelets when case series written	Weaning regime of prednisolone. Eltrombopag was discontinued
Case 5	Vaccine-associated ITP	Headaches and mucocutaneous bleeding	Platelet count: 26×10^9/L. D-dimer: *not elevated.* Anti-PF4 antibodies: 0.734	IVIg Dexamethasone Prednisolone	8 days (relapsed on day 15)	Weaning regime of prednisolone
Case 6	Vaccine-associated ITP	Petechiae	Platelet count: 16×10^9/L. D-dimer: *not elevated.* Anti PF4 antibodies: 0.070	IVIg Dexamethasone	7 days	Full recovery; off treatment
Case 7	Vaccine-associated ITP	Petechiae and mucocutaneous bleeding	Platelet count: 1×10^9/L. D-dimer: *not elevated.* Anti-PF4 antibodies: 0.172	IVIg Dexamethasone 2nd dose IVIg	28 days	Full recovery; off treatment

single test captures a diagnosis of VITT or "vaccine-associated ITP." Instead, a constellation of biochemical tests and clinical observations are required, and it remains important that the emphasis is on early detection and management.

3.2. The Management of VITT and "Vaccine-Associated ITP" at Our Centre. The treatment of VITT includes the management of any thrombus and suppressing the immune response. For the initial management of the immune response, 1 g/kg of IVIg is advised [21]. If the patient is showing progression of thrombosis or the platelet count fails to rise, options include further doses of IVIg, corticosteroids, plasma exchange, and rituximab [21]. Alongside the medical management, the surgical treatment of thrombosis in VITT includes embolectomy/thrombectomy, fasciotomy, or amputation (which occurred in Case 1), as has been described in several other cases [22–25].

One patient (Case 2) was started on anticoagulation for pre-VITT/probable VITT (without evidence of thrombosis), as there was suspicion of a high risk of impending thrombosis from the laboratory results. This is in line with current NICE guidance [21], who advocates prophylactic anticoagulation for those with VITT without thrombosis, especially while anti-PF4 antibodies are still present. By contrast, some of the patients with "vaccine-associated ITP" had detectable anti-PF4 antibodies, but as they primarily presented with a bleeding phenotype, they were not given anticoagulation. It is unclear moving forward whether these patients, especially those with detectable anti-PF4 antibodies, remain at risk of thrombosis.

Patients with VITT require ongoing follow-up, both initially with frequent blood tests (every 2–3 days for the first weeks) [21] and in a specialist hematology clinic. This will allow patients not only to be cared for in their recovery but also to be monitored for biochemical signs of relapse. None of the cases of VITT in this series had further episodes of thrombosis or thrombocytopenia. However, of those with "vaccine-associated ITP," several patients had relapses necessitating further therapy. Given the variability in presentations that have been observed at our center and the fact that it is as of yet unclear if VITT and "vaccine-associated ITP" are a spectrum of pathology, follow-up in a thrombosis clinic or with a hematologist with a special interest would be most appropriate to manage diagnostic uncertainty and to provide advice when considering further vaccinations against COVID-19.

In summary, the cases presented at our center have demonstrated the heterogeneity that exists in post-COVID-19 vaccine-related immune-mediated complications. Further data collected going forward will aid in the understanding of whether VITT and "vaccine-associated ITP" exist on a "spectrum" or are two distinct entities.

Consent

Verbal and written consent was obtained for all patients in this case series.

Disclosure

The views expressed in this publication are those of the authors and not necessarily those of the NIHR, NHS, or the Department of Health and Social Care. David Palmer, Lauren Davis, and Helena Sivaloganathan are co-first authors.

Acknowledgments

Helena Sivaloganathan, Academic Clinical Fellow in Haematology, NIHR27003, was funded by the National Institute for Health Research (NIHR).

References

[1] S. Pavord, W. Lester, M. Makris, M. Scully, and B. Hunt, "Guidance from the expert haematology panel (ehp) on covid-19 vaccine-induced immune thrombocytopenia and thrombosis (vitt)," 2021, https://b-s-h.org.uk/about-us/news/guidance-produced-by-the-expert-haematology-panel-ehp-focussed-on-vaccine-induced-thrombosis-and-thrombocytopenia-vitt/.

[2] S. Pavord, M. Scully, B. J. Hunt et al., "Clinical features of vaccine-induced immune thrombocytopenia and thrombosis," *New England Journal of Medicine*, vol. 385, no. 18, pp. 1680–1689, 2021.

[3] M. Franchini, G. M. Liumbruno, and M. Pezzo, "COVID-19 Vaccine-associated Immune Thrombosis and Thrombocytopenia (VITT): diagnostic and therapeutic recommendations for a new syndrome," *European Journal of Haematology*, vol. 107, no. 2, pp. 173–180, 2021.

[4] M. Lavin, P. T. Elder, D. O'Keeffe et al., "Vaccine-induced immune thrombotic thrombocytopenia (VITT)–a novel clinico-pathological entity with heterogeneous clinical presentations," *British Journal of Haematology*, vol. 195, no. 1, pp. 76–84, 2021.

[5] S. Sangli, A. Virani, N. Cheronis et al., "Thrombosis with thrombocytopenia after the messenger RNA-1273 vaccine," *Annals of Internal Medicine*, vol. 174, no. 10, pp. 1480–1482, 2021.

[6] R. J. Perry, A. Tamborska, B. Singh et al., "Cerebral venous thrombosis after vaccination against COVID-19 in the UK: a multicentre cohort study," *The Lancet*, vol. 398, no. 10306, pp. 1147–1156, 2021.

[7] M. Koch, S. Fuld, J. M. Middeke, J. Fantana, S. Von Bonin, and J. Beyer-Westendorf, "Secondary immune thrombocytopenia (ITP) associated with ChAdOx1 COVID-19 vaccination–A case report," *The Open*, vol. 05, no. 03, pp. e315–e318, 2021.

[8] A. Greinacher, K. Selleng, and T. E. Warkentin, "Autoimmune heparin-induced thrombocytopenia," *Journal of Thrombosis and Haemostasis*, vol. 15, no. 11, pp. 2099–2114, 2017.

[9] T. E. Warkentin, M. Makris, R. M. Jay, and J. G. Kelton, "A spontaneous prothrombotic disorder resembling heparin-induced thrombocytopenia," *The American Journal of Medicine*, vol. 121, no. 7, pp. 632–636, 2008.

[10] F. Salih, L. Schönborn, S. Kohler et al., "Vaccine-induced thrombocytopenia with severe headache," *New England Journal of Medicine*, vol. 385, pp. 2103–2105, 2021.

[11] F. A. Klok, M. Pai, M. V. Huisman, and M. Makris, "Vaccine-induced immune thrombotic thrombocytopenia," *The Lancet Haematology*, vol. 9, no. 1, pp. e73–e80, 2022.

[12] S. Bonato, A. Artoni, A. Lecchi et al., "Massive cerebral venous thrombosis due to vaccine-induced immune thrombotic thrombocytopenia," *Haematologica*, vol. 1, no. 11, pp. 3021–3024, 2021.

[13] P. R. Mehta, S. Apap Mangion, M. Benger et al., "Cerebral venous sinus thrombosis and thrombocytopenia after COVID-19 vaccination–A report of two UK cases," *Brain, Behavior, and Immunity*, vol. 95, no. 95, pp. 514–517, 2021.

[14] R. Marcucci and M. Marietta, "Vaccine-induced thrombotic thrombocytopenia: the elusive link between thrombosis and adenovirus-based SARS-CoV-2 vaccines," *Intern Emerg Med*, vol. 16, no. 5, pp. 1113–1119, 2021.

[15] I. Elalamy, G. Gerotziafas, S. Alamowitch et al., "SARS-CoV-2 vaccine and thrombosis: an expert consensus on vaccine-induced immune thrombotic thrombocytopenia," *Thrombosis & Haemostasis*, vol. 121, no. 8, pp. 982–991, 2021.

[16] O. Tarawneh and H. Tarawneh, "Immune thrombocytopenia in a 22-year-old post Covid-19 vaccine," *American journal of haematology*, vol. 96, 2021.

[17] M. Jawed, A. Khalid, M. Rubin, R. Shafiq, and N. Cemalovic, "Acute Immune Thrombocytopenia (ITP) following COVID-19 vaccination in a patient with previously stable ITP," *Open Forum Infectious Diseases*, vol. 8, no. 7, p. 343, 2021.

[18] O. Fueyo-Rodriguez, B. Valente-Acosta, R. Jimenez-Soto et al., "Secondary immune thrombocytopenia supposedly attributable to COVID-19 vaccination," *BMJ Case Reports*, vol. 14, no. 5, 2021.

[19] T. A. Nevzorova, E. R. Mordakhanova, A. G. Daminova et al., "Platelet factor 4-containing immune complexes induce platelet activation followed by calpain-dependent platelet death," *Cell death discovery*, vol. 5, no. 1, pp. 106–112, 2019.

[20] A. Cuker, "Clinical and laboratory diagnosis of heparin-induced thrombocytopenia: an integrated approach," *Seminars in Thrombosis and Hemostasis*, vol. 40, no. 1, pp. 106–114, 2013.

[21] S. Pavord, B. J. Hunt, D. Horner, S. Bewley, and J. Karpusheff, "Vaccine induced immune thrombocytopenia and thrombosis: summary of nice guidance," 2021, https://www.bmj.com/content/375/bmj.n2195.

[22] S. Lioudaki, N. Kontopodis, C. Pontikoglou et al., "Multiple sites of arterial thrombosis in a 35-year old patient after ChAdOx1 (AstraZeneca) vaccination, requiring emergent

femoral and carotid surgical thrombectomy," *Annals of Vascular Surgery*, vol. 79, no. 79, pp. 438.e1–438.e4, 2022.
[23] M. Vierstraete and T. Sabbe, "Aortic thrombosis and acute limb ischemia after ChAdOx1 nCov-19 (Oxford-AstraZeneca) vaccination: a case of vaccine-induced thrombocytopenia and thrombosis (VITT)," *Acta Chirurgica Belgica*, vol. 24, pp. 1–4, 2021.
[24] M. M. Alsmady, R. A. Al-Qaryouti, N. G. Sultan, O. I. Khrais, and H. Khrais, "Upper limb ischemia due to arterial thrombosis after COVID-19 vaccination," *Case Reports in Medicine*, no. 9, pp. 1–4, 2022.
[25] Y. Goereci, N. N. Kleineberg, M. Madlener et al., "Successful treatment of thromboses of major arteries after ChAdOx1 nCov-19 vaccination," *Neurological Research and Practice*, vol. 3, no. 1, pp. 52–54, 2021.

5

Immune Thrombocytopenic Purpura (ITP) as an Uncommon Extraintestinal Complication of Crohn's Disease: Case Vignette and Systematic Literature Review

Raisa Epistola,[1] Tiffanie Do,[1] Ritika Vankina,[2] Daniel Wu,[2] James Yeh,[2] Michael W. Fleischman,[3,4] and Jennifer M. Lee[2]

[1]*Harbor-UCLA Medical Center, Department of Medicine, Torrance, CA, USA*
[2]*Harbor-UCLA Medical Center, Department of Medicine, Division of Hematology & Medical Oncology, Torrance, CA, USA*
[3]*Harbor-UCLA Medical Center, Department of Medicine, Division of Gastroenterology, Torrance, CA, USA*
[4]*University of California Los Angeles Division of Digestive Diseases, Los Angeles, CA, USA*

Correspondence should be addressed to Raisa Epistola; repistola@dhs.lacounty.gov

Academic Editor: Salah Aref

While the association of immune thrombocytopenic purpura (ITP) and inflammatory bowel disease (IBD) has been described in a few case reports, management of ITP as an extraintestinal manifestation of Crohn's disease (CD) is less studied. There are approximately a dozen cases describing the management of patients dually diagnosed with CD/ITP. Previous reports postulated that the mechanism of ITP in CD was through the presence of circulating immune complexes in the serum and antigenic mimicry due to increased mucosal permeability in active colitis, versus increased mucosal production of TH1-type proinflammatory cytokines during CD flares, which may account for remission of ITP with surgery for CD. We present a case of a 27-year-old man who presented with medically refractory CD and ITP who responded to surgical management with colectomy and splenectomy, along with a systematic review of the literature. These cases suggest that colectomy should be considered in the treatment of medically refractory ITP among patients with concomitant CD.

1. Introduction

Immune thrombocytopenic purpura (ITP) is characterized by the presence of autoantibodies against platelet surface antigens leading to immune-mediated platelet destruction. While the occurrence of ITP and inflammatory bowel disease (IBD), including Crohn's disease (CD) and ulcerative colitis (UC), has been described in a limited number of case reports, the association of ITP as an extraintestinal manifestation of Crohn's disease has been sparsely reported [1]. Chronic inflammation, chronic intestinal bleeding, iron malabsorption, impaired dietary intake, and inadequate erythropoietin production contribute to anemia as a frequent finding in CD patients [2]. The humoral and cellular immune mechanisms that contribute to the onset of IBD suggest the association with ITP is not coincidental. Since the first reported cases of ITP associated with Crohn's disease in the late 1980s, there have been 13 case reports that have described treatment of ITP in Crohn's disease [3–5]. We present a case that queries the treatment choice for ITP in a patient with active Crohn's disease flare through postulated immune mechanisms.

2. Case Description

A 27-year-old man with a history of CD and ITP lost to follow-up for two years presented with two to three days of dark, bloody diarrhea, nausea, and nonbloody, nonbilious vomiting. Physical exam was notable for mild periumbilical tenderness; no hepatosplenomegaly was present.

The patient had been diagnosed with Crohn's disease seven years prior to this admission and had known moderate to severe colonic disease. He was diagnosed with ITP during a Crohn's disease flare four years prior to this presentation, was treated with IV methylprednisolone, and discharged on a prednisone taper. The direct antiglobulin test (Coombs) was negative; d-dimer, fibrinogen, C3, and C4 levels were within normal limits. Serologic studies for ANA, ANCA, viral hepatitis panel, and HIV were also negative. He did not undergo a bone marrow biopsy at time of ITP diagnosis.

On admission, laboratory results were notable for platelets of 18,000 per microliter (normal 160,000–360,000 per microliter), ESR of 49 mm/hr (normal 0.00–12 mm/hr), and CRP of 8.04 mg/L (normal 0.00–0.74 mg/L). He was started on methylprednisolone 20 mg IV every 8 hours and given 2 units of platelets, with platelet count improvement to 51,000 per microliter. He subsequently received intravenous immunoglobulin (IVIG) 1 g/kg daily for two days. He continued to experience bloody diarrhea and underwent esophagogastroduodenoscopy and flexible sigmoidoscopy, which revealed significant body and fundus gastropathy as well as moderate to severe proctosigmoiditis (Figure 1). He had a prior history of thrombocytopenia with adalimumab and infliximab, so he received a 390 mg IV loading dose of ustekinumab for his Crohn's disease flare. Antibody testing for anti-infliximab was negative during this hospitalization. His platelet count briefly responded to combined corticosteroids and IVIG but subsequently declined (Figure 2). He received rituximab on days 10 and 17 but had persistent thrombocytopenia. On hospital day 24, CRP increased to 5.99 mm/hr (from 0.09 mm/hr on hospital day 15), and symptoms for colitis persisted. Given his transfusion-dependent thrombocytopenia refractory to medical therapy, the patient underwent splenectomy. Due to persistent symptoms of bloody diarrhea and cramping, the patient concurrently underwent total colectomy with end ileostomy.

Following surgery, the patient's platelet count improved without transfusion support to 571,000 per microliter by the date of discharge. Pathologic review of the resected colon demonstrated changes consistent with chronic inflammatory disease, with severe disease activity. Five months following discharge, he has been maintained on ustekinumab and 6-mercaptopurine and has not had a Crohn's disease flare. His platelets remained stable at 170,000 per microliter without additional medical management for his ITP.

3. Discussion

Immune thrombocytopenic purpura may present as an extraintestinal manifestation of Crohn's disease. While there are at least 40 case reports describing the association of ITP and ulcerative colitis (UC) in the literature [6], there are fewer reports of dual diagnoses among Crohn's patients, particularly adults. While the prevalence of ITP among patients with ulcerative colitis is estimated at 0.1%–0.48%, the prevalence of patients with ITP and Crohn's disease is not known [8]. Given the relative dearth of information on the association of Crohn's disease and ITP, we performed a comprehensive literature search of the Medline database between March–May 2019. Keywords used included "Crohn's disease," "idiopathic thrombocytopenic purpura," "immune thrombocytopenic purpura," and "ITP." Titles and abstracts were reviewed to identify cases. References of included articles were reviewed to identify additional cases. The literature search identified 12 case reports of concomitant Crohn's disease and ITP and 1 small case-control study of IBD patients with autoimmune cytopenias, including ITP (Table 1).

Of the 13 case reports identified in our search, 12 cases demonstrated coexisting ITP and CD flare, suggesting that the two disease processes run in parallel. The parallel occurrence of these two processes was also seen in the one case-control study ($n = 40$ cases with coexisting IBD and autoimmune cytopenias; $n = 160$ controls with IBD alone) which reported 64% of IBD patients who presented with concomitant ITP and IBD flares. Compared to controls with IBD alone, there was a significantly higher frequency of extraintestinal manifestations and increased likelihood for severe acute flares among dual diagnosis patients, further supporting that autoimmune cytopenias such as ITP may be an extraintestinal manifestation of IBD [1].

Although the precise pathophysiology of concomitant ITP and Crohn's disease remains unclear, previous literature postulated the mechanism of ITP in Crohn's disease through the presence of circulating immune complexes in the serum and antigenic mimicry due to increased mucosal permeability in active colitis [8, 9]. Platelet surface antigens may carry similar peptide sequences as bacterial glycoproteins found in the gut; inflammation during IBD flare increases exposure to these antigens, resulting in antigenic cross-reactivity [10]. All but two cases identified in our literature review presented without colonic involvement. A preponderance of colonic involvement of CD has also been reported in the pediatric literature, suggesting that inflammation of the colon and/or dysregulation of colonic immunity contributes to the pathogenesis of CD-associated ITP [17, 18]. Bowel surgery could result in decreased exposure to cross-reactive antigens, and thus reduced ITP activity. Another postulated mechanism is mucosal production of TH1-type proinflammatory cytokines (IL-2 and IFN-gamma), which have been shown to be elevated in patients with ITP. Colectomy may reduce the production of these cytokines and thus reduce platelet destruction [18, 19].

The 2019 American Society of Hematology (ASH) guidelines on management of immune thrombocytopenic purpura recommend first-line therapy with corticosteroids, IVIG, or anti-D immunoglobulin as they have the quickest initial response [20]. Despite treatment with both corticosteroids and IVIG, our patient had no response and continued to be transfusion-dependent. In a typical patient with ITP unresponsive to initial corticosteroid therapy, ASH guidelines recommend thrombopoietin receptor agonists (TPO-RA), rituximab, and splenectomy as subsequent treatment options [20].

Our patient had persistent bloody diarrhea, abdominal pain, and transfusion-dependent thrombocytopenia for 24 days despite maximal medical therapy for CD. Because his CD did not improve over this prolonged period, he was offered a colectomy, as per the American College of Gastroenterology's (ACG) guidelines for medically refractory

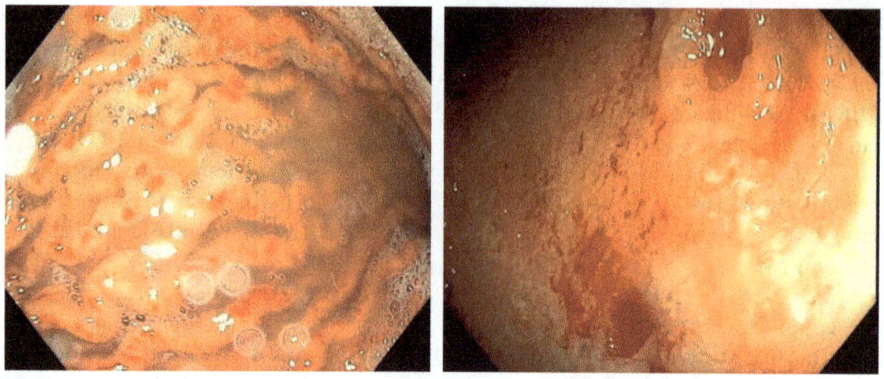

FIGURE 1: Left panel: upper endoscopy showing gastropathy. Right panel: flexible sigmoidoscopy showing moderate to severe proctosigmoiditis, Mayo Score-3.

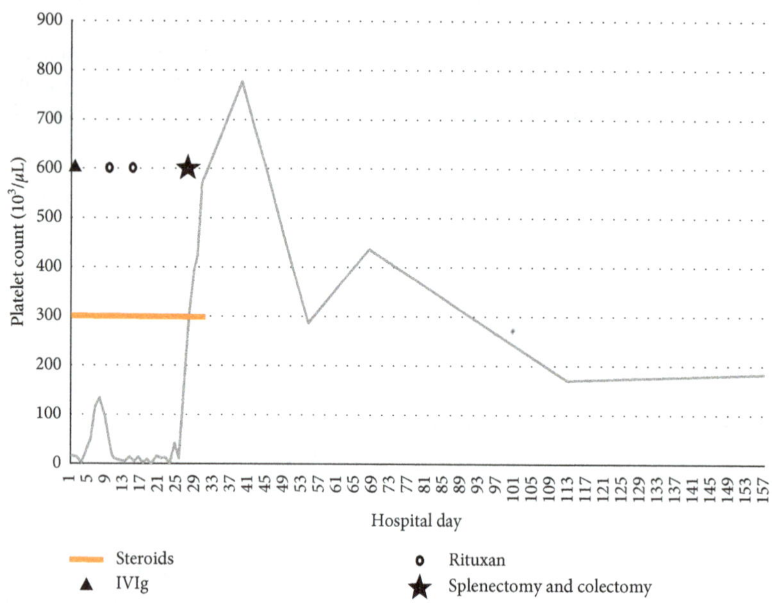

FIGURE 2: Platelet count trend and treatments. The patient was treated initially with steroids from day 1 to day 29 with concurrent IVIG on day 3 and 4 where there was a slight increase in platelets. Rituximab was given on day 10 and 17 with no drastic change in platelet count. Following splenectomy and colectomy on day 25, the platelet count increased without further treatment or platelet transfusions. The patient was discharged on day 29 without steroids.

CD [21]. The patient expressed a desire to control his illnesses with minimal long-term medications, so he was offered a splenectomy over TPO-RA therapy. He underwent both colectomy and splenectomy on hospital day 24. After surgery, the patient's hematochezia resolved, as did his thrombocytopenia, and he did not require further platelet transfusions after surgery.

Our literature review identified one case of ITP that was refractory to steroids and briefly responded to splenectomy; five months after splenectomy, the ITP recurred with a CD flare. The patient then underwent colectomy, after which his thrombocytopenia resolved [5]. Another case report documented medically refractory ITP that responded to bowel resection alone [16].

A case-control study of patients with IBD and autoimmune cytopenias included 25 patients with both IBD and ITP. This group comprised of 13 patients (52%) with a diagnosis of CD and 12 patients (48%) with a diagnosis of UC. Of these 25 patients with ITP, 15 were given steroids and 7 (46.7%) achieved a complete response with steroids alone. 4 (16%) received rituximab as second-line therapy, but these patients did not have a complete response. There were also six cases of IBD and autoimmune cytopenia (four of whom had ITP) who received rituximab. Of this group, four of six showed some response to rituximab; however, the only patient that achieved a complete response had a dual diagnosis of CD and autoimmune hemolytic anemia, not ITP. In the three cases with IBD and ITP treated with infliximab, a complete response was achieved for both disease processes. This study also reported two cases with IBD/ITP who underwent radical surgery (ileocecal resection and total colectomy) and achieved remission of ITP, though it is not reported whether these two cases received steroids or rituximab prior to surgery. Although this case-control study

TABLE 1: Case reports of Crohn's disease and immune thrombocytopenic purpura.

Title	Sex	Age	Interval between diagnoses	Concomitant CD and ITP flare	Location of Crohn's disease	Treatment (medical)	Treatment (surgical)	Outcome
Kosmo et al [5]	F	65	35 years	Yes	Colon	Steroids	Splenectomy, resection of rectal stump with terminal ileostomy	Refractory to steroids, resolved with surgical treatment
Manzano et al [7]	M	54	Simultaneous	Yes	Pancolitis with ileal involvement	Steroids	None	Resolved
Arruda et al [3]	M	43	2 weeks	Yes	Colon	Steroids	None	Resolved
Baudard et al [4]	F	19	Simultaneous	Yes	Duodenum, ileum, colon	IV steroids, IVIG	Splenectomy	CD symptoms improved; ITP refractory to medical and surgical treatment, patient lost to follow-up
Boyne and Dye [8]	F	17	9 years	Yes	Pancolitis without ileal involvement	IVIG, cyclosporine, steroids	None	Resolution of both ITP and CD symptoms
Selby et al [9]	M	15	5 months	Yes	Proximal colon	IV steroids, IVIG	None	ITP resolved with some residual CD symptoms on discharge
Kuloğlu et al [10]	M	5	1.5 years	No	Gastroesophageal, sigmoid	Steroids, IVIG	Splenectomy	CD responded to steroids, ITP medically refractory requiring splenectomy
Tsibouris et al [11]	M	44	Simultaneous	Yes	Ileocecal, sigmoid	IV steroids with azathioprine maintenance for Crohn's disease	None	Resolution
Germandis et al [12]	F	69	18 months	Yes	Ileocolonic	IVIG, steroids, ciprofloxacin, metronidazole, azathioprine, infliximab	None	Both CD and ITP symptoms resolved with infliximab, refractory to other therapies
De Rossi et al [13]	M	41	10 years	Yes	Ileum	IV steroids, ciprofloxacin, metonidazole infliximab	Surgical fistula sanitation and protective ileostomy	Anaphylaxis to infliximab; resolution of ITP and Crohn's disease following both medical and surgical treatment
Shaaban and Maroules [14]	M	57	Simultaneous	Yes	Gastric	IV steroids with mesalamine maintenance for Crohn's disease	None	Resolution
El Rassy et al [15] (2015)	F	25	Not reported	Yes	Ileocecal	Steroids, IVIG, rituximab, eltrombopag, methotrexate	Splenectomy	Resolution of ITP with eltrombopag, incomplete control of CD symptoms on methotrexate

Table 1: Continued.

Title	Sex	Age	Interval between diagnoses	Concomitant CD and ITP flare	Location of Crohn's disease	Treatment (medical)	Treatment (surgical)	Outcome
Mizuno et al [16]	M	32	18 years	Yes	Ileocecal	IVIG, steroids, infliximab, azathioprine	Ileocecal resection	CD & ITP medically refractory, but both resolved with surgical treatment

demonstrated varying responses to rituximab and infliximab, the small sample size queries the efficacy of nonsteroidal medical therapies in dual diagnosis patients [1].

The studies described above also bring to light the uncertainty of optimal surgical management of medically refractory ITP in the setting of Crohn's disease flare. In this context, our case queries further management of additional colectomy/bowel resection in cases of ITP during active Crohn's disease unresponsive to medical therapy.

ITP is a rare, but known, extraintestinal manifestation of CD. Treatment of ITP-associated Crohn's disease can be managed medically with steroids, IVIG, and biologics (i.e., rituximab and infliximab); however, our case adds to the small body of evidence suggesting the efficacy of colonic resection as part of definitive treatment of ITP associated with Crohn's disease.

References

[1] M. Uzzan, L. Galicier, J.-M. Gornet et al., "Autoimmune cytopenias associated with inflammatory bowel diseases: insights from a multicenter retrospective cohort," *Digestive and Liver Disease*, vol. 49, no. 4, pp. 397–404, 2017.

[2] C. Gasché, W. Reinisch, H. Lochs et al., "Anemia in Crohn's disease," *Digestive Diseases and Sciences*, vol. 39, no. 9, pp. 1930–1934, 1994.

[3] V. R. Arruda, C. G. Montes, A. Seva-Pereira, and J. M. Annicchino-Bizzacchi, "Association of severe autoimmune thrombocytopenic purpura and Crohn's disease," *The American journal of gastroenterology*, vol. 92, no. 10, pp. 1948-1949, 1997.

[4] M. Baudard, T. Molina, K. Benfiguig, J. P. Bethoux, and R. Zittoun, "Idiopathic thrombocytopenic purpura associated with Crohn's disease," *Haematologica*, vol. 83, no. 1, pp. 92-93, 1998.

[5] M. A. Kosmo, G. Bordin, P. Tani, and R. McMillan, "Immune thrombocytopenia and Crohn's disease," *Annals of Internal Medicine*, vol. 104, no. 1, p. 136, 1986.

[6] S. Chandra, S. Finn, and E. Obah, "Immune thrombocytopenic purpura in ulcerative colitis: a case report and systematic review," *Journal of Community Hospital Internal Medicine Perspectives*, vol. 4, no. 2, p. 23386, 2014.

[7] M. L. Manzano, C. Yela, G. Castellano, S. Rodriguez, and J. A. Solis, "Idiopathic thrombocytopenic purpura and pancytopenia in a patient with Crohn's disease: a new association," *The American Journal of Gastroenterology*, vol. 91, no. 8, pp. 1678-1679, 1996.

[8] M. S. Boyne and K. R. Dye, "Crohn's colitis and idiopathic thrombocytopenic purpura," *Postgraduate Medical Journal*, vol. 76, no. 895, pp. 299–301, 2000.

[9] L. A. Selby, D. Hess, H. Shashidar, W. J. S. de Villiers, and L. A. Selby, "Crohn's disease, infliximab and idiopathic thrombocytopenic purpura," *Inflammatory Bowel Diseases*, vol. 10, no. 5, pp. 698–700, 2004.

[10] Z. Kuloğlu, A. Kansu, F. Demirçeken, T. İleri, M. Ertem, and N. Girgin, "The association of chronic recurrent immune thrombocytopenic purpura and Crohn's disease," *Inflammatory Bowel Diseases*, vol. 11, no. 10, pp. 950-951, 2005.

[11] P. Tsibouris, A. N. Kapsoritakis, E. Bouronikou, M. Boulbou, D. Kyriakou, and S. P. Potamianos, "Crohn's disease associated with severe autoimmune thrombocytopenic purpura," *Inflammatory Bowel Diseases*, vol. 12, no. 12, pp. 1188-1189, 2006.

[12] G. Germanidis, G. Lazaraki, S. Gintikas, D. Karayannis, K. Mikoudi, and M. Sion, "Refractory Crohn-associated acute immune thrombocytopenic purpura treated with infliximab," *European Journal of Internal Medicine*, vol. 18, no. 4, pp. 344–346, 2007.

[13] T. M. De Rossi, N. Krauss, R. E. Voll et al., "Long-term partial remission of AutoImmune thrombocytopenia in a patient treated with the anti-tumor necrosis factor-alpha antibody infliximab for refractory fistulizing Crohn's disease," *Digestion*, vol. 78, no. 4, pp. 195–200, 2008.

[14] H. Shaaban and M. Maroules, "A rare case of gastric Crohn's disease associated with immune thrombocytopenic purpura," *Journal of Crohn's and Colitis*, vol. 7, no. 9, pp. e401–e402, 2013.

[15] E. El Rassy, H. R. Kourie, W. Nehme et al., "Successful eltrombopag treatment of refractory idiopathic thrombocytopenic purpura associated with Crohn disease," *Clinics and Research in Hepatology and Gastroenterology*, vol. 39, no. 2, pp. e23–e24, 2015.

[16] S. Mizuno, M. Naganuma, and T. Kanai, "Idiopathic thrombocytopenic purpura responsive to surgery for crohn's disease," *Inflammatory Bowel Diseases*, vol. 25, no. 3, p. e26, 2019.

[17] N. Crespo Madrid, C. Ruiz Hernández, L. Giraldo Escobar, G. Pujol Muncunill, and J. Martín de Carpi, "Co-existence of Crohn's disease and primary immune thrombocytopenia and its implications in treatment," *Anales de Pediatría (English Edition)*, vol. 83, no. 6, pp. 433–435, 2015.

[18] L. M. Higuchi, S. Joffe, E. J. Neufeld et al., "Inflammatory bowel disease associated with immune thrombocytopenic purpura in children," *Journal of Pediatric Gastroenterology and Nutrition*, vol. 33, no. 5, pp. 582–587, 2001.

[19] M. Nie, Y. Liu, X.-x. Li et al., "PD-1/PD-L pathway potentially involved in ITP immunopathogenesis," *Thrombosis and Haemostasis*, vol. 119, no. 5, pp. 758–765, 2019.

[20] C. Neunert, D. R. Terrell, D. M. Arnold et al., "American Society of Hematology 2019 guidelines for immune thrombocytopenia," *Blood Advances*, vol. 3, no. 23, pp. 3829–3866, 2019.

[21] G. R. Lichtenstein, E. V. Loftus, K. L. Isaacs, M. D. Regueiro, L. B. Gerson, and B. E. Sands, "ACG clinical guideline: management of Crohn's disease in adults," *American Journal of Gastroenterology*, vol. 113, no. 4, pp. 481–517, 2018.

6

Aplasia in Chronic Phase CML Post-TKI Therapy: A Management Dilemma

Jeremy L. Ramdial,[1] Luis E. Aguirre,[2] Robert A. Ali,[1] Ronan Swords,[1] and Mark Goodman[1]

[1]*Department of Hematology/Oncology, Sylvester Comprehensive Cancer Center, University of Miami Miller School of Medicine, Miami, FL, USA*
[2]*Department of Internal Medicine, University of Miami Miller School of Medicine, Miami, FL, USA*

Correspondence should be addressed to Mark Goodman; mgoodman@med.miami.edu

Academic Editor: Pier P. Piccaluga

Transient cytopenias and bone marrow hypoplasia commonly occur during treatment of CML with TKIs (tyrosine kinase inhibitors). This is usually related to the eradication of CML clones that initially compose the majority of hematopoietic cells in the bone marrow at the time of diagnosis. With continuation of effective therapy, normal blood counts return as normal hematopoiesis is restored and CML clones are reduced. Though rare and more unusual than myelodysplastic syndrome (MDS), isolated instances of persistent marrow aplasia have been documented with chronic use of TKIs. We describe two such instances of chronic phase CML where no significant reduction of CML clones was achieved following treatment with TKIs, but bone marrow aplasia occurred resulting in persistent dysfunctional hematopoiesis. Due to prolonged aplasia/hypoplasia, such patients are no longer amenable to TKI treatment. CML progression to accelerated or blast phase in that setting would likely be fatal.

1. Background

TKI-induced marrow aplasia is a rarely described and poorly characterized entity. Known accounts of this interesting phenomenon remain scarce throughout the literature and highlight how challenging their management can be. The consequences can be devastating for afflicted patients. An extensive review of the literature using Pubmed and Trip database with the words "Aplasia," "Chronic phase," "CML," and "TKI/Tyrosine kinase inhibitors" revealed only a handful of published case descriptions. It is with this in mind that we illustrate two local cases of chronic phase CML complicated with aplasia post-TKI therapy. To the extent of our knowledge, these cases represent the first reported instances in which patients developed this complication without having exhibited any meaningful response to therapy. We hope that public awareness of these 2 cases will contribute to expand current knowledge of this phenomenon and ultimately help bring further insight into this process.

2. Case Presentation

2.1. Case 1. A 64-year-old male with no comorbidities presented to our institution complaining of chronic fatigue and malaise in the setting of underlying hematologic abnormalities. On presentation, preliminary studies were significant for profound leukocytosis of $323 \times 10^3/\mu L$ and platelet count of $428 \times 10^3/\mu L$ with 5% blasts and 10% basophils in peripheral blood. CT scan of the abdomen revealed massive splenomegaly with an enlarged spleen measuring 24.5 cm in its largest craniocaudal dimensions. Further workup was consistent with chronic phase Ph (+) CML with a breakpoint at p210 and JAK2 negative status. The Sokal index was 2.1 and consistent with high risk disease (which translated to two-year survival rate of 65% and median survival estimated at 2.5 years). The EUTOS score obtained prior to starting TKI therapy was 132 and compatible with high-risk disease (5-year progression-free survival of 82% and complete cytogenic response (CCyR) of

66% at 18 months with a 31% likelihood of not achieving CCyR). Bone marrow FISH showed 81% BCR-ABL transcripts for which he was started on imatinib, achieving hematological response by the 3rd week of treatment and suboptimal cytological response by month 7. The clinical course was complicated by therapy-related pancytopenia/ aplastic anemia on month 8. Consequently, imatinib was held for 2 months which allowed his counts to fully recover by month 11.

Routine studies done at follow-up showed marked leukocytosis. Repeat BM biopsy was consistent with chronic phase CML with 5% blasts. Cytogenetics showed t(9; 22) and 3q inversion with 95% BCR-ABL transcripts, and the patient was started on dasatinib. By the 12th month of therapy, decision was made to treat him as accelerated phase due to clonal evolution, with consideration for potential allogeneic HSCT once response to dasatinib had been achieved. He was maintained on TKI therapy until month 15 when repeat FISH from peripheral blood showed 79% BCR-ABL transcripts with underlying severe pancytopenia. Dasatinib was held until counts recovered on Neupogen and biweekly transfusion of blood products and restarted subsequently at 80 mg.

Bone marrow biopsy on month 16 showed marked hypocellularity secondary to panmyeloid hypoplasia. Bone marrow cytogenetics demonstrated t(9; 22), inv(3) (q21q26), and 36% BCR-ABL transcripts. Dasatinib was reduced to 70 mg with additional reduction to 50 mg PO daily by month 17 due to persistent pancytopenia. Peripheral blood FISH on month 19 showed 70% BCR-ABL transcripts which led to discontinuation of Dasatinib and institution of omacetaxine by month 21.

On month 25, the patient was admitted to undergo allogeneic MUD/BMT. He was conditioned with Flu/Bu/ ATG and received stem cell infusion with successful engrafting on day +15. His post-transplant course was marked by a number of complications including CMV viremia, an episode of seizures attributed to posterior reversible encephalopathy (PRES) and development of myeloid sarcoma discovered incidentally on imaging as a paraspinal mass. BM biopsy at follow-up showed increased percentage of blasts, and he was started on ponatinib 45 mg daily.

2.2. Case 2. A 50-year-old male presented to our institution for evaluation of persistent leukocytosis of $26 \times 10^3/\mu L$, newfound thrombocytosis with platelet count of $1042 \times 10^3/\mu L$, and markedly elevated LDH. He had originally noted symptoms of progressive fatigue, weight loss, and general malaise over a period of 6 months. On presentation, the preliminary studies also showed 2% blasts and 5% basophils in peripheral blood. CT scan of the abdomen revealed splenomegaly with an enlarged spleen measuring 16 cm in its largest dimensions. Bone marrow biopsy and additional workup were consistent with chronic phase Ph (+) CML with 137.2% BCR-ABL transcripts, JAK2 negative status, and a breakpoint at p210. The Sokal index was 1.4 and consistent with high-risk disease. The EUTOS score obtained prior to initiation of TKI therapy was 63 and compatible with low-risk disease (5-year progression-free survival of 90% with probability of achieving complete cytogenic response (CCyR) at 18 months of 86% and likelihood of not achieving CCyR of 18%.

Two months after his original presentation, he was started on imatinib therapy at 400 mg QD. Nevertheless, and due to unforeseen circumstances, he was unable to get treatment during months 3 to 4. He returned to clinic on month 5. Imatinib was restarted at a lower dose of 200 mg due to reported GI toxicity. The patient endorsed compliance from months 5 to 10 resulting in hematological response. On month 11, repeat assessment of peripheral blood showed 190% BCR-ABL transcripts. The patient was lost again to follow-up until month 15.

Repeat analysis prior to restarting imatinib showed 190.9% BCR-ABL transcripts. After 3 months on TKI therapy, BCR-ABL transcripts had decreased to 90%. On month 19, he was switched to dasantinib due to suboptimal response. By the end of month 24, treatment was switched to nilotinib due to interim development of intolerance to dasatinib.

On month 26, a repeat biopsy while on nilotinib showed chronic phase CML with a hypocellular marrow with trilineage hypoplasia. Cytogenetic analysis showed trisomy 8 and t(9 : 22), a 46 XY karyotype and negative ABL1 kinase domain mutation. After 4 months of treatment, his counts normalized with the exception of persistent mild thrombocytopenia. Nilotinib dose was reduced from 400 mg to 200 mg due to development of worsening cytopenias, but his counts continued to deteriorate over time, prompting hospital admission on month 33 with flow cytometry showing 7% blasts. He was discharged after transfusion of platelets but was readmitted a few weeks later for rectal bleeding in the setting of pancytopenia. Repeat bone marrow biopsy showed a hypocellular marrow with stromal edema and no significant hematopoiesis consistent with therapy effect. Blasts were not increased. Given these results, he continued on nilotinib for one more month.

A repeat biopsy conducted on month 34 showed variable cellularity with left shifted granulopoiesis, focal megakaryocytic hyperplasia, dysmegakaripoiesis, stromal fibrosis, and plasmacytosis with 5% blasts. BCR-ABL transcripts were 95%. TKI therapy was promptly discontinued on month 35 after concluding that persistent cytopenias were a consequence of nilotinib treatment rather than disease progression.

Repeat marrow biopsy on month 37 showed a normocellular marrow with left-shifted myelopoiesis and no blasts. Cytogenetics confirmed 42% BCR-ABL transcripts.

Over the next months, the patient developed therapy-related aplastic anemia with severe pancytopenia. His counts eventually improved with eltrombopag while undergoing studies for allogeneic HSCT. Follow-up bone marrow biopsy two months after eltrombopag therapy showed a hypocellular marrow with 10–15% lymphoblasts suggestive of lymphoid blast phase CML. Studies showed persistent BCR-ABL transcripts (8% by PCR and 22% by FISH with no other cytogenetic abnormalities). He stopped responding to

Table 1: Description of reported cases of TKI-related Bone Marrow Hypoplasia/Aplasia.

	Demographics	Phase of CML	TKI therapy	Timeline for cytopenias	Bone marrow biopsy	Clinical course
Lokeshwar et al. [4]	46 yo, male	Chronic phase CML	Imatinib 400 mg/d. Prior treatments: busulfan, IFNα + low-dose Ara-C, hydroxyurea.	Pancytopenia at week 6.	D56: severely hypoplastic (5%) and fatty; no significant fibrosis. Blast cells not appreciable.	Admitted for febrile neutropenia secondary to gastroenteritis and *Escherichia coli* bacteremia. She clinically declined with the development of bilateral pulmonary infiltrates. The patient passed, with postmortem confirming pulmonary mucormycosis.
Sumi et al. [5]	73 yo, female	Chronic phase CML	Imaitinib 400 mg/d. Prior treatments: IFNα, hydroxyurea, busulfan.	Pancytopenia at week 17 GIV neutropenia at day 35 GIII thrombocytopenia at day 122.	D87: severe hypocellularity.	Supportive care: transfusion PRBC, platelet; filgrastim.
Khan et al. [6]	51 yo, male	Chronic phase CML	Imatinib 400 mg daily initially, then dose reduced to 300 mg daily, then 200 mg daily for thrombocytopenia.	Anemia and thrombocytopenia at week 13, progressing to pancytopenia by week 19.	D126: slightly depressed cellularity.	Deceased: pulmonary tuberculosis, liver failure, worsening pancytopenia. Passed away despite supportive care.
Song et al. [7]	77 yo, male	Chronic phase CML	Imatinib 400 mg PO daily, dose reduced to 300 mg secondary to patient intolerance, then eventually discontinued. Nilotinib 400 mg po BID.	CCR after 9 months of imatinib therapy. No evidence of pancytopenia. Pancytopenia at week 8 of nilotinib therapy.	D252 (imatinib): CCR D56 (nilotinib): <5% normal cellularity. Fatty tissue without myelofibrosis or adipocyte deposition. No chromosomal abnormalities.	Four months after discontinuation of nilotinib, the patient remained in CCR, in the absence of further CML-specific therapy. Hematologic parameters did not recover by this time.
Poudyal et al. [3]	35 yo, male	Chronic phase CML	Imatinib 400 mg po daily. Rechallenged with 300 mg po daily after recovery of PRCA. Eventually switched to Nilotinib 400 mg po BID, then dose-reduced to 200 mg po BID secondary to recurrence of PRCA.	Anemia with reticulopenia at week 16. Anemia recurred with rechallenge of imatinib 300 mg, at week 8. Anemia recurred with nilotinib 400 mg BID, at day 40.	Three BMBx performed, each prompted by anemia while on TKI. Each BMBx demonstrated PRCA.	PRCA developed with initial dose of imatinib 400 mg daily. Discontinuation of TKI and initiation of prednisone 1 mg/kg resulted in recovery of marrow by D21. Rechallenge with imatinib 300 mg daily also resulted in recurrence of PRCA but was steroid refractory. Oral cyclosporine facilitated marrow recovery. Nilotinib 400 mg po BID was initiated, but PRCA recurred. Nilotinib was held and cyclosporine continued, with recovery of counts. Nilotinib was resumed at 200 mg BID, with continuous cyclosporine. There were no further declines in hemoglobin.

Table 1: Continued.

	Demographics	Phase of CML	TKI therapy	Timeline for cytopenias	Bone marrow biopsy	Clinical course
Estephan et al. [8]	53 yo, female	Chronic phase CML	Nilotinib 300 mg po BID. Discontinued secondary to pancytopenia. Switched to Dasatinib 50 mg daily once, cytopenias recovered.	Pancytopenia at week 10.	D70: hypocellular (<5%) with decreased trilineage hematopoiesis (panhypoplasia) and no residual CML. D140: mormocellular marrow (40%) and trilineage hematopoiesis. No left shift in maturation or increased blasts. Cyteogenetics 46XX.	Romiplostim initiated with development of pancytopenia. By 3 months, intervals between transfusions lengthened. By 5 months, repeat BMBx demonstrated recovery. Dasatinib started with good cytogenetic response.
Prodduturi et al. [9]	49 yo, male	Chronic phase CML	Imatinib 400 mg po daily. Therapy switched as milestones not achieved at 7 months. Dasatinib 100 mg po daily. Discontinued due to anaphylactic reaction. Nilotinib 400 mg po BID, then daily, then 200 mg daily. Dose reduced and eventually discontinued secondary to cytopenias.	Pancytopenia with nilotinib 400 mg BID at month 6, but with CCR. Pancytopenia recurred after 1 month of dose-reduced nilotinib 200 mg daily.	D168 (nilotinib 400 mg BID): 5–10% cellularity; CCR D364 (nilotinib 400 mg BID): 5% cellularity; CCR D56 (discontinuation of nilotinib): 40% cellularity, Ph^+ in 13/20 metaphases D30 (Nilotinib 200 mg daily): <5% cellularity; Ph^+ in 12/20 metaphases.	Milestones not achieved after 7 months of Imatinib 400 mg daily. Anaphylaxis to Dasatinib 100 mg precluded further use. Initially started on nilotinib 400 mg po BID which was decreased to daily secondary to cytopenias. BMBx showed progression, and dose was escalated to twice daily. BMBx at 6 months, then after further 7 months, it showed 5% cellularity but CCR. Marrow recovered following discontinuation of nilotinib but also with disease progression. Thereafter, resumption of nilotinib at 200 mg daily resulted in pancytopenia after 1 month, with persistent disease. All CML-directed therapy discontinued with recovery of peripheral counts.

TKI, tyrosine kinase inhibitor; IFNα, interferon alfa; GIII, grade III; GIV, grade IV; CCR, complete cytogenetic remission; CHR, complete hematologic response; PRCA, pure red cell aplasia; BMBx, bone marrow biopsy.

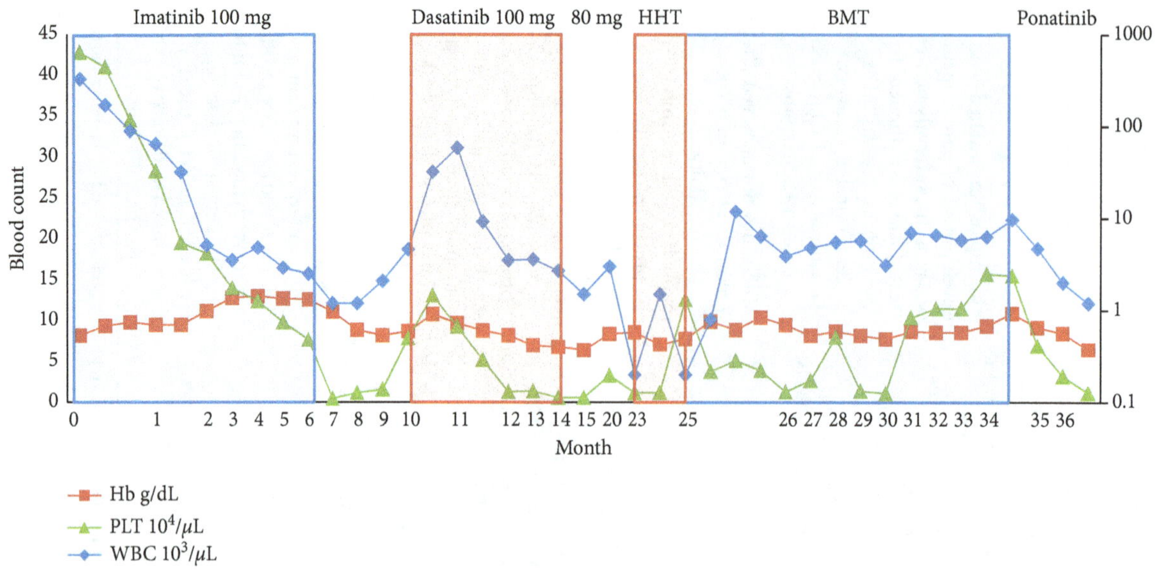

FIGURE 1: Hematologic parameters in patients with CML treated with imatinib, dasatinib, subsequent BMT, and ponatinib following relapse. White blood cells (WBC), hemoglobin (Hb), and platelets (PLTs) are depicted over a 36-month period until the last day of patient follow-up. The graph is divided into seven frames: (1) initial response to imatinib 100 mg followed by (2) discontinuation due to pancytopenia. (3) Treatment was switched to dasatinib 100 mg followed by (5) subsequent reductions in dosing in the setting of persistent pancytopenia. (6) The patient was switched to omacetaxine due to proven panmyeloid hypoplasia leading to (8) BMT. (9) The patient was started on ponatinib due to relapsed disease.

eltrombopag and became markedly thrombocytopenic. His condition declined precipitously culminating with a hemorrhagic stroke on month 45 and profuse hemorrhage leading to death.

3. Discussion

In CML, cellular proliferation and clonal expansion are driven by constitutively active BCR-ABL tyrosine kinase [1]. TKIs such as imatinib, nilotinib, and dasatanib have become the mainstay of therapy for Ph + CML by exerting selective inhibition of the BCR-ABL fusion protein through competitive binding at the ATP-binding site [2]. Continuous use of these drugs has been shown to achieve durable response in patients, and therefore awareness of their associated complications and methods to treat them becomes important.

Cytopenias are known to occur during treatment of CML. In 2016, Poudyal et al. described a patient who developed pure red cell aplasia (PRCA) from treatment with imatinib and nilotinib [3]. Sumi, Khan, Estephan, Prodduturi, Lokeshwar, and Song have each described patients developing aplasia after exposure to single BCR-ABL TKI (Table 1) [4–9].

Figures 1 and 2 show the trend of the hematologic parameters of patients 1 and 2 over their course of treatment with TKIs. In general, there are three reasons for therapy-related cytopenic events in CML. First, there is transient bone marrow hypoplasia at the onset of therapy related to reduction in CML clones during a time where normal hematopoiesis has not yet been restored. In this case, bone marrow hypoplasia/aplasia is usually accompanied by marked reduction of CML clones as judged by cytogenetics, FISH, and PCR for BCR-ABL. This was not the case in our two patients as aplasia was not associated with significant reduction in CML markers. Second, during therapy, some patients may develop new cytogenetic abnormalities (most commonly trisomy 8), suggesting development of myelodysplastic syndrome (MDS). In these instances, there is no marrow aplasia either. Third, some patients may develop into a blast phase and present with cytopenias. In these cases, marrows are also not aplastic.

While the patients described in our case series also developed aplasia, they never achieved cytological remission, in contrary to all other published reports. As such, both of our patients did poorly. It is important to notice, however, that both of them were identified as high-risk patients according to their Sokal scores (2.1 and 1.4 for patients 1 and 2, respectively). Indexes above 1.2 are considered high risk which translates to a two-year survival rate of 65% and estimated median survival of 2.5 years. Based on the Sokal score alone, these data mirror the well-known fact that patients with high risk disease are less prone to achieve cytological remission. High-risk patients who develop recurrent cytopenias on treatment that require dosing adjustments and sequential exposure to different TKIs may be more prone to develop aplasia.

There was less of an association between EUTOS scores (high risk for patient 1 and low risk for patient 2) and risk of developing marrow aplasia after TKI treatment. Both of them failed to achieve cytological remission. The reason for this disparity between our patients' Sokal and EUTOS risk stratification lies in fact that the data analyzed to develop these prognostic models were obtained from derivation studies conducted in radical different treatment eras [10, 11]. Given that the original study by Sokal and

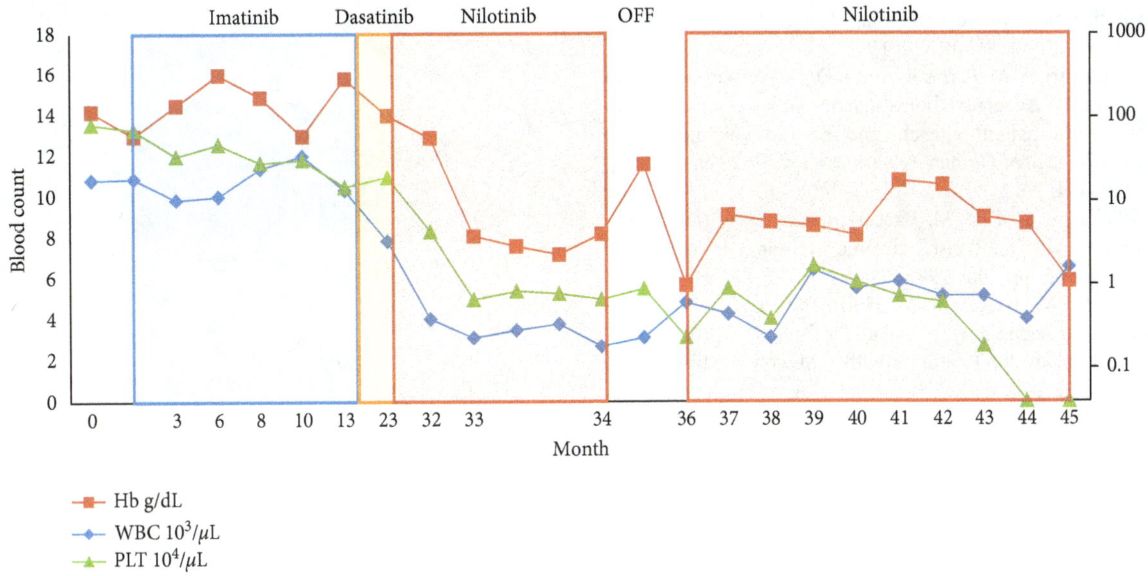

Figure 2: Hematologic parameters in patients with CML treated with imatinib, dasatinib, and subsequent nilotinib. White blood cells (WBC), hemoglobin (Hb), and platelets (PLTs) are depicted over a 45-month period until patient's death. The graph is divided into five frames: (1) initiation of imatinib and lack of adequate response due to noncompliance. Subsequent dose adjustments and continuation of treatment until month 18. (2) Initiation of dasatinib following discontinuation of imatinib due to lack of proper response. (3) Treatment was switched to nilotinib on month 23 due to persistent cytopenias and intolerable side effects. Bone marrow biopsy on month 25 revealed trilineage hypoplasia. (5) Discontinuation of nilotinib on month 34 due to persistent pancytopenia and marrow fibrosis attributed to TKI. (6) Decision to resume nilotinib with plan for urgent BMT frustrated by complications leading to death of the patient on month 45.

colleagues was conducted in 1984 in the pre-imatinib era and that treatment with TKIs has radically changed the prognosis of patients with CML since their introduction, the Sokal score may no longer be a strong predictor of the outcome in these patients according to a number of experts [11]. The EUTOS score may be a better predictor of outcome in CML after treatment with TKIs, as validated by Hoffman, Tribelli, Breccia, Uz, and Yahng, respectively [11–17], but there are also at least 3 studies (Marin, Jabbour, and Yamamoto) that question its validity [18–20]. This issue is still a matter of active debate.

4. Conclusion

Small molecule tyrosine kinase inhibitors have revolutionized the treatment of chronic myeloid leukemia. Transient myelosuppression is a common adverse event seen in patients taking TKIs; however, severe and prolonged pancytopenia together with BM aplasia secondary to TKI therapy is uncommon and only found in a handful of case reports. High-risk patients with Sokal scores greater than 1.2 who develop recurrent cytopenias on treatment that requires dosing adjustments and sequential exposure to different TKIs may be more prone to develop marrow aplasia.

Our cases describe the possible outcomes in these patients, with one of them able to undergo transplant by 24 months and the other unfortunately passing by month 45. Early recognition of this phenomenon followed by prompt transplant referral may prove to be crucial in order to prevent catastrophic consequences.

References

[1] B. J. Druker, F. Guilhot, S. G. O'Brien et al., "Five-year follow-up of patients receiving imatinib for chronic myeloid leukemia," *New England Journal of Medicine*, vol. 355, no. 23, pp. 2408–2417, 2006.

[2] B. J. Druker, S. Tamura, E. Buchdunger et al., "Effects of a selective inhibitor of the Abl tyrosine kinase on the growth of Bcr-Abl positive cells," *Nature Medicine*, vol. 2, no. 5, pp. 561-566, 1996.

[3] B. S. Poudyal, S. Tuladhar, and B. Gyawali, "TKI-induced pure red cell aplasia: first case report of pure red cell aplasia with both imatinib and nilotinib," *ESMO Open*, vol. 1, no. 3, article e000058, 2016.

[4] N. Lokeshwar, L. Kumar, and M. Kumari, "Severe bone marrow aplasia following imatinib mesylate in a patient with chronic myelogenous leukemia," *Leukemia & Lymphoma*, vol. 46, no. 5, pp. 781–784, 2005.

[5] M. Sumi, T. Tauchi, T. Shimamoto et al., "Chronic myeloid leukemia associated with sustained severe pancytopenia after imatinib mesylate therapy," *Rinsho Ketsueki*, vol. 43, no. 9, pp. 868–870, 2002.

[6] K. A. Khan, A. Junaid, N. S. Siddiqui, K. Mukhtar, and S. Siddiqui, "Imatinib-related bone marrow aplasia after complete cytogenetic response in chronic myeloid leukemia," *Journal of College of Physicians and Surgeons Pakistan*, vol. 18, no. 3, pp. 176–178, 2008.

[7] M.-K. Song, Y.-J. Choi, Y.-M. Seol et al., "Nilotinib-induced bone marrow aplasia," *European Journal of Haematology*, vol. 83, no. 2, pp. 161-162, 2009.

[8] F. Estephan, H. J. Rogers, V. Visconte et al., "Spontaneous recovery of severe nilotinib-induced bone marrow aplasia and successful retreatment with dasatinib in a patient with chronic

phase chronic myeloid leukemia," *Leukemia & Lymphoma*, vol. 56, no. 3, pp. 811–813, 2015.

[9] P. Prodduturi, A. M. Perry, P. Aoun, D. D. Weisenburger, and M. Akhtari, "Recurrent bone marrow aplasia secondary to nilotinib in a patient with chronic myeloid leukemia: a case report," *Journal of Oncology Pharmacy Practice*, vol. 18, no. 4, pp. 440–444, 2012.

[10] J. E. Sokal, E. B. Cox, M. Baccarani et al., "Prognostic discrimination in "good-risk" chronic granulocytic leukemia," *Blood*, vol. 63, pp. 789–799, 1984.

[11] J. Hasford, M. Baccarani, V. Hoffmann et al., "Predicting complete cytogenetic response and subsequent progression-free survival in 2060 patients with CML on imatinib treatment: the EUTOS score," *Blood*, vol. 118, no. 3, pp. 686–692, 2011.

[12] V. S. Hoffmann, J. Mayer, A. G. Turkina et al., "EUTOS score is also valid in CML patients not involved in clinical studies," *Blood*, vol. 120, p. 3759, 2012.

[13] V. S. Hoffmann, M. Baccarani, D. Lindoerfer et al., "The EUTOS prognostic score: review and validation in 1288 patients with CML treated frontline with imatinib," *Leukemia*, vol. 27, no. 10, pp. 2016–2022, 2013.

[14] M. Tiribelli, M. Bonifacio, E. Calistri et al., "EUTOS score identifies cases with poor outcome in patients with early chronic phase chronic myeloid leukemia, though not predictive for optimal response to imatinib," *Blood*, vol. 120, p. 3778, 2012.

[15] M. Breccia, P. Finsinger, G. Loglisci et al., "The EUTOS score identifies chronic myeloid leukeamia patients with poor prognosis treated with imatinib first or second line," *Leukemia Research*, vol. 36, no. 9, pp. e209–e210, 2012.

[16] B. Uz, Y. Buyukasik, H. Atay et al., "EUTOS CML prognostic scoring system predicts ELN-based 'event-free survival' better than Euro/Hasford and Sokal systems in CML patients receiving front-line imatinib mesylate," *Hematology*, vol. 18, no. 5, pp. 247–252, 2013.

[17] S. A. Yahng, E. J. Jang, S. Y. Choi et al., "Comparison of Sokal, Hasford and EUTOS scores in terms of long-term treatment outcome according to the risks in each prognostic model: a single center data analyzed in 255 early chronic phase chronic myeloid leukemia patients treated with frontline imatinib mesylate," *Blood*, vol. 120, p. 2794, 2012.

[18] D. Marin, A. R. Ibrahim, and J. M. Goldman, "European Treatment and Outcome Study (EUTOS) score for chronic myeloid leukemia still requires more confirmation," *Journal of Clinical Oncology*, vol. 29, no. 29, pp. 3944-3945, 2011.

[19] E. Jabbour, J. Cortes, A. Nazha et al., "EUTOS score is not predictive for survival and outcome in patients with early chronic phase chronic myeloid leukemia treated with tyrosine kinase inhibitors: a single institution experience," *Blood*, vol. 119, no. 19, pp. 4524–4526, 2012.

[20] E. Yamamoto, S. Fujisawa, M. Hagihara et al., "European Treatment and Outcome Study Score does not predict imatinib treatment response and outcome in chronic myeloid leukemia patients," *Cancer Science*, vol. 105, no. 1, pp. 105–109, 2014.

7

Unexplained Hematocrit Increase after Therapeutic Phlebotomy in a Patient with Marked Erythrocytosis

Rushad Machhi, Ashley M. Cunningham, Kenneth Hennrick, Karen A. Schaser, Eliot C. Williams, and William Nicholas Rose

Department of Pathology and Laboratory Medicine, University of Wisconsin Hospital, 600 Highland Ave, D4/250, Madison 53792, WI, USA

Correspondence should be addressed to William Nicholas Rose; wrose@uwhealth.org

Academic Editor: Kostas Konstantopoulos

We report a patient with hereditary erythrocytosis who underwent a therapeutic phlebotomy and had a post-phlebotomy hematocrit that was higher than the pre-phlebotomy hematocrit. We could not discern a reason for this hematocrit increase after phlebotomy. Instead of performing another phlebotomy, we performed an automated red cell depletion via an apheresis instrument. This procedure is essentially a red cell exchange, but 5% albumin is used as the replacement fluid instead of red blood cells. The patient's hematocrit decreased from 80% to 39% after three consecutive daily red cell depletion procedures. We share our experience to report the unusual finding of a patient's hematocrit that increased with phlebotomy and to raise awareness of the red cell depletion procedure.

1. Introduction

Erythrocytosis, or polycythemia, is an elevation of the red blood cell (RBC) mass often recognized through increases in the hemoglobin (Hgb) concentration or hematocrit (Hct). The WHO defines polycythemia as a Hgb concentration or Hct greater than 16.5 g/dL or 49% for males, respectively, or 16.0 g/dL or 48% for females, respectively [1]. The majority of erythrocytosis is incidentally discovered in asymptomatic individuals. However, symptoms and manifestations of erythrocytosis can be quite variable and are typically due to the excess RBC burden resulting in hyperviscosity. Mild symptoms can include fatigue, headaches, and plethora. More severe manifestations, while uncommon, include venous thromboembolism (VTE), myocardial infarction (MI), and cerebrovascular accident (CVA) [2].

Erythrocytosis is often classified into primary and secondary erythrocytosis. Primary erythrocytosis involves alteration in the erythropoietin (EPO) receptor (EpoR) either through an acquired or congenital process [3]. Patients with primary erythrocytosis generally have low levels of EPO and normal oxygen dissociation curves [4]. The most common acquired process is polycythemia vera, which is driven by a somatic mutation in the JAK2 signaling pathway of the EpoR [5]. Less common is hereditary erythrocytosis, which involves a congenital mutation of the EpoR.

Common mutations in hereditary erythrocytosis involve the SHP-1 docking site, which turns off EPO signaling. Patients with hereditary erythrocytosis will have a wild type JAK2 gene [3]. Secondary erythrocytosis, meanwhile, is driven largely by an increase in EPO. Generally, patients will have elevated or inappropriately normal levels of EPO [4]. Common causes of secondary erythrocytosis include chronic hypoxia, EPO producing tumors, and increased androgens. Congenital causes such as 2,3 BPG deficiency, methemoglobinemia, and genetic mutations involving the hypoxia inducing factor (HIF) pathway are less common [3].

The management of secondary erythrocytosis usually requires treating the underlying cause. The management of both primary erythrocytosis and hereditary causes of secondary erythrocytosis usually requires directly decreasing the RBC burden [6]. To that end, the goal of treatment is not only to provide symptomatic relief but also to lower the risk of mortality from the major complications of erythrocytosis. Lowering the hematocrit to a goal of less than 45% has been shown to decrease mortality from major cardiac or thromboembolic events [7].

The mainstay of treatment is therapeutic phlebotomy. Depending on patient size and ability to tolerate an acute decrease in hematocrit, about 500 mL to 1000 mL of whole blood is removed by weighing 500 g to 1000 g, respectively, on a tared blood bag on a scale. In essentially all cases that we have experienced or read about, a therapeutic phlebotomy decreases the hematocrit. If the hematocrit is not lowered enough or if the patient requires frequent intervals of phlebotomy, erythrocytapheresis or red cell depletion (RCD) is an effective and safe alternative. Here, we present the case of a patient with hereditary erythrocytosis whose hematocrit increased after phlebotomy, a finding that appears to be unreported, and then decreased significantly following successive RCDs.

2. Case Presentation

A 45-year-old female with a past medical history of hereditary erythrocytosis, juvenile rheumatoid arthritis, and thrombocytopenia presented to the University of Wisconsin Hospital (UWH) with altered mental status, dyspnea, and dysphagia. Chest X-ray showed infiltrates suggestive of pneumonia, and the patient was positive for influenza A. She was admitted and started on a 5-day course of oseltamivir. On admission, her Hct reached a high of 78%, and her Hgb was 22.6 g/dL. The patient had previously been evaluated for hereditary erythrocytosis with negative testing for JAK2 gene exon 14, a normal oxygen dissociation curve, and no significant cardiopulmonary abnormalities. Her EPO levels had been consistently elevated, but the significance of this finding was never clearly found.

After adequate rehydration, a 350 mL therapeutic phlebotomy was performed. However, a post-phlebotomy Hct revealed an increase to 80%. Based on this increase and her small body habitus (patient weight 31.8 kg on admission), the decision to proceed with RCD was made.

RCD was performed via centrifugal apheresis using the Cobe Spectra apheresis system through an internal jugular (IJ) vein hemodialysis line. While RCD is rarely performed, a program for RCD already existed as a program in this machine. The replacement fluid was 5% albumin. No “rinse back” of the whole blood that remained in the machine at the end was performed. The manufacturer, Terumo BCT, was contacted and recommended that the Hct not be lowered by more than 22% per session. However, given her small body habitus and significantly elevated Hct, the decision was made to set the Hct target to 50%. The first RCD lowered her Hct from 80% to 61%. The following day a second RCD with a Hct target of 35% was performed that lowered her Hct to 48%. A third and final RCD was completed the next day with a Hct target of 35% that lowered her Hct from 50% to 39%. About 600 mL of RBCs was removed during each session with an inlet speed of 20 mL/min and whole blood to anticoagulant ratio of 13 : 1. There were no complications or adverse reactions during the procedures. The patient was discharged shortly after completing her RCDs with outpatient follow-up and a plan for regular 500 mL therapeutic phlebotomies.

3. Discussion

The key reportable phenomenon was not the use of RCD, which is unusual but reported, but rather the increase in the hematocrit after therapeutic phlebotomy. If this has happened with any regularity, we were not able to find reports of it in our literature search. The main teaching message that we wish to communicate is that if a therapeutic phlebotomy non-intuitively increases your patient’s hematocrit, consider this strategy as one option: do not repeat the phlebotomy but do a RCD. Our rationale was that performing another phlebotomy might have increased her hematocrit even higher, and a second increase in hematocrit, however unlikely or unexplainable, seemed like a risk that was unwarranted.

We concede that we do not know why this happened. We can speculate about several possible factors. Perhaps one or more hematocrit results of 78% and 80% were spurious. That is, we speculate that perhaps the hematocrit loses accuracy at the extremes of measurement as the values greatly exceed or recede from the linear or reportable range. After all, the hematocrit is calculated from the MCV and RBC count, so perhaps an extreme RBC count introduces imprecision and/or inaccuracy.

Perhaps the phlebotomy removed relatively more non-RBC fluid and relatively less RBC mass than the proportions that were present in the patient. We can speculate that there may be a rheological explanation that is beyond our expertise. Perhaps when the hematocrit blood becomes that high and the blood becomes that viscous, the physical characteristics of the blood are such that a routine phlebotomy can lead to, for example, relatively more plasma loss and less RBC loss than one would predict. Perhaps one plausible factor is the smaller gauge venous access needle in peripheral access phlebotomy compared to the larger gauge venous access device that was used for the RCDs.

Perhaps the 78% was spuriously low instead of the 80% being spuriously high. For both theories, we have no evidence for or against them, but perhaps the 78% result was relatively diluted by hydration in the patient’s body and/or a relatively higher ratio of EDTA anticoagulant to patient sample. Alternatively, the 80% could have been spuriously high from the 2 opposite factors: relative dehydration and/or a relatively lower ratio of anticoagulant to patient sample.

Finally, perhaps the instrument’s coefficient of variation was such that 78% and 80% overlap to some degree. This is also beyond our expertise, but we have anecdotal experience with lab test that yields slightly different results when they are repeated nearly simultaneously using the same specimen. Perhaps other factors could explain the increase. We do not claim to have provided an exhaustive list of hypotheses from the fields of laboratory medicine, rheology, or other fields. We stress that our focus is simply to raise awareness of existence of automated red cell depletion and to consider using it if phlebotomy is ineffective for any reason.

The exact etiology of this patient's erythrocytosis is not known with complete clarity. In short, we labeled her with the diagnosis of presumed hereditary erythrocytosis not otherwise specified. Our rationale was that the erythrocytosis appeared to be lifelong and no overt external stimuli appeared to be causing it.

One can suggest additional testing to clarify a specific mutation or labeled syndrome. We admit that we did not go as far as one could in terms of genetic testing for diagnostic or research purposes. Although this patient has not had the full array of genetic testing done to confirm the exact etiology of her hereditary erythrocytosis, based on her chronically elevated EPO levels and normal dissociation curve, this is highly suggestive of a defect in her HIF pathway. Mutations in this pathway commonly arise from the VHL, EGLN2, or EPAS1 genes [4].

As is often the case, we judged that a battery of genetic tests would not be worth the large expense when the result would not be likely to change our management. That is, the probability that any one of these mutations would be found was very low. Also, more importantly, even if one of these mutations had been found, the treatment strategy would almost certainly be the same: to reduce RBC mass via therapeutic phlebotomy (and/or RCD) and, depending on risk stratification, to reduce thrombosis risk (for example, with aspirin). Thus, we judged that we had obtained a sufficient amount of actionable diagnostic information while minimizing the costs.

RCD has been known to be a safe procedure for severe erythrocytosis for many years. In other words, the procedure exists as an option in the most popular therapeutic apheresis machines, but many specialists may not have ever used it and may not be aware of it. Therapeutic apheresis machines and the specialists that use and medically manage them may not be available in all centers. But if the option is available nearby, consider it if your patient has severe erythrocytosis that requires acute treatment, especially if therapeutic phlebotomy is inadequate.

The American Society for Apheresis (ASFA) in their 2019 guidelines reiterated the use of RCD for PV and hereditary erythrocytosis, specifically stating that it can be a useful alternative to phlebotomy in cases where the patient is a high bleeding risk or if red cell reduction is rapidly needed prior to a surgery [6]. RCD treatment has been shown to increase the interval needed between red cell depleting therapies when compared to therapeutic phlebotomy [8].

Furthermore, the complication rate of RCDs has been shown to be as low as 7%, and the complications are usually benign (e.g., mild hypocalcemia from the citrate anticoagulant) [9]. However, IJ line placement usually poses greater risks than RCD itself. Thus, the aggregate risks and benefits of line placement plus RCD should be considered as a bundle. In addition, RCD treatment can cost up to three times more than therapeutic phlebotomy, and this cost is only slightly offset by the increased interval between treatment [10]. Nevertheless, as observed in our case presented here that was expanded from our previous abstract, RCD is a potential option for a patient with severe erythrocytosis that does not respond to therapeutic phlebotomy [11].

References

[1] E. Campo, N. L. Harris, E. S. Jaffe et al., *WHO Classification of Tumours of Haematopoietic and Lymphoid Tissues*, BookBaby, Portland, OR, USA, 2008.

[2] M. S. Aljabry, "Primary familial and congenital polycythemia; the forgotten entity," *Journal of Applied Hematology*, vol. 9, no. 2, 2018.

[3] M. F. McMullin, "Diagnostic workflow for hereditary erythrocytosis and thrombocytosis," *Hematology 2014, the American Society of Hematology Education Program Book*, no. 1, pp. 391–396, 2019.

[4] J. L. Oliveira, "Algorithmic evaluation of hereditary erythrocytosis: pathways and caveats," *The International Journal of Literary Humanities*, vol. 41, pp. 89–94, 2019.

[5] W. J. Hong and J. Gotlib, "Hereditary erythrocytosis, thrombocytosis and neutrophilia," *Best Practice & Research Clinical Haematology*, vol. 27, no. 2, pp. 95–106, 2014.

[6] A. Padmanabhan, L. Connelly Smith, N. Aqui et al., "Guidelines on the use of therapeutic apheresis in clinical practice–evidence based approach from the Writing Committee of the American Society for Apheresis: the eighth special issue," *Journal of Clinical Apheresis*, vol. 34, no. 3, pp. 171–354, 2019.

[7] R. Marchioli, G. Finazzi, G. Specchia et al., "Cardiovascular events and intensity of treatment in polycythemia vera," *New England Journal of Medicine*, vol. 368, no. 1, pp. 22–33, 2013.

[8] S. Vecchio, P. Leonardo, V. Musuraca, A. R. D'Ettoris, and W. Geremicca, "A comparison of the results obtained with traditional phlebotomy and with therapeutic erythrocytapheresis in patients with erythrocytosis," *Blood Transfusion*, vol. 5, no. 1, pp. 20–23, 2007.

[9] I. Parra Salinas, V. Recasens Flores, M. Á. Montañés, and J. A. García-Erce, "Therapeutic erythroapheresis: experience in patients with polycythemia vera and secondary erythrocytosis," *Medicina Clínica*, vol. 154, no. 1, pp. 16–19, 2020.

[10] L. Teofili, C. G. Valentini, E. Rossi, and V. De Stefano, "Indications and use of therapeutic phlebotomy in polycythemia vera: which role for erythrocytapheresis?" *Leukemia*, vol. 33, no. 1, pp. 279–281, 2019.

[11] A. Cunningham, K. Hennrick, K. Schaser, E. Williams, and W. Rose, "Red cell depletion for a patient with hereditary erythrocytosis after unsuccessful therapeutic phlebotomy: 88," *Journal of Clinical Apheresis*, vol. 29, p. 1, 2014.

Successful Management of Immune Thrombocytopenia Presenting with Lethal Alveolar Hemorrhage

Keiki Nagaharu[1,2] **Masahiro Masuya,**[1] **Keiki Kawakami**[2] **and Naoyuki Katayama**[1]

[1]*Department of Hematology and Oncology, Mie University Graduate School of Medicine, Edobashi 2-174, Tsu, Mie Prefecture 514-8507, Japan*
[2]*Department of Hematology and Oncology, Suzuka General Hospital, Yamanohana 1275-53, Suzuka, Mie Prefecture 513-8630, Japan*

Correspondence should be addressed to Keiki Nagaharu; keiki.nagaharu@gmail.com

Academic Editor: Tomás J. González-López

Immune thrombocytopenic purpura (ITP) typically presents with bleeding due to immunologic thrombocytopenia. Severe hemorrhage due to ITP is sometimes lethal, and the urgent recovery of platelets is necessary. In addition to conventional therapeutic strategies, romiplostim shows promising efficacy for chronic ITP. However, there is little evidence for the utilization of this treatment for acute ITP or acute exacerbation of chronic ITP. We report the case details of three elderly ITP patients presenting with lethal diffuse alveolar hemorrhage. These patients had the following underlying pulmonary diseases: case 1, nontuberculous mycobacterial infection and sarcoidosis; case 2, cryptogenic organizing pneumonia; case 3, pulmonary emphysema. These patients recovered following treatment with romiplostim at a higher dose (10 μg/kg), in addition to conventional therapies including corticosteroids and high-dose intravenous immunoglobulin. In summary, the addition of romiplostim resulted in earlier recovery of thrombocytopenia than has been previously reported. Our three cases suggest that early romiplostim at a higher dose could be an efficacious therapeutic option for acute ITP patients with severe lethal bleeding.

1. Introduction

Immune thrombocytopenic purpura (ITP) is a hematological disorder characterized by thrombocytopenia due to immunological mechanisms. Lethal bleeding symptoms (e.g., intracranial, gastrointestinal, and diffuse alveolar hemorrhage (DAH)) have been reported as severe complications in ITP [1]. Standard first-line therapy for ITP is corticosteroids, with or without high-dose intravenous immunoglobulin (IVIG). In cases refractory to these therapies, splenectomy or treatment with rituximab is recommended [2–4]. Recently, romiplostim has been reported as an additional strategy [5]. In chronic ITP, weekly subcutaneous administration of romiplostim increased the platelet count without significant adverse effects [6, 7]. However, few reports have focused on early care with romiplostim for newly diagnosed patients or cases of acute exacerbation of ITP [8, 9]. We report three elderly ITP patients presenting with lethal DAH. These cases were successfully treated with romiplostim at a higher dose, in addition to conventional therapies. Through our cases, we suggest the efficacy of romiplostim at a higher dose against lethal hemorrhage.

2. Case Presentation

2.1. Case 1. A 65-year-old male was admitted to our hospital because of ecchymosis on both lower extremities. Three years before admission, he was diagnosed with ITP by laboratory tests, including antibodies against platelet glycoprotein (GP) IIb/IIIa and GP IV, and bone marrow aspiration. He had been treated successfully with corticosteroids. History included nontuberculosis mycobacterial infection. Previous treatment included prednisolone

(PSL; 5 mg/day), clarithromycin, rifampicin, and ethambutol hydrochloride. Two weeks before admission, routine laboratory examination showed normal platelet counts (PC; 185×10^9/l).

On admission, laboratory findings showed a PC of 3.0×10^9/l. Biochemical parameters and coagulation values were within the normal limit. Antibodies against *Helicobacter pylori*, hepatitis C virus (HCV), hepatitis B virus (HBV), and human immunodeficiency virus (HIV) were negative. We diagnosed him with acute exacerbation of chronic ITP. The clinical course is shown in Supplementary Figure 1.

He was treated immediately with high-dose IVIG, PSL (40 mg/day, p.o.), and romiplostim (1 μg/kg). During the next four days, he developed respiratory failure; PaO_2/FiO_2 ratio was approximately 250. On the fourth day of hospitalization, computed tomography (CT) revealed ground-glass opacities (GGOs) with marginal infiltration in both lung fields, on the basis of which a diagnosis of alveolar hemorrhage was made. His dyspnea worsened gradually, and noninvasive positive pressure ventilation (NPPV) was initiated.

On the 11th day of hospitalization, a higher dose of romiplostim (10 μg/kg) was initiated together with pulsed doses of methyl-PSL (1000 mg/day for 3 days) and a second cycle of IVIG. His PC recovered by the 21st day of hospitalization, and he was discharged without any complications. The patient's PC has remained normal whilst being treated with 12.5 mg of PSL daily for 12 months, without recurrence of alveolar hemorrhage.

2.2. Case 2. A 71-year-old male was referred to our hospital because of gingival bleeding, hemoptysis, and dyspnea. His past medical history included acute HBV infection during the pediatric period, which resolved without any prolonged hepatic disorders. Three months prior to admission, chest radiography showed a consolidation in the right lung field. Two days before admission, he underwent transbronchial lung biopsy and was diagnosed with cryptogenic organizing pneumonia.

The patient's PC was low (6.0×10^9/l) at admission, despite a normal PC (224×10^9/l) at 12 days before admission. Platelet-associated IgG increased to 81.7 ng/10^7 cells, and tests for antibodies against GP IIb/IIIa and GP Ia/IIa were positive. Serological tests for *H. pylori*, HCV, and, HIV were negative but positive for anti-HBs antibody, without viremia. Bone marrow examination showed an increased number of megakaryocytes, without apparent malignancy. CT at admission revealed pulmonary bilateral GGOs. The patient was diagnosed as having acute ITP with alveolar hemorrhage.

High-dose IVIG was started with PSL (0.5 mg/kg, p.o.); however, he developed dyspnea on the second day of hospitalization (Supplementary Figure 1). Given the risk for respiratory failure, a higher dose of romiplostim (10 μg/kg/w) was initiated. Nine days after admission, his PC increased to 9.0×10^9/l and respiratory symptoms resolved. On the 30th day after admission, he was discharged without any complications.

2.3. Case 3. A 71-year-old male was admitted because of dyspnea and hemoptysis. He had a history of Stevens–Johnson syndrome due to salazosulfapyridine and pulmonary emphysema. On admission, he developed severe respiratory failure (P/F ratio: 100) and NPPV support was initiated. His PC was low ($2.0 \times 10^9/\mu$l) at admission but had been normal (158×10^9/l) two months before. Laboratory tests showed high PA-IgG (605.8 ng/10^7 cells), and serological tests for *H. pylori*, HCV, HBV, and HIV were negative. Bone marrow examination revealed an increase in the number of megakaryocytes without malignancies. CT on the day of admission revealed GGOs with no evidence of infection. He was diagnosed as having acute ITP with alveolar hemorrhage.

The patient was treated with methyl-PSL pulse therapy (1000 mg daily for 5 days) and IVIG (Supplemental Figure 1). Rapid progression of severe respiratory failure occurred over the next two days; hence, we added romiplostim at a higher dose (10 μg/kg weekly). Four days after initiating treatment, his PC increased to 25×10^9/l and hemoptysis and dyspnea resolved. Despite tapering of the PSL dose, there was no recurrence of thrombocytopenia.

3. Discussion

The causes of DAH are heterogeneous: vasculitis, drug-induced lung injury, stem cell transplantation, infection, trauma, coagulopathy, and thrombocytopenia [10, 11]. The prognosis of thrombocytopenia-related DAH is especially poor [12]. ITP patients with DAH are rare although are described in several case reports [13–17]. Although these cases have no apparent relationship with pulmonary diseases, our three patients had underlying pulmonary diseases, in addition to thrombocytopenia. Clinicians should consider the importance of DAH in ITP with underlying lung diseases.

IVIG and corticosteroids are reported to result in recovery in approximately 2 days and 2–5 days, respectively [1]. Alternative strategies including splenectomy and/or thrombopoietin receptor agonists should be considered in refractory cases. The usual initiation dose of romiplostim is 1.0 μg/kg, and dose adjustment is necessary to achieve PC responses. The standard initiation dose is not sufficient in many cases. Indeed, Shirasugi et al. reported that treatment with an initial dose of 3 to 6 μg/kg promotes more rapid platelet recovery compared with that of 1.0 μg/kg in chronic ITP [18]. In addition, Contis et al. showed that higher doses (6–9 μg/kg) of romiplostim might be needed in patients with severe acute or persistent ITP, who are refractory to conventional therapies [8]. These findings indicated that the higher dose is effective for lethal cases.

Our cases showed a more rapid response, compared with previous cases with available clinical data [15–17] (Figure 1). Despite having a much higher platelet count (600 to 1000×10^9/l) after treatment (Supplementary Figure 1), no vascular thrombosis was observed in all cases. These cases indicated that early and higher doses of romiplostim can be effective for ITP with lethal hemorrhage. Further investigations will be needed to establish the appropriate dose

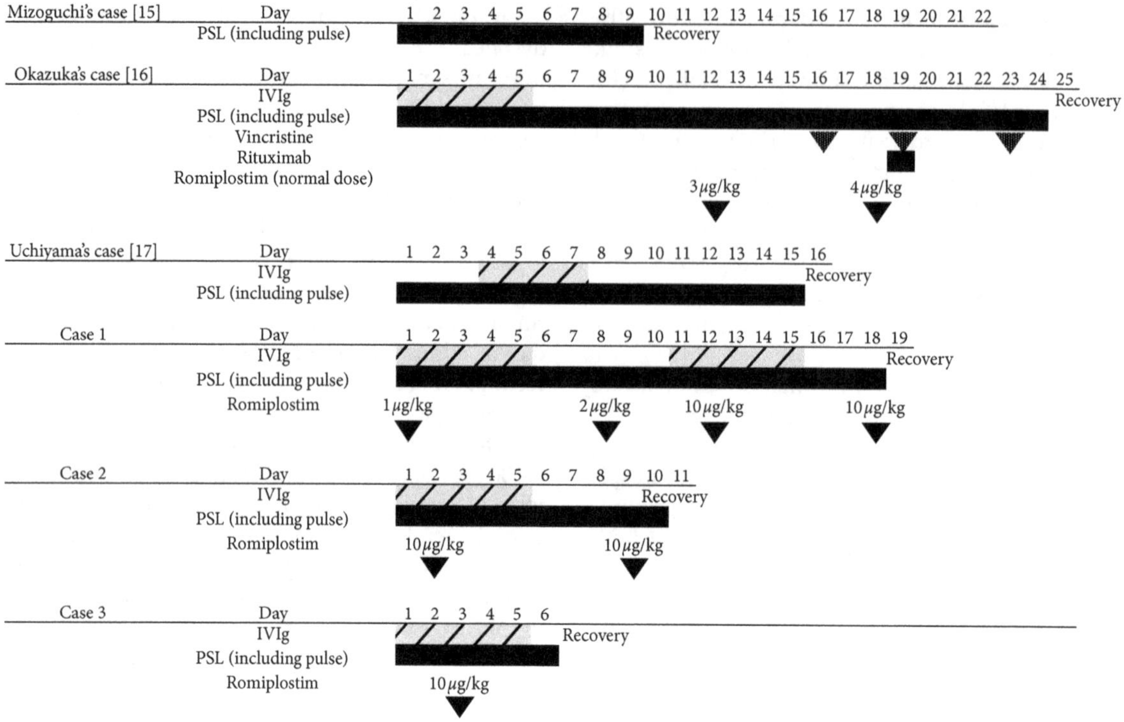

FIGURE 1: Literature review of the cases with DAH due to ITP. Recovery is defined as a platelet count of more than 100×10^9/l.

of romiplostim for patients with ITP presenting with lethal hemorrhage.

Acknowledgments

We would like to thank Editage (http://www.editage.jp) for English language editing.

References

[1] D. M. Arnold, "Bleeding complications in immune thrombocytopenia," *Hematology American Society of Hematology Education Program*, vol. 2015, no. 1, pp. 237–242, 2015.

[2] Z. Zhou and R. Yang, "Rituximab treatment for chronic refractory idiopathic thrombocytopenic purpura," *Critical Reviews in Oncology/Hematology*, vol. 65, no. 1, pp. 21–31, 2008.

[3] W. A. Hammond, E. M. Rodriguez, Z. Li et al., "Splenectomy or rituximab in steroid-refractory immune thrombocytopenia (ITP): the mayo clinic experience," *Blood*, vol. 128, p. 3735, 2016.

[4] S. Chaturvedi, D. M. Arnold, and K. R. McCrae, "Splenectomy for immune thrombocytopenia: down but not out," *Blood*, vol. 131, no. 11, pp. 1172–1182, 2018.

[5] C. Neunert, W. Lim, M. Crowther, A. Cohen, L. Solberg Jr., and M. A. Crowther, "The American Society of Hematology 2011 evidence-based practice guideline for immune thrombocytopenia," *Blood*, vol. 117, no. 16, pp. 4190–4207, 2011.

[6] D. J. Kuter, M. Rummel, R. Boccia et al., "Romiplostim or standard of care in patients with immune thrombocytopenia," *New England Journal of Medicine*, vol. 363, no. 20, pp. 1889–1899, 2010.

[7] J. B. Bussel, D. J. Kuter, V. Pullarkat, R. M. Lyons, M. Guo, and J. L. Nichol, "Safety and efficacy of long-term treatment with romiplostim in thrombocytopenic patients with chronic ITP," *Blood*, vol. 113, no. 10, pp. 2161–2171, 2009.

[8] A. Contis, E. Lazaro, C. Greib, J.-L. Pellegrin, and J.-F. Viallard, "Romiplostim as early treatment for refractory primary immune thrombocytopenia," *International Journal of Hematology*, vol. 98, no. 5, pp. 520–524, 2013.

[9] G. Tagariello, R. Sartori, P. Radossi, N. Maschio, R. Risato, and R. Stasi, "Romiplostim for the early management of severe immune thrombocytopenia unresponsive to conventional treatment," *British Journal of Haematology*, vol. 157, no. 2, pp. 256–258, 2012.

[10] N. de Prost, A. Parrot, C. Picard et al., "Diffuse alveolar haemorrhage: factors associated with in-hospital and long-term mortality," *European Respiratory Journal*, vol. 35, no. 6, pp. 1303–1311, 2010.

[11] F. M. von Ranke, G. Zanetti, B. Hochhegger, and E. Marchiori, "Infectious diseases causing diffuse alveolar hemorrhage in immunocompetent patients: a state-of-the-art review," *Lung*, vol. 191, no. 1, pp. 9–18, 2013.

[12] C. Rabe, B. Appenrodt, C. Hoff et al., "Severe respiratory failure due to diffuse alveolar hemorrhage: clinical characteristics and outcome of intensive care," *Journal of Critical Care*, vol. 25, no. 2, pp. 230–235, 2010.

[13] S. Das, S. Cherian, W. Hamarneh et al., "Diffuse alveolar hemorrhage secondary to idiopathic thrombocytopenic purpura; an extremely rare presentation," *Chest*, vol. 142, no. 4, p. 469A, 2012.

[14] H. R. T. Hashmi, S. Venkatram, and G. Diaz-Fuentes, "A case report of an elderly woman with thrombocytopenia and bilateral lung infiltrates," *Medicine*, vol. 94, no. 50, article e2235, 2015.

[15] M. Mizoguchi, K. Kazuhiro, M. Naoto, K. Fukutani, and M. Yukio, "A case of idiopathic thrombocytopenic purpura

involving diffuse alveolar hemorrhage," *Journal of the Yonago Medical Association*, vol. 67, no. 1-2, pp. 9–16, 2016.

[16] K. Okazuka, M. Masuko, Y. Matsuo et al., "Successful treatment of severe newly diagnosed immune thrombocytopenia involving an alveolar hemorrhage with combination therapy consisting of romiplostim, rituximab and vincristine," *Internal Medicine*, vol. 52, no. 11, pp. 1239–1242, 2013.

[17] M. Uchiyama, A. Hattori, T. Tanaka et al., "Acute idiopathic thrombocytopenic purpura complicated with diffuse alveolar hemorrhage in an elderly patient," *Internal Medicine*, vol. 48, no. 16, pp. 1449–1452, 2009.

[18] Y. Shirasugi, K. Ando, S. Hashino et al., "A phase II, open-label, sequential-cohort, dose-escalation study of romiplostim in Japanese patients with chronic immune thrombocytopenic purpura," *International Journal of Hematology*, vol. 90, no. 2, pp. 157–165, 2009.

De Novo Mutation of the ADAMTS13 Gene with Mesenteric Ischemia in an Infant with Congenital Thrombotic Thrombocytopenic Purpura

Ibrahim Alharbi,[1,2] Sarah Alqarni,[3] Wed Khayyat,[3] and Amirah Almatrafi[3]

[1]*Department of Pediatrics, Umm Al-Qura University, Makkah, Saudi Arabia*
[2]*King Fahad Armed Forces Hospital, Jeddah, Saudi Arabia*
[3]*Umm Al-Qura University, Makkah, Saudi Arabia*

Correspondence should be addressed to Amirah Almatrafi; amiraalmatrafi1997@gmail.com

Academic Editor: Saveria Capria

Introduction. Congenital thrombotic thrombocytopenic purpura (cTTP) is a rare autosomal recessive disease characterized by ADAMTS13 deficiency or a severe decrease in its activity that is caused by homozygous or combined heterozygous mutations in its encoding gene. Here, we describe a de novo genetic mutation of the ADAMTS13 gene and a rare complication of cTTP in a neonate. *Case Presentation.* A full-term baby boy developed tachypnea, bradycardia, and oxygen desaturation at 2 h of life and was shifted to the newborn intensive care unit. He was oliguric in the first 24 h of life and had one episode of epistaxis. Blood-stained urine was observed in the urine catheter, and a coffee-ground-colored fluid was drained from the orogastric tube. Histopathological analysis revealed gastric perforation with features of ischemic insult. On day 8, genetic analysis confirmed the diagnosis of autosomal recessive familial thrombotic thrombocytopenic purpura and revealed a unique homozygous deletion mutation on exon 23 of ADAMTS13: c.2883del p.(Cys962Alafs*3). *Conclusion.* cTTP is a rare life-threatening autosomal recessive disease with a high mortality rate. Early detection and initiation of aggressive treatment with plasma infusion could be a life-saving strategy in such cases.

1. Introduction

Congenital thrombotic thrombocytopenic purpura (cTTP), which is also known as Upshaw–Schulman syndrome, is a rare life-threatening autosomal recessive disease. It is caused by mutations on a disintegrin and metalloproteinase with a thrombospondin type 1 motif member 13 (ADAMTS13). In comparison to acquired TTP, cTTP is less common and has an incidence of 1/1000,000 individuals annually worldwide [1]. cTTP is often associated with multiorgan involvement: it not only mainly involves the central nervous system but also results in myocardial and renal impairment [2]. A variety of mutations have been found to cause cTTP [3–7]. In this paper, we present a de novo genetic mutation of the ADAMTS13 gene that has never been reported before in a patient with gastric ischemia and perforation, which are unusual secondary complications of cTTP.

2. Case Presentation

The patient was a full-term baby boy born via normal spontaneous vaginal delivery. His birth weight was 2.718 kg, and the Apgar score was 9 and 10 at 1 min and 5 min, respectively. He was born to consanguineous parents and did not have a family history of hematological disease or similar conditions. At 2 h after delivery, he developed tachypnea, bradycardia, and oxygen desaturation, and he was shifted to the neonatal intensive care unit. The neonate had oliguria in the first 24 h of life, and he also had one episode of epistaxis. Blood-stained urine was observed in the urine catheter, and a coffee-ground-colored fluid was drained from the orogastric tube. Complete blood count performed at the age of 2 h revealed a platelet count of <8.5 (according to both automated and manual examination), a white blood cell count of 36.40×10^9/L, a hemoglobin level of 21.7 g/dl, and a hematocrit value of 63.9%. Based on a consultation with a hematologist, TTP was suspected due to unexplained thrombocytopenia. A full septic workup was carried out, and based on the findings, he was intravenously administered antibiotics. The patient's lactic acid level was 3.2 mmol/L, and his bone profile was normal. Furthermore, the total bilirubin level was 348.4 μmol/L, and renal function profile showed that his urea level was 8.2 mmol/L (which is higher than normal for his age) and creatinine level was 178 μmol/L (which is also much higher than normal for his age).

Two days later, abdominal distention was noticed. Abdominal radiography showed the presence of a large pneumoperitoneum along with spontaneous gastric perforation. An urgent pediatric surgery consultation was requested, and total gastrectomy and feeding jejunostomy were performed. Histopathological analysis revealed gastric perforation with features of ischemic insult.

On day 8 of life, genetic analysis confirmed the diagnosis of autosomal recessive familial TTP or cTTP. A unique homozygous deletion mutation was found on exon 23 of ADAMTS13: c.2883del p.(Cys962Alafs*3). The patient received fresh frozen plasma twice a day for eight days and then once daily for three days.

3. Outcome and Follow-Up

Two months later, the jejunostomy tube got spontaneously dislodged on two occasions, and the abdomen became tense. Abdomen ultrasound examination showed focally dilated small bowel loops with extensive pneumatosis in the right side of the abdomen and associated extensive portal venous gas, minimal complex free fluid, and diminished peristalsis. There were no indications of cTTP recurrence. The patient was then continued weekly infusions of Fresh Frozen Plasma (FFP) 10 ml/kg IV over 1-2 hours. These plasma infusions are meant to keep ADAMTS13 at a trough level >1% and to keep platelet count >100. However, when there is an infection, we sometimes increase FFP to 3 times per week and even once daily if platelet count dropped <100. All these measures kept the baby free of symptoms for prolonged periods of time (30–60 days sometimes).

Throughout the disease course, the patient exhibited classical signs of cTTP, for instance, developmental delay, failure to thrive, renal injury, bladder hematoma, and high blood pressure. His condition further deteriorated, and he had three episodes of sepsis, pneumonia, and severe intractable pulmonary hemorrhage. The patient eventually succumbed to these complications and died at the age of 6 months.

4. Discussion

The glycoprotein Von Willebrand Factor (vWF) is released by endothelial cells at the site of vascular injury, where it acts as a bridging molecule for the activation of the coagulation cascade. ADAMTS13 is an important plasma metalloproteinase that plays a role in degrading large vWF multimers under normal physiological conditions [8]. The underlying pathophysiology of cTTP is a result of ADAMTS13 deficiency or a severe decrease in its activity. Such deficiency or defects in ADAMTS13 are caused by homozygous or combined heterozygous mutations, which result in the adhesion of nondegraded and ultralarge multimers of vWF that eventually cause platelet aggregation and microangiopathic hemolytic anemia [1]. The diverse nonspecific presentation of the disease ranges from acute onset of symptoms in the neonatal period, as observed in the present case, to an asymptomatic presentation that is triggered by stressors such as surgery, pregnancy, and infection [9]. Additionally, the overlapping symptoms of cTTP, immune thrombocytopenic purpura, and hemolytic uremic syndrome sometimes result in delays in the diagnosis of cTTP [10]. cTTP should be suspected in neonates with a clinical presentation of jaundice, thrombocytopenia, and severe anemia requiring exchange blood transfusion [4]. This condition can also present with life-threatening widespread multiorgan systemic thromboses and related complications, such as stroke, renal injuries, and myocardial involvement. If medical intervention is delayed, the mortality can be as high as 90% or higher [6]. In the present case, the patient had mesenteric ischemia and perforation. The findings so far indicate that the severity of the systemic involvement varies according to the ADAMTS13 level.

Management of cTTP is controversial. There is no international consensus on the proper management of such rare cases. All the available evidence is based on anecdotal evidence, case reports, and case series. A recent literature review recommended plasma infusion over plasma exchange for the management of acute episodes in infants and children with confirmed cTTP [11]. However, there is no consensus on the best prophylactic regimen. Some papers advocate FFP infusions on a weekly basis or every 10 days to maintain ADAMTS13 at trough levels of >1–3% [12], while others recommend the use of plasma-derived factors that are rich in ADAMTS13, such as KOATE-DVI [13]. In this case report, we have described a new mutation in the ADAMTS13 gene. It will add to the database of more than 150 mutations that have been reported in the gene encoding ADAMTS13 [14].

5. Conclusions

cTTP is a rare life-threatening autosomal recessive disease with a high mortality rate. It is caused by a mutation in the gene encoding for the ADAMTS13 protein. In neonates presenting with early onset of severe anemia, jaundice, thrombocytopenia and/or renal dysfunction, and neurological manifestations, physicians need to consider cTTP as a potential diagnosis. Timely initiation of aggressive treatment with plasma infusion could be a life-saving strategy in such cases.

References

[1] L. A. Lotta, I. Garagiola, R. Palla, A. Cairo, and F. Peyvandi, "ADAMTS13mutations and polymorphisms in congenital thrombotic thrombocytopenic purpura," *Human Mutation*, vol. 31, no. 1, pp. 11–19, 2010.

[2] V. M. Brandenburg, S. Gaertner, K. Lindemann-Docter et al., "Underestimated complications in thrombotic thrombocytopenic purpura--haemolytic uraemic syndrome," *Nephrology Dialysis Transplantation*, vol. 19, no. 8, pp. 2142–2146, 2004.

[3] Z. A. Hing, T. Schiller, A. Wu et al., "Multiplein silicotools predict phenotypic manifestations in congenital thrombotic thrombocytopenic purpura," *British Journal of Haematology*, vol. 160, no. 6, pp. 825–837, 2013.

[4] R. S. Camilleri, M. Scully, M. Thomas et al., "A phenotype-genotype correlation of ADAMTS13 mutations in congenital thrombotic thrombocytopenic purpura patients treated in the United Kingdom," *Journal of Thrombosis and Haemostasis*, vol. 10, no. 9, pp. 1792–1801, 2012.

[5] G. G. Levy, W. C. Nichols, E. C. Lian et al., "Mutations in a member of the ADAMTS gene family cause thrombotic thrombocytopenic purpura," *Nature*, vol. 413, no. 6855, pp. 488–494, 2001.

[6] H. A. van Dorland, M. M. Taleghani, K. Sakai et al., "The international hereditary thrombotic thrombocytopenic purpura registry: key findings at enrollment until 2017," *Haematologica*, vol. 104, no. 10, pp. 2107–2115, 2019.

[7] K. Kokame, M. Matsumoto, K. Soejima et al., "Mutations and common polymorphisms in ADAMTS13 gene responsible for von Willebrand factor-cleaving protease activity," *Proceedings of the National Academy of Sciences*, vol. 99, no. 18, pp. 11902–11907, 2002.

[8] D. Sharma, S. Shastri, A. Pandita, and P. Sharma, "Congenital thrombotic thrombocytopenic purpura: Upshaw-Schulman syndrome: a cause of neonatal death and review of literature," *The Journal of Maternal-Fetal & Neonatal Medicine*, vol. 29, no. 12, pp. 1977–1979, 2016.

[9] M. Scully, B. J. Hunt, S. Benjamin et al., "Guidelines on the diagnosis and management of thrombotic thrombocytopenic purpura and other thrombotic microangiopathies," *British Journal of Haematology*, vol. 158, no. 3, pp. 323–335, 2012.

[10] A. Klukowska, E. Niewiadomska, U. Budde, F. Oyen, and R. Schneppenheim, "Difficulties in diagnosing congenital thrombotic thrombocytopenic purpura," *Journal of Pediatric Hematology/Oncology*, vol. 32, no. 2, pp. 103–107, 2010.

[11] J. N. George and A. Cuker, "Hereditary thrombotic thrombocytopenic purpura (TTP)," *New England Journal of Medicine*, vol. 24, 2017.

[12] L. M. Aledort, T. C. Singleton, and P. J. Ulsh, "Treatment of congenital thrombotic thrombocytopenia purpura: a new paradigm," *Journal of Pediatric Hematology/Oncology*, vol. 39, no. 7, pp. 524–527, 2017.

[13] S. Naik and D. H. Mahoney, "Successful treatment of congenital TTP with a novel approach using plasma-derived factor VIII," *Journal of Pediatric Hematology/Oncology*, vol. 35, no. 7, pp. 551–553, 2013.

[14] L. Hou and Y. Du, "Two novel mutations in ADAMTS13 in a Chinese boy with congenital thrombocytopenic purpura: a case report," *BMC Medical Genetics*, vol. 21, no. 1, pp. 57–61, 2020.

10

Thrombosis as the First Manifestation of Granulomatosis with Polyangiitis Disease in an Adolescent

Mohsen Jari

Department of Pediatric Rheumatology, Imam Hossein Children's Hospital, Isfahan University of Medical Sciences, Isfahan, Iran

Correspondence should be addressed to Mohsen Jari; mjari14@yahoo.com

Academic Editor: Yusuke Shiozawa

Background. Granulomatosis with polyangiitis disease (GPA) is a rare vasculitis characterized by granulomatous inflammation of respiratory tracts, glomerulonephritis, and vasculitis of other organs. *Case Presentation.* A 13-year-old girl was referred due to swelling and pain on her left arm. The Doppler and compression ultrasonography showed noncompressible left brachial and axillary vein thrombosis. Sinus computed tomography (CT) demonstrated pansinusitis, and spiral chest CT showed alveolar hemorrhage. Laboratory tests showed hematuria, proteinuria, and highly positive antineutrophil cytoplasmic antibody (cANCA). Laboratory tests of coagulopathy were normal. The patient was recognized as a case of GPA. *Conclusion.* Although GPA is not frequently associated with thrombosis especially in children, this is the first report that shows thrombosis may be the first manifestation of GPA in an adolescent.

1. Introduction

Thrombosis can occur in the artery or vein. Venous thrombosis is less common in children than in adults, but leads to more morbidity and mortality that emphasize timely diagnosis and therapy [1, 2]. Risk factors for thrombosis include central venous catheter (CVÇ), immobility, heart disease, coagulation disorders, congenital heart disease, trauma (especially fractures), cancer, surgery, infections, dehydration, shock, obesity, nephrotic syndrome, antiphospholipid antibody syndrome, and vasculitis [1–3]. Granulomatosis with polyangiitis disease (GPA), formerly Wegener's granulomatosis, is a chronic vasculitis. Thrombosis is a rare manifestation of this disease especially in children and adolescents [2, 3].

2. Case Presentation

A 13-year-old girl was admitted to the pediatric rheumatology ward of Imam Hossein Children's Hospital, Isfahan University of Medical Sciences, due to swelling and pain on her left arm 3 days prior to admission. Since 3 months, she had fatigue, bloody nasal discharge, and cough.

On physical examination, she was alert, and her blood pressure and temperature were within normal limit. Her body weight was 43 kg. There were no abnormalities on heart and lung examination. There was no lymphadenopathy or hepatosplenomegaly. There was swelling on her left arm without any sign of inflammation. The size of her left vs. right arm and left vs. right forearm was 28 cm vs. 23 cm and 18 cm vs. 17 cm, respectively.

The radial and brachial pulses on the left were reduced. The laboratory examinations showed anemia (hemoglobin, 8.3 g/dL); leukocytosis (white blood count, 19500/mm^3 (lymphocytes 24%)); thrombocytosis (platelets = 530.000/mm^3); elevation of estimated sedimentation rate (ESR = 105 mm/hr) and C-reactive protein (CRP = 97 mg/L); prothrombin time (PT), 13.0 seconds; INR, 1.1; activated partial thromboplastin time (aPTT), 32.3 seconds; and d-dimer 5.8 mg/L (normal <0.3 mg/L). The serum levels of protein C, protein S, antithrombin III, and factor V Leiden were normal. Renal function and electrolytes were within normal limits. Peripheral blood smear was normal.

Urinalysis showed proteinuria 3+ and hematuria 4+, and 24-hour urine showed proteinuria (750 mg/24 hrs). Antinuclear antibody (ANA) was negative, and antiphospholipid antibodies, anti-DNA antibody, and serum complement levels were normal. Antineutrophil cytoplasmic antibody (ANCA) was highly positive (cANCA = 450 U/ml, Nl <25 U/ml).

The Doppler and compression ultrasonography showed noncompressible and completely occlusive thrombosis of left brachial and axillary veins (noncompressible venous segment, lack of flow augmentation with calf squeeze, and increased flow in superficial veins). Sinus computed tomography (CT) demonstrated mucosal thickening and pansinusitis, and spiral chest CT showed minimal alveolar hemorrhage.

According to the EULAR/PRINTO//PRES criteria, the patient was recognized as a case of GPA, and the treatment started by prescribing subcutaneous enoxaparin and pulse methylprednisolone 30 mg/kg/d (max 1 gr) for three days. Then, in the fourth day of treatment, intravenous infusion (IV) with cyclophosphamide 500 mg/m^2 was given. The patient was discharged in the fifth day given oral prednisolone 2 mg/kg/d and enoxaparin. After a one-week follow-up, the Doppler and compression ultrasonography of left brachial and axillary veins was normal. Enoxaparin was continued (for three months), and IV cyclophosphamide, oral prednisolone, and azathioprine were continued based on EULAR/PRINTO//PRES criteria.

3. Discussion

Granulomatosis with polyangiitis disease (GPA) is not frequently associated with thrombosis. There are few reports of intracranial thrombosis of large and small vessels in adults and children. These events have been occurred due to intracranial vasculitis or extension of granulomatous lesions from the nasal cavity [1, 2]. Few recent reports of thrombosis at other organs have been described in some adults, that are very rare in children and adolescents [3–6]. Systematic studies of factors contributing to hypercoagulability in these patients were not reported.

GPA is a antineutrophil cytoplasmic antibody- (ANCA-) associated vasculitis (AAV) characterized by necrotizing inflammation of small vessels and the presence of ANCA directed to specific antigens, particularly proteinase 3 (PR3-ANCA) and myeloperoxidase (MPO-ANCA). This disease [7] primarily affects the small vessels of the skin, lungs, and kidneys. During AAV, proinflammatory cytokines are elevated in the serum of these patients.

Circulating tumor necrosis factor (TNF) is a major factor of atherothrombotic events in AAV [8, 9].

Pathogenesis of thrombosis in AAV including endothelial cell dysfunction and interaction between neutrophils (activated by TNFα and ANCA) and with consequent massive oxidative stress finally lead to atherothrombotic complications [10]. TNF can increase gene expression of procoagulant proteins, such as tissue factor. Anti-PR3 antibodies can increase the expression of tissue factor [11]. Recently, reports demonstrated that neutrophils are able to release extracellular nucleic acids associated with histones and granular proteins capable of entrapping bacterial agents [12, 13].

These mechanisms may explain why in patients with GPA thrombosis occurred during the initial stage of disease or when inflammation was not yet controlled.

4. Conclusion

Although GPA and other AAV are not frequently associated with thrombosis especially in children and adolescents, thrombosis may be the first manifestation of GPA.

Consent

Written informed consent form has been provided by the parents to have the case details published.

References

[1] C. X. Tang, U. J. Schoepf, S. M. Chowdhury, M. A. Fox, L. J. Zhang, and G. M. Lu, "Multidetector computed tomography pulmonary angiography in childhood acute pulmonary embolism," *Pediatric Radiology*, vol. 45, no. 10, p. 1431, 2015.

[2] A. N. C. Santana, A. M. Ab'Saber, W. R. Teodoro, V. L. Capelozzi, and C. S. V. Barbas, "Trombose em artérias pulmonares pequenas e médias em granulomatose de Wegener: um estudo com microscopia confocal por varredura a laser," *Jornal Brasileiro de Pneumologia*, vol. 36, no. 6, pp. 724–730, 2010.

[3] P. Lamprecht, K. Holl-Ulrich, and S. Wieczorek, "Venous thromboembolism in Wegener's granulomatosis," *The Journal of Rheumatology*, vol. 34, no. 12, pp. 2323–2325, 2007.

[4] M. Mortazavi and H. Nasri, "Granulomatosis with polyangiitis (Wegener's) presenting as the right ventricular masses: a case report and review of the literature," *Journal of Nephropathology*, vol. 1, no. 1, 2012.

[5] J. C. Jennette, R. J. Falk, P. A. Bacon et al., "2012 revised international chapel hill consensus conference nomenclature of vasculitides," *Arthritis & Rheumatism*, vol. 65, no. 1, pp. 1–11, 2013.

[6] M. F. Meyer, A. Schnabel, H. Schatz, and W. L. Gross, "Lack of association between antiphospholipid antibodies and thrombocytopenia in patients with Wegener's granulomatosis," *Seminars in Arthritis and Rheumatism*, vol. 31, no. 1, pp. 4–11, 2001.

[7] C. G. M. Kallenberg, "Key advances in the clinical approach to ANCA-associated vasculitis," *Nature Reviews Rheumatology*, vol. 10, no. 8, pp. 484–493, 2014.

[8] J. C. Jennette, R. J. Falk, P. Hu, and H. Xiao, "Pathogenesis of antineutrophil cytoplasmic autoantibody-associated small-vessel vasculitis," *Annual Review of Pathology: Mechanisms of Disease*, vol. 8, no. 1, pp. 139–160, 2013.

[9] D. P. Thomas and H. R. Roberts, "Hypercoagulability in venous and arterial thrombosis," *Annals of Internal Medicine*, vol. 126, no. 8, pp. 638–644, 1997.

[10] I. L. Noronha, C. Krüger, K. Andrassy, E. Ritz, and R. Waldherr, "In situ production of TNF-α, IL-1β and IL-2R in ANCA-positive glomerulonephritis," *Kidney International*, vol. 43, no. 3, pp. 682–692, 1993.

[11] M. De Bandt, V. Ollivier, C. Babin-Chevaye et al., "Induction of interleukin-1 and subsequent tissue factor expression by anti-proteinase 3 antibodies in human umbilical vein endothelial cells," *Arthritis & Rheumatism*, vol. 40, no. 11, pp. 2030–2038, 1997.

[12] K. Kambas, A. Chrysanthopoulou, D. Vassilopoulos et al., "Tissue factor expression in neutrophil extracellular traps and neutrophil derived microparticles in antineutrophil cytoplasmic antibody associated vasculitis may promote thromboinflammation and the thrombophilic state associated with the disease," *Annals of the Rheumatic Diseases*, vol. 73, no. 10, pp. 1854–1863, 2014.

[13] S. Sangaletti, C. Tripodo, C. Chiodoni et al., "Neutrophil extracellular traps mediate transfer of cytoplasmic neutrophil antigens to myeloid dendritic cells toward ANCA induction and associated autoimmunity," *Blood*, vol. 120, no. 15, pp. 3007–3018, 2012.

11

Hemoadsorption Treatment with CytoSorb® in Probable Hemophagocytic Lymphohistiocytosis: A Role as Adjunctive Therapy?

Samuele Ceruti,[1] **Andrea Glotta**,[1] **Harriet Adamson**,[2] **Romano Mauri**,[1] **and Zsolt Molnar**[2,3,4,5]

[1]*Critical Care Department, Clinica Luganese Moncucco, Lugano, Switzerland*
[2]*CytoSorbents Europe GmbH, Berlin, Germany*
[3]*Centre for Translational Medicine, Semmelweis University, Budapest, Hungary*
[4]*Department of Anaesthesiology and Intensive Therapy, Poznan University of Medical Sciences, Poznan, Poland*
[5]*Department of Anaesthesiology and Intensive Therapy, Semmelweis University, Budapest, Hungary*

Correspondence should be addressed to Samuele Ceruti; samuele.ceruti@moncucco.ch

Academic Editor: Sudhir Tauro

Acute hemophagocytic lymphohistiocytosis (HLH) is a life-threatening disease, with an annual incidence of 1 : 800,000 people. The disease is characterized by a cytokine storm, with concomitant macrophage and natural killer (NK) cell activation; death can occur from multiple organ failure or complications such as bleeding diathesis. Therefore, HLH treatment remains a challenging one. We hereby present a case of a 76-year-old man with severe HLH in whom hemoadsorption was successfully applied. Due to the failure of the immunomodulatory therapy , continuous venovenous hemodiafiltration therapy with the CytoSorb® adsorber was successfully applied for 48 hours. Upon therapy discontinuation, the biological and clinical condition reverted, unfortunately evolving towards the patient's death.

1. Introduction

Acute hemophagocytic lymphohistiocytosis (HLH) is a highly fatal disease, with an incidence of 1 : 800,000 cases each year [1]. Reactive or secondary hemophagocytosis more frequently affects adults in response to an infectious stimulus, usually involving immune dysfunction [2]. The disease is characterized by a specific cytokine burst, in particular of the IFN-gamma, interleukin (IL) 6 and IL-18, and CD25 [3], associated with macrophage and NK-cell activation [4]. Death can occur due to tissue destruction, multiple organ failure, or complications such as bleeding diathesis [5]. Despite advances in critical care over the past decades, HLH treatment remains a challenging one. Hereby, we present a case of severe HLH in a complex scenario in whom hemoadsorption therapy was successfully used.

2. Case Report

2.1. Investigation. A 76-year-old man was admitted tothe Intensive Care Unit (ICU) for abdominal septic shock due to perforation of the colon; an obstructive colonic adenocarcinoma with metastatic lymph node spread was diagnosed immediately after the emergency laparotomy. Rapid resolution of the septic shock was managed after an emergency hemicolectomy followed by treatment with meropenem, vancomycin, and supportive treatment in ICU. However, on day 3, the patient developed refractory fever (around 40°C), altered level of consciousness (Glasgow Coma Scale 7/15), anemia (hemoglobin 6.8 g/dL), and thrombocytopenia (platelets 20 G/L) despite multiple replacements with blood products and hemodynamic support. Blood cultures remained negative during the entire ICU stay. Clinical course was further complicated by hemorrhagic shock for a massive right hemothorax (2,500 mL) as a result of a severe refractory thrombocytopenia, requiring fluid administration and high doses of norepinephrine (around 0.34 μg/kg/min). Differential diagnosis was performed, which excluded other diseases. Heparin-induced thrombocytopenia [6] was excluded as a result of a low 4T-score pretest probability and the absence of anti-PF_4 antibodies. Disseminated intravascular coagulation was also excluded due to relatively high fibrinogen levels and normal PT/aPTT according to the International Society of Thrombosis and Haemostasis (ISTH) score [7]. Thrombotic microangiopathy was excluded because of a negative schistocytes identification on smear evaluation at medium microscope magnification that was double checked [8]. Catastrophic antiphospholipid syndrome was also excluded as antiphospholipid antibodies were not identified [9]. High levels of serum ferritin (14,299 ng/mL), hypertriglyceridemia (4.49 mmol/L), and lactate dehydrogenase (LDH) elevation (1,354 U/L) supported the possibility of acute HLH. This was further reinforced by the H-score [10], which strongly suggested an acute HLH most likely triggered by septic shock due to the active cancer (Figure 1); bone marrow aspirate could not be obtained at this stage.

2.2. Diagnosis. Due to the high active infectious risk plus the diagnosis of metastatic colonic carcinoma, it was not feasible to proceed with the recommended immunomodulatory therapy with etoposide and corticosteroids, cyclosporin A, followed by bone marrow transplantation, according to the HLH-94 protocol [11]. Therefore, we started an alternative treatment of a 5-day cycle of immunoglobulin IV, which unfortunately failed to show any benefit. His clinical condition continued to deteriorate, with high norepinephrine doses, GCS around 6-7/15 points, and a continuous worsening of the inflammation and cell damage indices.

2.3. Treatment. Therefore, on day 7, an empiric hemoadsorption with the predialyzer CytoSorb® (Ultraflux AV 1000S filter) was started in combination with a neutral fluid balance [12]. A total of 48 hours of continuous hemoadsorption was performed, with each of the two adsorbers running for 24 hours.

2.4. Follow-Up and Outcome. From the start of the extracorporeal blood purification therapy, the patient's clinical and biochemical parameters improved, including creatinine (from 100 to 57 μmol/L, Table 1); the patient regained consciousness (GCS 14/15) allowing endotracheal tube removal and complete norepinephrine cessation together with albumin replacement; inflammatory biomarker levels also improved (Table 1 and Figure 2), especially IFNγ (from 14.9 to 3.8 ng/mL, −74.5%), IL-8 (from 1137 to 497 pg/mL, −56.29%), IL-6 (from 183.4 to 30.6 pg/mL, −83.32%), ferritin (from 12209 to 9616 ng/mL, −21.24%), and C reactive protein (CRP from 343 to 108 mg/L, −68.51%). After 48 hours, the hemoadsorption treatment was stopped. However, on the following day, an unexpected deterioration occurred with worsening of both the clinical and laboratory values (up to +164% compared to the last day of hemoadsorption, Table 1 and Figure 2). The sudden worsening and the already compromised patient's clinical conditions prevented any further therapeutic approach with the hemoadsorption treatment. Despite all efforts, the patient died four days later.

3. Discussion

Acute HLH is a life-threatening disease, with an estimated incidence of one per 800,000 people [1]. Reactive or secondary HLH more frequently affects adults following an infectious stimulus in the context of certain predisposing factors and usually involves the dysregulated immune response [2]. The phenomenon is often characterized by cytokine storm, especially of IFNγ, IL-6, and IL-8 [3] with concomitant macrophage and NK-cell activation [4]. Death can occur due to tissue destruction, multiple organ failure, or complications such as bleeding diathesis [5]. In our case, the combination of septic shock, surgery inflicted tissue damage, and hemorrhagic shock led to an overwhelming inflammatory response, resulting in high ferritin levels and potentially fatal cytokine storm [13].

Sometimes, the recommended first-line therapy with etoposide and steroids may be contraindicated or associated with high risks, as is the case with a recent septic shock. Support with the CytoSorb® adsorber could be a valid treatment as a salvage therapy since it may remove both general inflammatory cytokines and the specific HLH cytokines (especially IL-8 and CD25). Clinical improvement and better survival rates could be the consequences [14].

In an HLH German registry concerning 137 patients, CytoSorb® has been applied as a rescue therapy in just 3 cases [14]. Although these data have been mainly demonstrated in the context of septic shock, some relevant trials have shown how hemoadsorption can be applied as an effective therapy compared to simple continuous venovenous hemodiafiltration (CVVHDF) for the removal of inflammatory cytokines and reducing high-dose catecholamine infusions, with quick reductions in procalcitonin (PCT) and C-reactive protein (CRP) levels [15,16]. The efficacy of CytoSorb® therapy in septic shock has not yet been proven in randomized controlled trials (RCT); the only two published RCTs demonstrated significant reductions in inflammatory cytokines in the treatment group, but this did not translate into an improvement in clinical outcomes [17,18]. Nevertheless, as compared to any type of dialysis or hemofiltration, hemoadsorption with CytoSorb® is fundamentally different: the cartridge contains biocompatible polymer beads, which allows a huge adsorption surface area as compared to dialysis filters, with an adsorption spectrum of up to 60 kDa [19].

Due to the rarity of HLH, data are scarce. As cytokines certainly play a pathogenic role in HLH [3,4], they could play a pivotal role in the observed high mortality rate [5]; hence, it has sound pathophysiological rationale to use

The diagnosis of HLH can be established if Criterion 1 or 2 is fulfilled
1. A molecular diagnosis constinstent with HLH

2. Diagnostic criteria for HLH fulfilled (5 of the 8 criteria below):
- Fever
- Splenomegaly
- Cytopenias (affecting 2 or 3 lineages in the peripheral blood)
    - Hemoglobin < 90 g/L
    - Platelets < 100 * 10^9/L
    - Neutrophils < 1.0 * 10^9/L
- Hypertrigliceridemia and/or Hypofibrinogemia
    - Fasting triglyceride > 3.0 mmol/L
    - Fibrinogen < 1.5 g/L
- Hemophagocytosis in bone marrow or spleen or lymph nodes. No evidences of malignancy
- Low or no NK cells activity
- Ferritin > 500 ug/L
- sCD25 (i.e. soluble IL2 receptor) > 2400 U/mL

Parameter	No. of points (scoring criteria)
Known underlying immunosuppression*	0 (no) or 18 (yes)
Temperature (°C)	0 (< 38.4°C), 33 (38.4 - 39.4) or 49 (> 39.4)
Organomegaly	0 (no), 23 (hepatomegaly or splenomegaly) or 38 (hepatomegaly and splenomegaly)
No, of Cytopenias**	0 (1 lineage), 24 (2 lineages) or 34 (3 lineages)
Ferritin (ug/L)	0 (< 2000), 35 (2000-6000) or 60 (> 5000)
Trygliceryde (mmol/L)	0 (< 1.5), 44 (1.5 - 4) or 64 (> 4)
Fibrinogen (g/L)	0 (> 2.5) or 30 (< 2.5)
Aspartate aminotransferase (U/L)	0 (< 30) or 19 (> 30)
Hemophagocytosis on bone marrow aspirate	0 (no) or 35 (yes)

* HIV positive or receiving long-term immunosuppressive therapy (i.e. glucocorticoids, cyclosporine A, azathioprine)

** Defined as a hemoglobin level of 9.2 g/L and/or a leukocyte count < 5 * 10^9/L and/or a platelet count < 110 * 10^9/L

FIGURE 1: H-score calculator (H-score calculator redraw ([13])): the probability of HLH increases with the increase of score. The best cutoff value was 169, which corresponds to an accuracy of 90% (sensitivity of 93%, specificity of 86%). In this case report, patient presented a H-index of 229 points (96–99% of probability).

TABLE 1: Laboratory characteristics.

	Normal values	Day 5	Day 6	Day 7	Day 8	Day 9	Day 10	Day 11	Day 12	Day 13
Hematology										
Hemoglobin	14.0–18.0 (g/dL)	9.2	9.3	9.5	10.0	8.2	7.5	8.0		7.2
Red cells	4.5–6.0 (G/L)	3.19	3.23	3.26	3.42	2.77	2.52	2.69		2.38
Leucocyte	4.0–10.0 (G/L)	3.4	4.0	4.6	7.2	4.2	3.6	2.3		3.4
Thrombocyte	150–450 (G/L)	53.0	44.0	49.0	49.0	34.0	33.0	26.0		30.0
Coagulation										
Quick	70–130 (%)	110.0	110.0	94.0	70.0					63.0
INR		0.98	0.98	1.04	1.16					1.22
aPTT	26–36 (sec)	32.0	34.0	35.0	33.0					42.0
Fibrinogen	1.7–4.1(g/L)	5.34	5.07	4.66	4.22					5.57
D-dimer	<500 (ng/mL)		>9000	>9000	>9000					>9000
Chemistry										
Creatinine	62–105 (μmol/L)	92.0	100.0	98.0	69.0	60.0	57.0	95.0		119.0
Albumin	35–52 (g/L)		19.0	22.0	19.0	27.0	32.0			22.0
Total bilirubin	<21 (μmol/L)	7.5	7.0	9.6	8.6	13.5	14.6	18.4		10.1
Ferritin	30–50 (ng/mL)	12209		11586	14299	9616		14231		25408
LDH	135–225 (U/L)		1159.0	1461.0	1354.0	1177.0	1292.0	1898.0		2099.0
CK	39–308 (U/L)		221.0	242.0	243.0	234.0	239.0	307.0		349.0
GOT	10–50 (U/L)		133.0	152.0	119.0	136.0	131.0	240.0		253.0
GPT	10–50 (U/L)		51.0	43.0	35.0	33.0	26.0	41.0		59.0
Lipase	13–60 (U/L)				77.0	85.0	356.0	183.0		28.0
Calcium	2.13–2.65 (nmol/L)				2.56	2.44	2.45			2.28
Phosphate	0.81–1.45 (nmol/L)				1.54	1.58	1.48	1.88		2.59
CRP	<5 (mg/L)	349	343	335	155	108	146			601
Procalcitonin	<0.05 (μmol/L)	1.21	1.16	1.49	1.74	1.56	1.18	1.3		15.1
Immunology										
IFNγ	<15 (ng/L)	9.8	14.9	11.2	3.3	3.8	9.6			
IL8	<31.2 (pg/mL)	963	1137		499	497	1064			
IL6	<6.4 (pg/mL)	79.5	67.4	183.4	45.1	30.6	807			

Laboratory characteristics. Days 7–9 correspond to CytoSorb® adsorbent application through CVVHDF.

hemoadsorption early in these patients. So far, studies concerning the effect of cytokine removal on mortality reduction are missing in general and certainly for such a rare disease as HLH. Therefore, our knowledge is limited to a few single case studies only [20,21]. Despite the negative eventual outcome, the current case report is one the first ones to show that at least temporary improvement of both clinical and biochemical parameters could

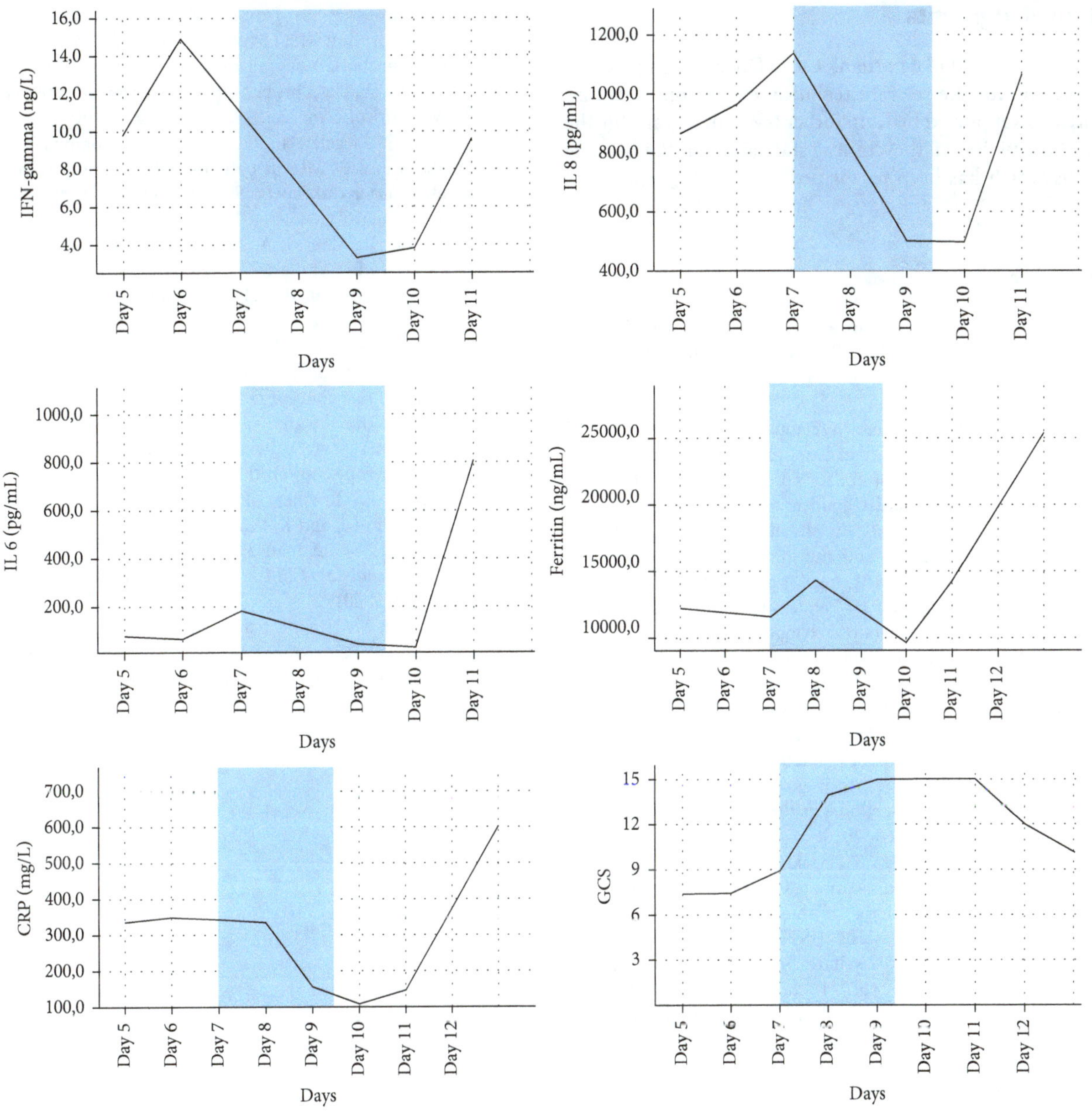

FIGURE 2: Temporal evolution of clinical and biological data: temporal evolution of IFN-gamma, interleukin (IL) 6 and IL8 cytokines' serum values, biological data like ferritin, C-reactive protein (CRP), and clinical data such as Glasgow Coma Scale (GCS). Days refer to the day of ICU treatment. Shaded blue areas are the days of CytoSorb® adsorbent application through CVVHDF.

be achieved within a matter of a couple of days. These data could be hypothesis generating for prospective studies in the future.

These data have been mainly demonstrated in the context of septic shock; some relevant trials have shown how hemoadsorption can be applied as an effective therapy compared to simple CVVHDF for the removal of inflammatory cytokines and reducing high-dose catecholamine infusions, with quick reductions in PCT and CRP levels [15,16]. CytoSorb® has been reported to be applied as a rescue therapy in 3 cases of HLH [14]. HLH in the context of sepsis presents a unique challenge as the treatment of HLH requires strong immunomodulation, which can potentially worsen sepsis. Our case report provides further support to the pathophysiological rationale that CytoSorb® could mitigate the cytokine storm with minimum immunomodulation; hence, it could provide an alternative therapeutic approach in this patient population.

Consent

The consent was obtained before data analysis.

Acknowledgments

The authors would like to thank Carlo Duca for his precious support and for the relevant technical evaluation. This case report was supported by CytoSorbents® with a grant for the scientific activity of the clinical staff and for the specific analysis which has been performed.

References

[1] M. Ramos-Casals, P. Brito-Zerón, A. López-Guillermo, M. A. Khamashta, and X. Bosch, "Adult haemophagocytic syndrome," *The Lancet*, vol. 383, no. 9927, pp. 1503–1516, 2014.

[2] M. B. Jordan, C. E. Allen, S. Weitzman, A. H. Filipovich, and K. L. McClain, "How i treat hemophagocytic lymphohistiocytosis," *Blood*, vol. 118, no. 15, pp. 4041–4052, 2011.

[3] E. S. Weiss, C. Girard-Guyonvarc'h, D. Holzinger et al., "Interleukin-18 diagnostically distinguishes and pathogenically promotes human and murine macrophage activation syndrome," *Blood*, vol. 131, no. 13, pp. 1442–1455, 2018.

[4] M. Aricò, C. Danesino, D. Pende, and L. Moretta, "Pathogenesis of haemophagocytic lymphohistiocytosis," *British Journal of Haematology*, vol. 114, no. 4, pp. 761–769, 2001.

[5] Z. K. Otrock and C. S. Eby, "Clinical characteristics, prognostic factors, and outcomes of adult patients with hemophagocytic lymphohistiocytosis," *American Journal of Hematology*, vol. 90, no. 3, pp. 220–224, 2015.

[6] T. E. Warkentin, "Heparin-induced thrombocytopenia in critically ill patients," *Seminars in Thrombosis and Hemostasis*, vol. 41, no. 1, pp. 49–60, 2015.

[7] H. Wada, E. C. Gabazza, H. Asakura et al., "Comparison of diagnostic criteria for disseminated intravascular coagulation (DIC): diagnostic criteria of the international society of thrombosis and hemostasis (ISTH) and of the Japanese ministry of health and welfare for overt DIC," *American Journal of Hematology*, vol. 74, no. 1, pp. 17–22, 2003.

[8] J. L. Vincent, P. Castro, B. J. Hunt et al., "Thrombocytopenia in the ICU: disseminated intravascular coagulation and thrombotic microangiopathies-what intensivists need to know," *Critical Care*, vol. 22, no. 1, p. 158, 2018.

[9] G. E. Westney and E. N. Harris, "Catastrophic antiphospholipid syndrome in the intensive care unit," *Critical Care Clinics*, vol. 18, no. 4, pp. 805–817, 2002.

[10] F. Debaugnies, B. Mahadeb, A. Ferster et al., "Performances of the H-score for diagnosis of hemophagocytic lymphohistiocytosis in adult and pediatric patients," *American Journal of Clinical Pathology*, vol. 145, no. 6, pp. 862–870, 2016.

[11] J.-I. Henter, A. C. Samuelsson-Horne, M. Aricò et al., "Treatment of hemophagocytic lymphohistiocytosis with HLH-94 immunochemotherapy and bone marrow transplantation," *Blood*, vol. 100, no. 7, pp. 2367–2373, 2002.

[12] "Cytosorbents—the adsorber," 2020, https://cytosorb-therapy.com/en/the-adsorber/.

[13] P. La Rosée, A. Horne, M. Hines et al., "Recommendations for the management of hemophagocytic lymphohistiocytosis in adults," *Blood*, vol. 133, no. 23, pp. 2465–2477, 2019.

[14] S. Birndt, T. Schenk, B. Heinevetter et al., "Hemophagocytic lymphohistiocytosis in adults: collaborative analysis of 137 cases of a nationwide German registry," *Journal of Cancer Research and Clinical Oncology*, vol. 146, no. 4, pp. 1065–1077, 2020.

[15] W. P. Brouwer, S. Duran, M. Kuijper, and C. Ince, "Hemoadsorption with CytoSorb shows a decreased observed versus expected 28-day all-cause mortality in ICU patients with septic shock: a propensity-score-weighted retrospective study," *Critical Care*, vol. 23, no. 1, p. 317, 2019.

[16] A. Akil, S. Ziegeler, J. Reichelt et al., "Combined use of CytoSorb and ECMO in patients with severe pneumogenic sepsis," *Thorac Cardiovasc Surg*, vol. 69, no. 3, pp. 246–251, 2020.

[17] E. C. Poli, L. Alberio, A. Bauer-Doerries et al., "Cytokine clearance with CytoSorb® during cardiac surgery: a pilot randomized controlled trial," *Critical Care*, vol. 23, pp. 1–12, 2019.

[18] F. Hawchar, I. László, N. Öveges, D. Trásy, Z. Ondrik, and Z. Molnar, "Extracorporeal cytokine adsorption in septic shock: a proof of concept randomized, controlled pilot study," *Journal of Critical Care*, vol. 49, pp. 172–178, 2019.

[19] "The adsorber—cytoSorbents Europe GmbH," 2021, https://cytosorb-therapy.com/en/the-adsorber/.

[20] C. Greil, F. Roether, P. La Rosée, B. Grimbacher, D. Duerschmied, and K. Warnatz, "Rescue of cytokine storm due to HLH by hemoadsorption in a CTLA4-deficient patient," *Journal of Clinical Immunology*, vol. 37, no. 3, pp. 273–276, 2017.

[21] S. Frimmel, M. Hinz, J. Schipper, S. Bogdanow, S. Mitzner, and S. Koball, "Cytokine adsorption is a promising tool in the therapy of hemophagocytic lymphohistiocytosis," *The International Journal of Artificial Organs*, vol. 42, no. 11, pp. 658–664, 2019.

12

Hemophagocytic Lymphohistiocytosis (HLH) in a Patient with Disseminated Histoplasmosis

Neeraja Swaminathan, Jorge M. Vinicius, and Jesse Serrins

Albert Einstein Medical Center, Philadelphia, PA 19141, USA

Correspondence should be addressed to Neeraja Swaminathan; swaminan@einstein.edu

Academic Editor: Kiyotaka Kawauchi

Hemophagocytic lymphohistiocytosis (HLH) is a rare condition characterized by an overwhelming inflammatory cascade activation which is often associated with rapid progression and high mortality. It may be familial with an underlying genetic mutation or triggered by infection, malignancy, and autoimmune disease. Disseminated histoplasmosis caused by histoplasma capsulatum is a granulomatous fungal disease seen typically in immunocompromised patients with varied clinical manifestations and requires long-term antifungal therapy. We present the case of a 61-year-old immunocompromised female with significant travel history who came with fever, pancytopenia, and liver failure raising suspicion for HLH that prompted a bone marrow biopsy procedure. Hemophagocytic figures consistent with HLH and numerous encapsulated fungi resembling histoplasma were visualized. She was treated with intravenous (IV) liposomal amphotericin B. Etoposide chemotherapy and interleukin-1 (IL-1) antagonist anakinra were deferred in order to limit her immunosuppression, and treatment was focused on antifungal therapy.

1. Introduction

Hemophagocytic lymphohistiocytosis is a life-threatening condition associated with an inflammatory cytokine surge leading to multiorgan failure. Acquired HLH is described typically in adult patients who have a clear trigger such as infection, malignancy, and autoimmune conditions. This serious condition needs prompt recognition and management; otherwise, mortality is extremely high. Diagnosis of HLH requires 5 out of the following criteria: fever, splenomegaly, cytopenia affecting >2 lineages, hypertriglyceridemia and/or hypofibrinogenemia, hemophagocytosis in the marrow/spleen/lymph node or liver, low or absent natural killer (NK) cell activity, high ferritin, and elevated soluble CD25 [1, 2]. Normally NK cells play a central role in the response to intracellular infections. In HLH, there is a defect in NK cell response which leads to a positive feedback loop of uncontrolled intracellular infection and ongoing immune activation [2, 3].

Histoplasmosis is an endemic mycosis that is common in many tropical countries, South America, and also in the Midwestern states of the US. Initial exposure is usually by inhalation of the conidia into the respiratory tract, and dissemination occurs usually due to reactivation of histoplasmosis secondary to immunosuppressive status. Diagnosis by urine antigen is the most sensitive (90% sensitivity) and rapid method. However, the gold standard is a fungal culture which may take several weeks to result. Lymph node/bone marrow biopsy to demonstrate the histoplasma yeast form is also useful to make a quick diagnosis [4–6]. Disseminated histoplasmosis has certainly been described in the past to be a trigger for HLH. However, in the setting of an underlying infection, the management approach for HLH has not been well defined. Disseminated histoplasmosis is a fulminant infection which needs long-term systemic antifungal therapy. Immunosuppressive therapy can potentially worsen the underlying infection especially since histoplasmosis is typically seen to affect immunosuppressed individuals such as those with HIV or taking chemotherapy [3–5]. In this case report, we would like to discuss diagnosis and management of HLH and the spectrum of presentation of disseminated histoplasmosis and its treatment.

2. Case Presentation

A 61-year-old female presented with past medical history of rheumatoid arthritis (RA) on long-term treatment with methotrexate and infliximab came with fevers, upper respiratory symptoms, fatigue, and myalgia for 1 week which notably began a few weeks after she returned from travel to Brazil and Panama. She was empirically managed with oseltamivir for suspected influenza; however, she had no improvement in her symptoms. She was admitted at a local hospital where she was noted to have significantly elevated liver enzymes along with thrombocytopenia, elevated international normalized ratio (INR), and creatinine. She was placed on broad-spectrum antibiotic coverage (piperacillin-tazobactam, vancomycin, doxycycline, and micafungin) at the outside hospital. In view of clinical deterioration, the patient was transferred. At presentation, she was noted to be alert and oriented, tachycardic, tachypneic, and normotensive. Chest radiography showed diffuse bilateral pulmonary infiltrates which was concerning for fluid versus multifocal pneumonia. She was pancytopenic, had elevated ferritin level, and her peripheral smear showed toxic granulations within the granulocytes, rare inclusions, and Dohle bodies.

Differentials considered for this patient who was a recent traveler, immunocompromised (due to RA treatment) presenting with pyrexia of unknown origin, pancytopenia, acute liver failure, and respiratory distress, included acute viral hepatitis (A, B, C, and E), cytomegalovirus (CMV), Epstein–Barr virus (EBV), etc. Apart from infections, possibility of malignancy or autoimmune etiology given the history of rheumatoid arthritis was also considered. She had computed tomography (CT) of the chest and abdomen which showed hepatomegaly, bilateral pleural effusions, extensive ground glassing, and septal thickening. In view of such a broad differential in a critically ill patient, she was continued on broad antibiotic coverage as noted above. Since she met 5 out of 8 criteria for HLH including peripheral smear findings concerning for possible hemophagocytosis, she was empirically initiated on IVIG 0.4 g/kg and dexamethasone 10 mg/m^2.

She had active bleeding from her IV-line site secondary to coagulopathy which was managed with blood product transfusions. Her respiratory status continued to worsen despite noninvasive ventilation, and she had significant hypoxia as a result of which she was intubated on day 4 of her admission. After she was clinically stabilized, she underwent a bone marrow biopsy. The aspirate smear was positive for hemophagocytosis (Figure 1). Additionally, it also showed some inclusions on the marrow that were highly suspicious for a fungal infection (Figure 2). Encapsulated organisms with narrow based budding positive on silver stain were confirmed which clinched the diagnosis of disseminated histoplasmosis (Figure 3). Urine histoplasma antigen was sent which was >25 U/mL. Giemsa staining, immunohistochemistry, and polymerase chain reaction (PCR) for leishmania were all negative. Cryptococcal antigen and HIV testing were also negative. Fungal cultures—blood and sputum—were sent, and the patient was started on IV liposomal amphotericin B (5 mg/kg) and all the other broad-spectrum empiric antibiotics were stopped.

Since the patient had HLH secondary to disseminated histoplasmosis, it was decided to limit immunosuppression, and therefore steroids were also discontinued. After initiation of amphotericin, the patient had steady and gradual clinical improvement along with improvement in her liver function tests and her leukocyte count (see Table 1).

Subsequently, the patient developed thrombocytopenia and petechial rash on her back and had increasing creatinine. In view of this, she was switched to itraconazole after 9 days of treatment with amphotericin. However, after discontinuation of amphotericin, there was further clinical deterioration and the patient had worsening shock and new fever spikes and developed gastrointestinal bleeding and disseminated intravascular coagulation (DIC). She was supported with blood products and was also started on vancomycin and cefepime in view of concern for new nosocomial infection. Since inadequate amphotericin treatment was also considered, it was resumed on day 17 of admission. Unfortunately, despite her initial hematological response and aggressive treatment measures, she had refractory shock and multiorgan failure and eventually succumbed on day 19 of her admission.

3. Discussion

Histoplasma capsulatum is a ubiquitous dimorphic fungus and usually presents as a pulmonary infection. However, in immunocompromised hosts such as HIV infected individuals, there can be systemic spread. Treatment with tumor necrosis factor (TNF) inhibitors such as infliximab can also lead to increased risk of opportunistic infections particularly granulomatous diseases such as histoplasmosis and tuberculosis. Symptoms of disseminated histoplasmosis usually include fever, fatigue, weight loss, hepatosplenomegaly, lymphadenopathy, skin lesions, and pancytopenia [4, 6–8]. There is considerable overlap of these symptoms with primary HLH, and the infection can itself trigger HLH. HLH simulates a variety of conditions such as sepsis, acute viral hepatitis, lymphoproliferative disorders, and thrombotic thrombocytopenic purpura, making it difficult to recognize. It is characterized by a hyperstimulated but ineffective immune response especially in the NK cells. It is because of this that intracellular pathogens such as EBV, CMV, coxiella, mycobacteria, and fungi are more likely to trigger HLH [9]. HLH is characterized by low/absent NK cell activity, defective cytotoxic cell function, and unopposed macrophage activity. These activated macrophages secrete ferritin. They also secrete soluble interleukin-2 (IL-2) receptor which is also referred to as CD 25. Elevated levels of ferritin and soluble CD25 can be used to distinguish it from other mimics [2, 3].

In this patient, prior to establishing histoplasmosis, there were other potential triggers to be considered for HLH such as her underlying rheumatoid arthritis or a malignancy. Although the patient had well controlled symptoms of her RA, her exact premorbid immunological status was not known since records of her CD4 and CD8 counts or

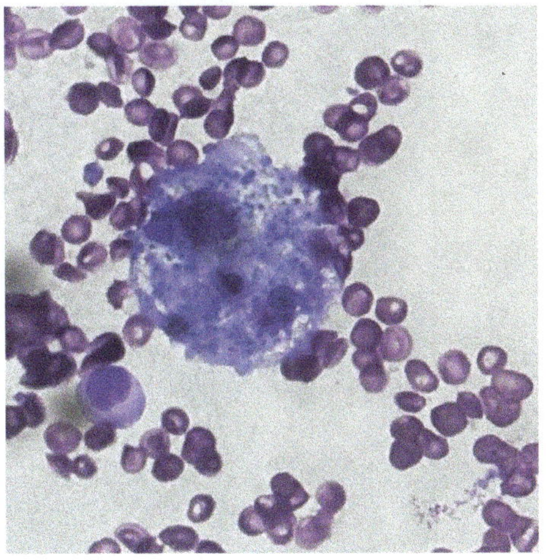

Figure 1: Hemophagocytosis on bone marrow smear (100x magnification).

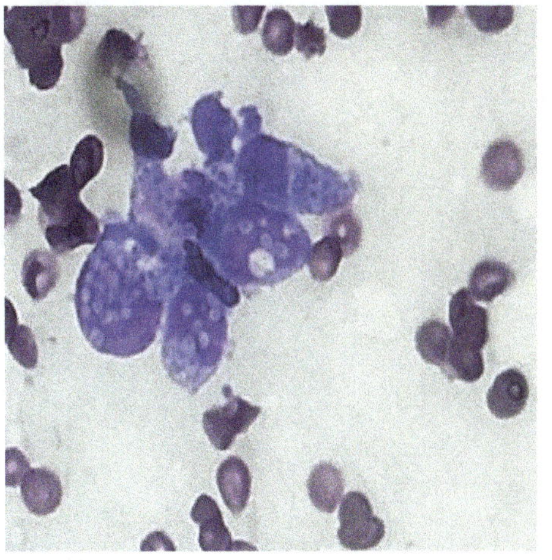

Figure 2: Encapsulated fungus in the cytoplasm of mononuclear cells on bone marrow smear (100x magnification).

immunoglobulin levels were unavailable. Hence, this patient received a 5-day course of IVIG and steroids. This was stopped after confirmation of the infection. Initiation of chemotherapy with etoposide and IL-1 antagonist therapy with anakinra for treatment of HLH were also considered but deferred because the patient had notable improvement clinically and in her laboratory parameters after initiation of amphotericin.

Guidelines from the Infectious Disease Society of America (IDSA) state that disseminated histoplasmosis requires at least 1-2 weeks of treatment with liposomal amphotericin B followed by maintenance itraconazole for 12 months [10]. After initial improvement, this patient developed rash, kidney injury, and thrombocytopenia which were attributed to amphotericin-related toxicity and the patient was switched to itraconazole after 9 days of amphotericin. However the patient continued to deteriorate and had DIC and overt gastrointestinal bleeding. It was unclear if this rapid decline was due to gastrointestinal histoplasmosis after premature discontinuation of amphotericin, progression of amphotericin treatment toxicity, or perhaps sepsis secondary to a new nosocomial infection acquired in the intensive care unit [11].

This patient received empiric antifungal treatment with micafungin. In hindsight, amphotericin B may have been a more prudent choice given its robust antifungal activity against histoplasma. However, this benefit needs to be weighed against the risks of its adverse effects including infusion reaction and nephrotoxicity. Ultimately, the choice of antifungal depends on which kind of mycosis is being suspected. In this immunocompromised patient who was also a returning traveler, there were several mycoses that were on the differential and it was challenging to prioritize one over the other.

There is limited data regarding the role of immunosuppressive therapy and IVIG in the setting of an underlying infection. In a prior review of 11 patients with histoplasma-associated HLH, of the 5 patients that received immunosuppression (including steroids, IVIG), 4 died. 2 out of the 5 who got no additional immunosuppression also died.

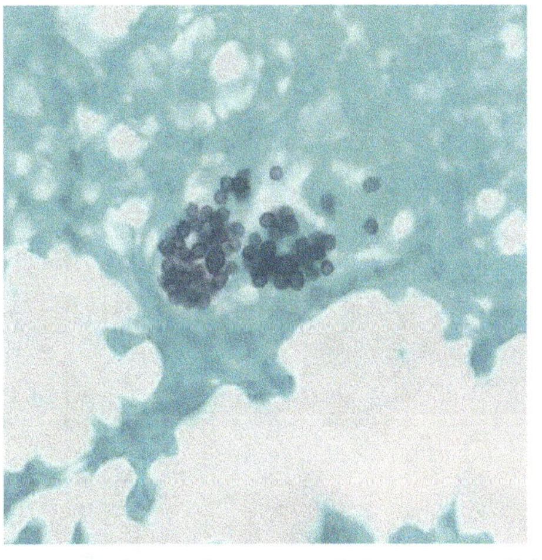

Figure 3: Budding fungus from intracellular to extracellular space on silver staining of mononuclear cells on bone marrow smear (100x magnification).

Although there were more survivors in the group that did not get immunosuppression, the authors note that the analysis was under powered [3]. In another review of 60 patients with histoplasma-associated HLH, 9 out of the 19 that died (47%) and 12 out of the 41 (29%) survivors had received etoposide or steroids/IVIG [12].

The HLH-2004 guidelines recommend treatment with etoposide, dexamethasone, cyclosporine A, and also intrathecal methotrexate as steroids in selected patients [1, 13]. However, these protocols largely pertain to primary HLH and are adapted from the pediatric population. At present, there is no consensus regarding continuation of chronic immunosuppression and also about initiating steroids or IVIG in those with an identified infectious trigger for HLH.

Thus, several pertinent clinical questions and challenges arose during the management of this patient such as role of immunosuppressive therapy in histoplasma-related HLH, optimal duration of amphotericin, and management of its toxicity.

Table 1: Patient's trend of laboratory values during course of admission.

Day	1	2	3	4	5	6	7	8	9	10	11	12	13	14	15	16	17	18	19
ALP (IU/L)	227	241	247	326	349	405	503	557	475	475	584	877	484	470	444	355	233	197	143
Total bilirubin (mg/dL)	7.5	9.4	10.2	9.9	8.9	9.3	8.7	8.4	6.8	5.9	5.7	7.1	5.8	5.2	5.6	4.4	4.3	4.2	3.7
Direct bilirubin (mg/dL)	6.0	7.0	8.0	7.1	6.6	6.4	6.1	6.2	5.2	4.7	4.6	5.5	4.3	2.9	4.1	3.2	3.1	3.2	2.8
ALT (IU/L)	272	340	466	405	366	428	446	400	328	242	247	246	185	172	142	105	75	55	39
AST (IU/L)	712	965	1827	1379	1319	1935	1718	1288	818	416	358	284	151	119	87	64	43	37	27
Ferritin (ng/mL)	>40,000	>40,000	>40,000	>40,000	>40,000	>40,000	>40,000	>40,000	>40,000	35548	16993	11886	8775	6157	4609	2990	1918	1521	1425
WBC ($\times10^3$/mcL)	2.73	2.91	2.97	1.70	1.41	2.62	5.25	9.67	9.64	9.96	10.73	11.81	11.37	10.66	9.87	9.29	7.52	9.44	9.79
Absolute lymphocyte count (cells/mm^3)	410							1793		1827		2350		1978		1858		1888	
Hemoglobin 0 (g/dL)	7.8	6.9	7.2	6.8	7.1	7.1	8.4	7.5	7.7	6.9	7.9	6.4	7.7	7.4	7.3	7.2	6.0	5.0	3.8
Platelet ($\times10^3$/mcL)	40	53	57	85	91	105	110	125	128	113	72	75	57	36	44	55	58	42	30
Fibrinogen (mg/dL)	78	60	90	120	206	353	293	292	296	294	220	201	217	181	172	183	273	177	91
INR	2.5	2.4	1.7	1.4	1.5	1.2	1.2	1.2	1.1	1.1	1.3	1.1	1.1	1.2	1.2	1.2	1.5	1.9	2

ALP, alkaline phosphatase; ALT, alanine transaminase; AST, aspartate transaminase; WBC, white blood cell.

4. Conclusion

This case report highlights the importance of being aware of HLH as a diagnosis in patients with fever of unknown origin especially when associated with pancytopenia and liver failure. Early recognition of a patient that meets diagnostic criteria for HLH and subsequently identifying a trigger and appropriately managing the same is vital in ensuring improved mortality outcomes in this otherwise fatal condition. Further studies are required to develop a robust treatment protocol for adult secondary HLH especially with regard to immunosuppressive therapy and IVIG in the setting of concomitant infection.

Consent

Since the patient is deceased, informed consent was obtained from the family member.

References

[1] J.-I. Henter, A. Horne, M. Aricó et al., "HLH-2004: diagnostic and therapeutic guidelines for hemophagocytic lymphohistiocytosis," *Pediatric Blood & Cancer*, vol. 48, no. 2, pp. 124–131, 2007.

[2] A. M. Schram and N. Berliner, "How I treat hemophagocytic lymphohistiocytosis in the adult patient," *Blood*, vol. 125, no. 19, pp. 2908 2914, 2015.

[3] J. L. Townsend, S. Shanbhag, J. Hancock, K. Bowman, and A. E. Nijhawan, "Histoplasmosis-induced hemophagocytic syndrome: a case series and review of the literature," *Open Forum Infectious Diseases*, vol. 2, no. 2, p. ofv055, 2015.

[4] S. Asanad, B. Cerk, and V. Ramirez, "Hemophagocytic lymphohistiocytosis (HLH) secondary to disseminated histoplasmosis in the setting of Acquired Immunodeficiency Syndrome (AIDS)," *Medical Mycology Case Reports*, vol. 20, pp. 15–17, 2018.

[5] A. D. Sonavane, P. B. Sonawane, S. V. Chandak, and P. M. Rathi, "Disseminated histoplasmosis with haemophagocytic lymphohistiocytosis in an immunocompetent host," *Journal of Clinical and Diagnostic Research*, vol. 10, no. 3, pp. OD03–OD05, 2016.

[6] M. Kashif, H. Tariq, M. Ijaz, and J. Gomez-Marquez, "Disseminated histoplasmosis and secondary hemophagocytic syndrome in a non-HIV patient," *Case Reports in Critical Care*, vol. 2015, Article ID 295735, 5 pages, 2015.

[7] M. M. Lo, J. Q. Mo, B. P. Dixon, and K. A. Czech, "Disseminated histoplasmosis associated with hemophagocytic lymphohistiocytosis in kidney transplant recipients," *American Journal of Transplantation*, vol. 10, no. 3, pp. 687–691, 2010.

[8] A. A. Castelli, D. G. Rosenthal, R. Bender Ignacio, and H. Y. Chu, "Hemophagocytic lymphohistiocytosis secondary to human immunodeficiency virus-associated histoplasmosis," *Open Forum Infectious Diseases*, vol. 2, no. 4, p. ofv140, 2015.

[9] N. G. Rouphael, N. J. Talati, C. Vaughan, K. Cunningham, R. Moreira, and C. Gould, "Infections associated with haemophagocytic syndrome," *The Lancet Infectious Diseases*, vol. 7, no. 12, pp. 814–822, 2007.

[10] L. J. Wheat, A. G. Freifeld, M. B. Kleiman et al., "Clinical practice guidelines for the management of patients with histoplasmosis: 2007 update by the Infectious Diseases Society of America," *Clinical Infectious Diseases*, vol. 45, no. 7, pp. 807–825, 2007.

[11] K. B. Pastakia, N. E. Brownson, D. A. Terle, and B. J. Poindexter, "Amphotericin B induced abnormalities in human platelets," *Molecular Pathology*, vol. 49, no. 5, pp. M301–M307, 1996.

[12] R. Jabr, W. El Atrouni, H. J. Male, and K. A. Hammoud, "Histoplasmosis-associated hemophagocytic lymphohistiocytosis: a review of the literature," *Canadian Journal of Infectious Diseases and Medical Microbiology*, vol. 2019, Article ID 7107326, 8 pages, 2019.

[13] S. Suman and A. Lenert, "Diagnostic dilemma of disseminated histoplasmosis mimicking hemophagocytosis lymphohistiocytosis in patient with rheumatoid arthritis on anti-TNF therapy: case report and review of the literature," *Case Reports in Rheumatology*, vol. 2019, Article ID 4169052, 3 pages, 2019.

13

Recurrent Gastrointestinal Hemorrhage in Children with Philadelphia-Positive B-Cell Acute Lymphoblastic Leukemia Treated with Dasatinib: Case Reports

Xin Liao,[1] **Yuxia Guo**,[1,2,3] **Yali Shen**,[1,3,4] **and Jianwen Xiao**[1,2,4]

[1]*Department of Hematology, Children's Hospital of Chongqing Medical University, Chongqing 400014, China*
[2]*Ministry of Education Key Laboratory of Child Development and Disorders, Chongqing 400014, China*
[3]*China International Science and Technology Cooperation Center for Child Development and Disorders, Chongqing 400014, China*
[4]*Chongqing Key Laboratory of Pediatrics, Chongqing 400014, China*

Correspondence should be addressed to Jianwen Xiao; tomahawk6502@sohu.com

Academic Editor: Pier Paolo Piccaluga

Dasatinib, a second-line tyrosine kinase inhibitor (TKI), has been widely used in chronic myeloid leukemia (CML) and Philadelphia-positive B-cell acute lymphoblastic leukemia (Ph + B-ALL). Although dasatinib has been well tolerated, side effects including hemorrhage are not rare. Cases of bleeding disorders ultimately result in thrombocytopenia, but platelet aggregation dysfunction induced by dasatinib has also been demonstrated in Ph + B-ALL and CML patients. We report three Chinese children with Ph + B-ALL who received a combination treatment of chemotherapy and dasatinib and developed gastrointestinal bleeding several months later. The platelet count and clotting tests were normal, and these patients presented with dasatinib-induced platelet dysfunction. These findings reveal that physicians should be aware of and carefully monitor for side effects, including bleeding disorders.

1. Introduction

Acute lymphoblastic leukemia (ALL) is the most common cancer in children, and precursor B-cell lymphoblastic leukemia (B-ALL) accounts for 70–75% of pediatric ALL cases [1]. Pediatric B-ALL with Philadelphia positivity (Ph + B-ALL) is relatively rare and accounts for less than 5% of childhood cases of B-ALL [2]. Historically, in both children and adults, Ph + B-ALL has been considered to have the worst prognosis of all B-ALL subtypes [2]. Since the introduction of tyrosine kinase inhibitors (TKIs), the outcome for Ph$^+$ B-ALL has gradually improved, and with a combination therapy of chemotherapy and TKIs, the 5-year event-free survival (EFS) rate of such patients has exceeded 80% [3]. Studies of Ph + B-ALL have revealed that the efficacy of dasatinib is superior to that of imatinib [4, 5], and the utilization of dasatinib in Ph + B-ALL is gradually increasing. Although TKIs were designed to target the fusion protein BCR-ABL1, they have shown some off-target inhibition of other tyrosine kinases [3], and it is important to recognize and manage adverse events caused by TKIs that share pathways in other organs.

In this article, we report three Ph + B-ALL children treated with dasatinib in which recurrent gastrointestinal (GI) hemorrhage was observed.

2. Case Reports

Three male patients were diagnosed with Ph + B-ALL between November 2016 and January 2018 at the Children's Hospital of Chongqing Medical University (CHCMU). The clinical characteristics and laboratory findings were collected and are listed in Table 1. Bone marrow (BM) samples were collected, and the diagnosis of Ph + B-ALL was confirmed

TABLE 1: Clinical characteristics and laboratory findings of the patients.

Clinical and laboratory findings	Patient 1	Patient 2	Patient 3
Age at diagnosis (m)	115	64	141
Clinical presentation	Bone pain, adenopathy, and hepatosplenomegaly	Fever, pale appearance, adenopathy, and hepatosplenomegaly	Pale appearance, ecchymosis, headache, adenopathy, and hepatosplenomegaly
WBC count ($\times 10^9$/L)	107.21	299.36	223.39
PLT count ($\times 10^9$/L)	140	20	22
Hb level (g/L)	126	58	88
Blasts in PB	0.86	0.95	0.89
BM smear	ALL-L_2	ALL-L_2	ALL-L_2
BM biopsy	B-ALL	B-ALL	B-ALL
Immunophenotype	Common B-ALL	Common B-ALL	Common B-ALL
Chromosomal karyotype	45, XY, −7, *t*(9;22)(q34;q11)	45, XY, −20, *t*(9;22)(q34;q11)	45, XY, −7, *t*(9;22)(q34;q11)
FISH for BCR-ABL1	(+), 90%	(+), 96%	(+), 85%
Fusion gene screening	BCR-ABL1(P210)	BCR-ABL1(P190)	BCR-ABL1(P210)
IS BCR-ABL1	1.049	0.743	0.126

WBC: white blood cell; PLT: platelet; Hb: hemoglobin; PB: peripheral blood; BM: bone marrow; FISH: fluorescence in situ hybridization.

according to WHO-2016 criteria [6]. The initial diagnosis of Ph + B-ALL was based on the FAB morphological classification detected by cytomorphological observation in the BM smear and biopsy. The immunophenotype was detected by flow cytometry (FCM) per protocol. The chromosomal karyotype was determined, and fluorescence in situ hybridization (FISH) was used to detect chromosomal translocations reported in the literature, including ETV6-RUNX1, MLL rearrangements, BCR-ABL1, C-MYC rearrangements, and PDGFRB rearrangements [7–9]. In total, 29 common fusion genes [10], including ETV6-RUNX1, MLL rearrangements, BCR-ABL1, TCF3-PBX1, and 27 Ph-like ALL fusion genes [11], were detected by multiplex nested reverse transcription polymerase chain reaction (multiplex RT-PCR), and positive BCR-ABL1 status was confirmed by real-time quantitative RT-PCR (qRT-PCR) [4].

Patients with Ph + B-ALL were treated as the intermediate risk group according to the CCCG-ALL-2015 protocol (the clinical trial began in 2015, registration number: ChiCTR-IPR-14005706). The protocol was divided into 4 phases: remission induction, consolidation, continuation, and maintenance. TKIs, including imatinib (300 mg/m^2 daily, CTTQ PHARMA, China) and dasatinib (60 mg/m^2 daily, CTTQ PHARMA, China), were administered randomly once the BCR-ABL1 fusion gene was confirmed. The three enrolled patients were administered imatinib, and treatment was suspended when the absolute neutrophil count (ANC) was $<0.5 \times 10^9$/L or severe infection occurred.

BM samples were obtained at different time points (TPs) throughout the duration of chemotherapy, and minimal residual disease (MRD) levels were monitored by FCM [12] at TP1 and TP2 (day 19 and day 46 of remission induction, respectively). FISH and qRT-PCR for BCR-ABL1 [13] were also performed at TP1 and TP2, and molecular remission monitored by qRT-PCR was achieved at TP2 for these patients. In the subsequent chemotherapy, FISH and qRT-PCR for BCR-ABL1 and mutation of ABL1 [13] were performed every six months, and the results were negative (Table 2).

The results of the clinical trial showed that the effect of dasatinib was superior to that of imatinib for the EFS rate (data have not been published), and the three patients were treated with a combination of dasatinib and chemotherapy instead of imatinib and chemotherapy. Changes in the type of TKI being administered occurred in the three patients at 24, 10, and 8 months after the initial administration of imatinib. The patients were admitted with consistent hemafecia and/or anemia 4 and 5 months later, when blood, white blood cells, and occult blood appeared in the stool, but stool cultures were negative. CMV and EBV were screened by PCR, and the results were negative. Platelet count, clotting tests (thrombin time, prothrombin time, international normalized ratio of prothrombin time, activated partial thromboplastin time, fibrinogen, and D-dimer), and coagulation factor (VII, VIII, IX, XI, XIII, and vW factor) tests were normal; platelet aggregation tests induced by adenosine diphosphate (ADP) were performed, and the results were abnormal (Table 3).

Endoscope and biopsy were refused by patient 1, and examinations were performed on patient 2 and patient 3. Patient 2 presented with ulcerative colitis under endoscopy, and infiltration of lymphocytes and eosinophils was detected under a microscope. Patient 3 presented with normal colonic mucosa under endoscopy, but eosinophilic infiltration was also found by histopathology. These data are shown in Figures 1 and 2.

Concerning comedications such as nonsteroidal anti-inflammatory drugs (NSAIDs), glucocorticoids, and traditional herbs were not administered before GI bleeding, and the side effects leading to hemafecia were suspected to be caused by chemotherapy and/or dasatinib. Chemotherapy was continued when GI hemorrhage vanished, and hemafecia did not reappear. Patients presented with hemafecia once dasatinib had been administered for 2–4 weeks even

TABLE 2: Results of MRD, FISH, and qRT-PCR analyses for the patients.

Time point	Laboratory findings	Patient 1	Patient 2	Patient 3
TP1	MRD	$<10^{-4}$	0.38%	1.38%
	FISH	Negative	Negative	Negative
	IS BCR-ABL1	0.012	0.015	0.0015
TP2	MRD	$<10^{-4}$	$<10^{-4}$	$<10^{-4}$
	FISH	Negative	Negative	Negative
	IS BCR-ABL1	Negative	Negative	Negative
Every 6 months after chemotherapy	FISH	Negative	Negative	Negative
	IS BCR-ABL1	Negative	Negative	Negative
	ABL1 mutation	Negative	Negative	Negative

TP: time point; MRD: minimal residual disease; FISH: fluorescence in situ hybridization.

TABLE 3: Laboratory findings for hemafecia status.

Results	Patient 1	Patient 2	Patient 3
Hb level (g/L)	127	127	70
PLT count ($\times10^9$/L)	206	255	197
Clotting tests	Normal	Normal	Normal
PLT function	Abnormal	Abnormal	Abnormal
Stool test	RBC (4+), WBC (+), OB (+)	RBC (5+), WBC (2+), OB (+)	RBC (2+), WBC (+), OB (+)

PLT: platelet; Hb: hemoglobin; ND: no data.

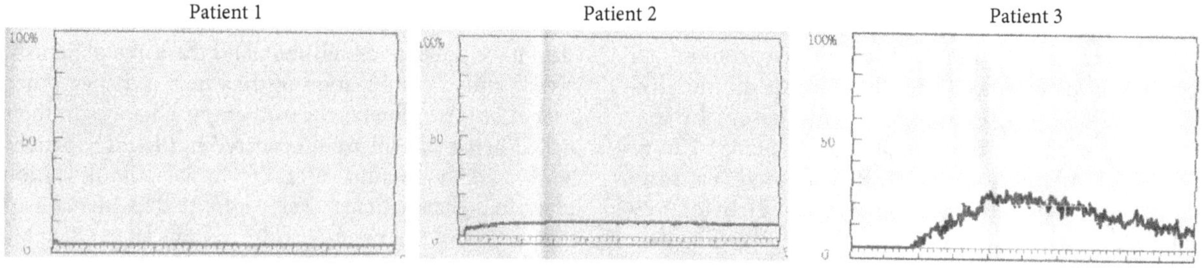

FIGURE 1: PLT function tests of the three patients.

when the initial dosage of dasatinib was reduced to 20 mg daily.

Dasatinib-induced GI hemorrhage in the Ph + B-ALL patients was confirmed. Chemotherapy was continued, and imatinib was carefully increased from a dosage of 100 mg/m^2 daily to 300 mg/m^2 daily; hemafecia disappeared. The patients remained in complete remission and underwent chemotherapy and imatinib treatment.

3. Discussion

Ph + B-ALL is a subtype of B-ALL in which blast cells are detected to have a translocation between BCR on chromosome 22 and the ABL1 oncogene on chromosome 9; this molecular subtype accounts for 2–4% of pediatric ALL cases and approximately 20% of adult ALL cases [1–4]. TKIs have been approved for the treatment of chronic myeloid leukemia (CML) and Ph + ALL [1], and the prognosis of Ph + B-ALL has improved since the introduction of combination treatments with TKIs and chemotherapy [2–5]. Imatinib and dasatinib are the most widely used TKIs in the Ph + B-ALL population.

Dasatinib had 325-fold greater potency than imatinib in cells transduced with the BCR-ABL fusion gene [2]. In addition, outstanding outcomes with the combination of dasatinib and chemotherapy were confirmed in a clinical trial, and the three patients in this report received dasatinib instead of imatinib. TKIs, including dasatinib, have several side effects, and toxicities occur in many organs and/or systems [14]. The majority of side effects induced by TKIs involve the hematological and endocrine systems.

With the widespread use of TKIs, bleeding complications induced by dasatinib have been reported in chronic myeloid leukemia patients [15–17] and Ph + B-ALL patients [18–20]. Adverse bleeding events have been reported in 26–40% of patients with CML or Ph + ALL who received dasatinib [2–4]. The majority of bleeding occurred in the GI tract, and the main reason for bleeding was thrombocytopenia due to myelosuppression or hematopoietic cell transplantation [19, 21], whereas GI hemorrhage in such patients with a normal platelet count is uncommon.

In this article, the patients presented with dasatinib-induced GI hemorrhage, and we think that bleeding was mainly due to abnormal platelet aggregation. It is well known that damaged platelet function leads to bleeding, whereas proteins targeted by dasatinib are implicated in the dynamic processes of platelet activation, likely contributing to the bleeding diathesis seen with dasatinib use [22].

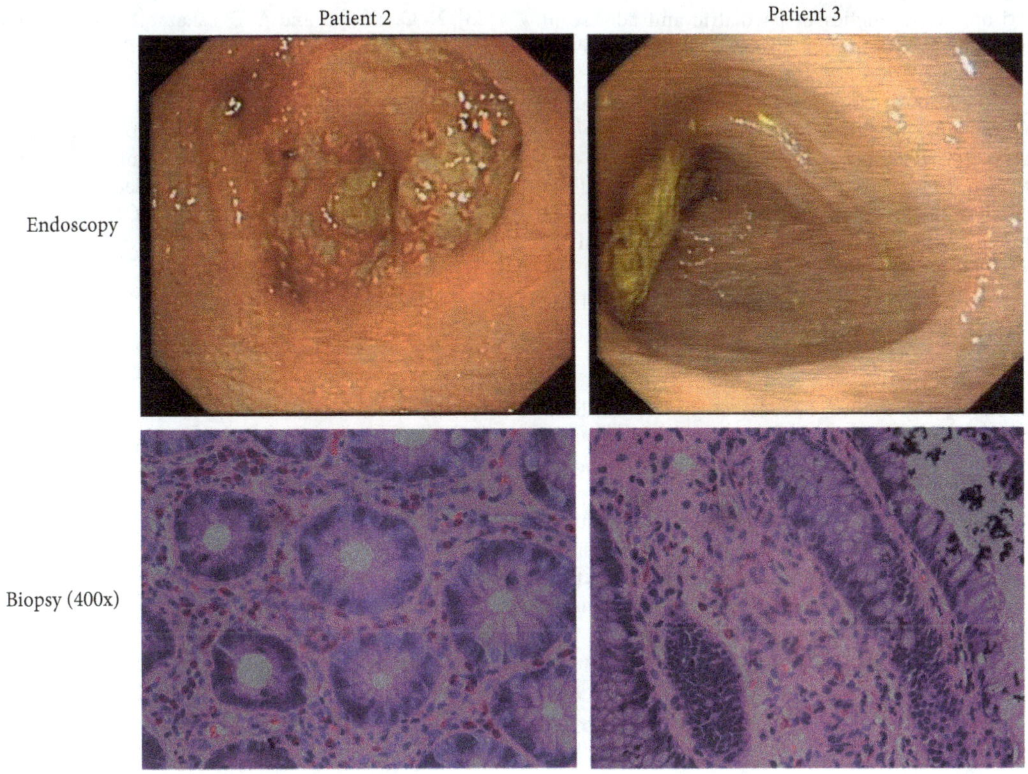

FIGURE 2: Endoscopy and biopsy results of the two patients.

Comedications that may lead to GI bleeding are common in leukemia patients [23], familiar drugs including NSAIDs, glucocorticoids, and traditional Chinese herbs had not been prescribed to the patients at least 2 weeks before the GI bleeding, and thus the role of comedications in the GI bleeding was excluded. Patient 2 had ulcerative colitis, which is uncommon during dasatinib treatment [24], and the underlying pathophysiology remains poorly understood. Dasatinib shows some off-target inhibition of other tyrosine kinases [3], and platelet-derived growth factor receptor (PDGFR) kinase is a potent target of dasatinib [14]. It has been reported that PDGFR-null mice have defective angiogenesis and capillary wall development, which lead to microaneurysm formation and hemorrhage [15].

In summary, we report three Chinese children with Ph + B-ALL who received a combination therapy of TKIs and chemotherapy. They presented with GI hemorrhage due to the side effects of dasatinib; GI hemorrhage disappeared when they were administered with imatinib. These cases reveal that platelet function should be monitored in patients who receive dasatinib.

Acknowledgments

The authors thank the patients and their parents for their cooperation and approval. This work was supported by research funding from the Children's Hospital of Chongqing Medical University and Chongqing Science and Technology Commission.

References

[1] W. Sun, J. Malvar, R. Sposto et al., "Outcome of children with multiply relapsed B-cell acute lymphoblastic leukemia: a therapeutic advances in childhood leukemia & lymphoma study," *Leukemia*, vol. 32, no. 11, pp. 2316–2325, 2018.

[2] K. R. Schultz, W. P. Bowman, A. Aledo et al., "Improved early event-free survival with imatinib in Philadelphia chromosome-positive acute lymphoblastic leukemia: a children's oncology group study," *Journal of Clinical Oncology*, vol. 27, no. 31, pp. 5175–5181, 2009.

[3] K. R. Schultz, N. A. Heerema, A. Carroll et al., "Long-term follow-up of imatinib in pediatric Philadelphia chromosome-positive acute lymphoblastic leukemia: Children's Oncology Group Study AALL0031," *Leukemia*, vol. 28, no. 7, pp. 1467–1471, 2014.

[4] F. Ravandi, J. L. Jorgensen, D. A. Thomas et al., "Detection of MRD may predict the outcome of patients with Philadelphia chromosome-positive ALL treated with tyrosine kinase inhibitors plus chemotherapy," *Blood*, vol. 122, no. 7, pp. 1214–1221, 2013.

[5] F. Ravandi, S. M. O'Brien, J. E. Cortes et al., "Long-term follow-up of a phase 2 study of chemotherapy plus dasatinib for the initial treatment of patients with Philadelphia chromosome-positive acute lymphoblastic leukemia," *Cancer*, vol. 121, no. 23, pp. 4158–4164, 2015.

[6] M. Cazzola, "Introduction to a review series: the 2016 revision of the WHO classification of tumors of hematopoietic and lymphoid tissues," *Blood*, vol. 127, no. 20, pp. 2361–2364, 2016.

[7] C. H. Dunphy, "Comprehensive review of adult acute myelogenous leukemia: cytomorphological, enzyme cytochemical, flow cytometric immunophenotypic, and cytogenetic findings," *Journal of Clinical Laboratory Analysis*, vol. 13, no. 1, pp. 19–26, 1999.

[8] C. J. Harrison, "Cytogenetics of paediatric and adolescent acute lymphoblastic leukaemia," *British Journal of Haematology*, vol. 144, no. 2, pp. 147–156, 2009.

[9] M. Shago, "Recurrent cytogenetic abnormalities in acute lymphoblastic leukemia," *Methods in Molecular Biology*, vol. 1541, pp. 257–278, 2017.

[10] J. Van Dongen, E. Macintyre, J. Gabert et al., "Standardized RT-PCR analysis of fusion gene transcripts from chromosome aberrations in acute leukemia for detection of minimal residual disease," *Leukemia*, vol. 13, no. 12, pp. 1901–1928, 1999.

[11] M. Z. Xu, Q. Y. Fang, X. Y. Gong et al., "Screening of adult Ph-like acute lymphoblastic leukemia by multiplex real-time quantitative PCR," *Zhonghua Xue Ye Xue Za Zhi*, vol. 38, no. 11, pp. 956–961, 2017.

[12] P. Theunissen, E. Mejstrikova, L. Sedek et al., "Standardized flow cytometry for highly sensitive MRD measurements in B-cell acute lymphoblastic leukemia," *Blood*, vol. 129, no. 3, pp. 347–357, 2017.

[13] A. Biondi, V. Gandemer, P. De Lorenzo et al., "Imatinib treatment of paediatric Philadelphia chromosome-positive acute lymphoblastic leukaemia (EsPhALL2010): a prospective, intergroup, open-label, single-arm clinical trial," *The Lancet Haematology*, vol. 5, no. 12, pp. e641–e652, 2018.

[14] U. Athale, N. Hijiya, B. C. Patterson et al., "Management of chronic myeloid leukemia in children and adolescents: recommendations from the children's oncology group CML working group," *Pediatric Blood & Cancer*, vol. 66, no. 9, Article ID e27827, 2019.

[15] N. Patodi, N. Sagar, Z. Rudzki, G. Langman, and N. Sharma, "Haemorrhagic colitis caused by dasatinib," *Case Reports in Hematology*, vol. 2012, Article ID 417106, 4 pages, 2012.

[16] D. N. Perdigoto, S. Lopes, F. Portela, M. A. Cipriano, and L. Tomé, "Dasatinib-induced colitis in a patient with chronic myelogenous leukemia," *GE–Portuguese Journal of Gastroenterology*, vol. 25, no. 4, pp. 198–200, 2018.

[17] M. M. Chisti, A. Khachani, G. R. Brahmanday, and J. Klamerus, "Dasatinib-induced haemorrhagic colitis in chronic myeloid leukaemia (CML) in blast crisis," *Case Reports*, vol. 2013, 2013.

[18] T. Shimokaze, T. Mitsui, H. Takeda et al., "Severe hemorrhagic colitis caused by dasatinib in Philadelphia chromosome-positive acute lymphoblastic leukemia," *Pediatric Hematology and Oncology*, vol. 26, no. 6, pp. 448–453, 2009.

[19] H.-Y. Yhim, H. S. Kim, N.-R. Lee, E.-K. Song, J.-Y. Kwak, and C.-Y. Yim, "Bilateral subdural hemorrhage as a serious adverse event of dasatinib in a patient with Philadelphia chromosome-positive acute lymphoblastic leukemia," *International Journal of Hematology*, vol. 95, no. 5, pp. 585–587, 2012.

[20] M. K. Mustafa Ali, M. M. Sabha, and K. H. Al-Rabi, "Spontaneous subdural hematoma in a patient with Philadelphia chromosome-positive acute lymphoblastic leukemia with normal platelet count after dasatinib treatment," *Platelets*, vol. 26, no. 5, pp. 491–494, 2015.

[21] I. Aldoss, K. Gaal, M. M. Al Malki et al., "Dasatinib-induced colitis after allogeneic stem cell transplantation for Philadelphia chromosome-positive acute lymphoblastic leukemia," *Biology of Blood and Marrow Transplantation*, vol. 22, no. 10, pp. 1900–1903, 2016.

[22] L. Kostos, K. Burbury, G. Srivastava, and H. M. Prince, "Gastrointestinal bleeding in a chronic myeloid leukaemia patient precipitated by dasatinib-induced platelet dysfunction: case report," *Platelets*, vol. 26, no. 8, pp. 809–811, 2015.

[23] N. O. Yurttas and A. E. Eskazan, "Tyrosine kinase inhibitor-associated platelet dysfunction: does this need to have a significant clinical impact?" *Clinical and Applied Thrombosis/Hemostasis*, vol. 25, 2019.

[24] A. E. Eskazan, I. Hatemi, S. Ongoren Aydin, M. C. Ar, and T. Soysal, "Acute colitis presenting with hematochezia in a patient with chronic myeloid leukemia during dasatinib therapy," *The Turkish Journal of Gastroenterology*, vol. 25, no. 1, p. 233, 2015.

14

Amoxicillin/Clavulanic Acid-Induced Agranulocytosis: A Case Report and Review of the Literature

Aristides Armas Villalba[1], **Marya Haq**[1], **Cunxian Zhang**[2,3] and **Jinen Thakkar**[1]

[1]*Internal Medicine Department, Kent County Hospital, Warren Alpert Medical School of Brown University, Providence, RI, USA*
[2]*Associate Professor of Pathology and Laboratory Medicine, Brown University, Providence, RI, USA*
[3]*Chief of Pathology, Kent County Hospital, Warwick, RI, USA*

Correspondence should be addressed to Aristides Armas Villalba; aristides_armas_villalba@brown.edu

Academic Editor: Kazunori Nakase

Amoxicillin/clavulanic acid is one of the widely prescribed antibiotics in the outpatient setting giving excellent antimicrobial coverage and relatively safe profile in terms of adverse reactions. Gastrointestinal and cutaneous reactions are among the commonly reported. Our goal is to describe a case of agranulocytosis induced by amoxicillin/clavulanic acid in a previously healthy patient and review prior reports with similar presentation.

1. Introduction

According to the Center for Disease Control and Prevention (CDC), 269.4 millions of antibiotic prescriptions were ordered in the outpatient setting within the United States of America in 2015. Amoxicillin is the most commonly prescribed antibiotic, and amoxicillin-clavulanate is the third most commonly prescribed [1].

There are drugs classically described as the potential cause of neutropenia or agranulocytosis, but amoxicillin/clavulanate is not included in the list. Since the development of the drug, the most common side effect or adverse reaction reported is diarrhea.

Here, we present a case about amoxicillin/clavulanate-induced agranulocytosis and review of the literature.

2. Case Report

A 49-year-old male patient without a significant past medical history presented to hospital with complaints of diarrhea. Five days prior to presentation, he developed a sore throat and consulted a local urgent care center where rapid influenza and streptococcal antigen testing were completed. Despite the negative results of both of these tests, he was prescribed amoxicillin/clavulanate (875/125 mg twice a day, day 5 on presentation to the hospital).

His symptoms persisted and progressed, with the addition of watery diarrhea to his complaints, at which point he presented to the emergency department. Initial physical exam was significant for a temperature of 38.7°C (101.7°F), with other vital signs within normal limits. Skin exam demonstrated a generalized macular and erythematous exanthema. The pharynx was found to be erythematous but without exudates, and chest auscultation demonstrated bilateral wheezing. The remainder of the physical exam was unremarkable.

Initial laboratory data reported hemoglobin 14.0 g/dL, hematocrit 40.6%, platelet count of $159 \times 10^3/mm^3$, and white blood cell count of $500/mm^3$. Considering the fever, physical examination and degree of neutropenia, the patient was admitted to the hospital with diagnosis of febrile neutropenia and started on broad-spectrum antibiotics immediately (vancomycin and piperacillin-tazobactam).

At the same time, blood cultures were drawn and the patient was started on filgrastim (granulocyte-colony stimulating factor) and continued on a daily basis. When he remained febrile and profoundly leukopenic, the hematology department was consulted for bone marrow aspirate and biopsy. On day three, marrow examination was done and reported a 40–60% cellularity with myeloid hypoplasia (myeloid to erythroid precursor ratio of 0.5 : 1) and increased blasts (Figure 1).

Despite a slowly rising leukocyte count, he continued to spike fevers for the first seven days of admission; on day nine of admission, his leukocyte count had normalized (Figure 2). Throughout the stay in hospital, extensive work-up for infectious and immunologic causes of agranulocytosis (Table 1) was done and revealed only a positive IgG result against parvovirus B19. Since the diagnosis was still a challenge, skin biopsy of the aforementioned rash was performed and reported perivascular and periadnexal lymphoplasmacytic inflammation.

His clinical condition continued to improve, with stable vital signs including lack of recurrence of fevers for the last four days of his inpatient stay, and as there were no further indications for either antibiotics or filgrastim, he was discharged home on day eleven of his hospital stay.

One week after discharge, he was seen in follow-up by his hematologist, with continued demonstration of a complete blood count within normal limits and no further concerning signs or symptoms.

3. Discussion

Classically, neutropenia is defined as an absolute blood neutrophil count less than two standard deviations below the normal mean, and agranulocytosis is often used to define severe neutropenia (below 0.5×10^9 cells/liter) [2]. The causes of neutropenia can be classified as a disorder in the production and distribution or turnover of neutrophils.

In terms of duration, neutropenia can be classified as transient or chronic, with three months being the cutoff point. The most common etiology of transient neutropenia is a viral infection [3].

Several studies have studied the incidence of drug-induced neutropenia, estimating it anywhere between 1.1 and 15.4 cases per million population around the world per year [4–6].

Interestingly, despite an extensive infectious work-up, no infectious etiology was identified in this patient with acute onset agranulocytosis or neutropenia. He did present to the emergency department six days after the onset of symptoms, but most infectious causes of agranulocytosis do not typically cause the persistent marrow suppression seen in this patient despite resolution of his symptoms.

Taking the extensive work-up, the presence of a maculopapular rash and the temporal association with exposure to amoxicillin-clavulanate, we concluded that his presentation was consistent with amoxicillin-clavulanate-induced agranulocytosis. On top of that, ferritin and C-reactice protein levels were found to be elevated, well know acute phase reactants that can be triggered by immune processes.

There are well-described nonchemotherapeutic medications associated with agranulocytosis, and the term is known as idiosyncratic drug-induced agranulocytosis.

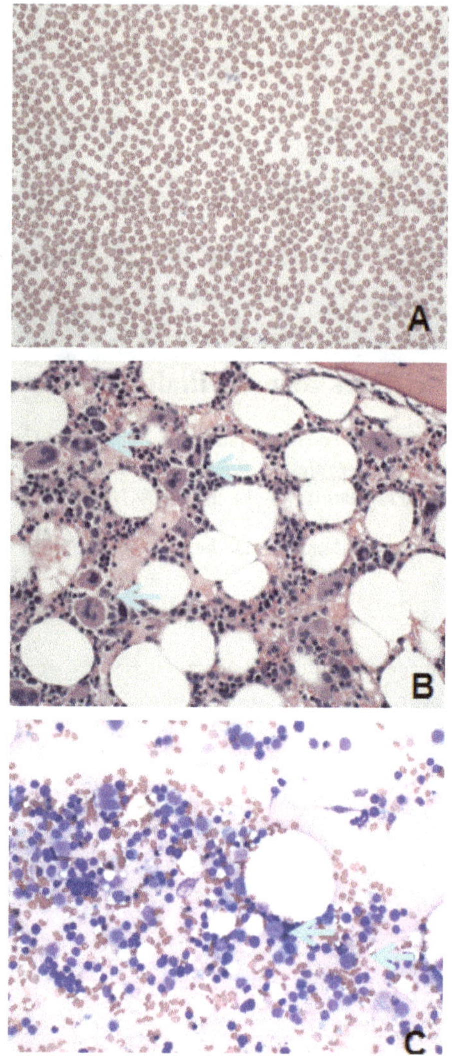

Figure 1: Peripheral blood smear and bone marrow studies. (a) Peripheral blood smear shows severe neutropenia with no neutrophils seen in this field (hematoxylin and eosin stain; ×400), (b) bone marrow biopsy with normal cellularity, increased megakaryocytes (blue arrows), and severe decrease in neutrophils (hematoxylin and eosin stain; ×400), and (c) bone marrow smear displays severely decreased segmented granulocytes and increased blasts (blue arrows; Wright–Giemsa stain ×400).

There are only two case reports associating amoxicillin-clavulanate with agranulocytosis, but unfortunately the investigations were not as thorough as our patient had, leading to multiple questions about whether it truly was the drug that caused the hematologic findings [5].

Briefly, the pathogenesis of the disease has been attributed to direct "toxic" effect of the medication (or a metabolite) and recently has been described an immune-mediated process. A widely accepted hypothesis explains that the drug can activate the immune system via haptens that later will induce direct damage to the cell or bone marrow itself [7, 8].

Our approach to this patient's management was to first exclude infections as a possible etiology, and the extensive work-up can be seen in Table 1. In the meantime, broad-spectrum

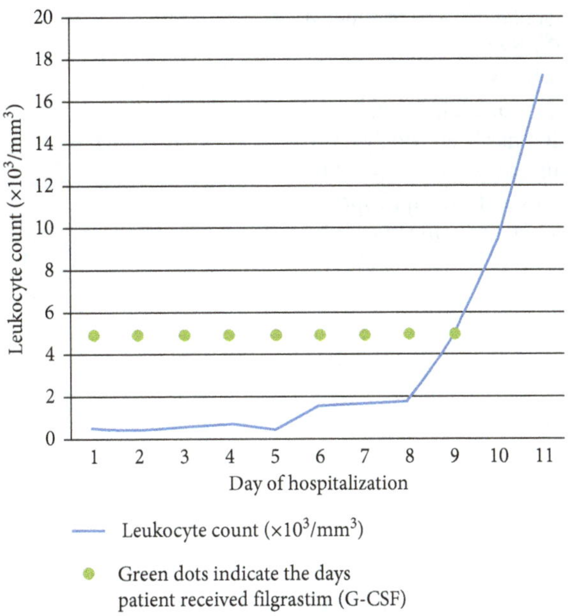

FIGURE 2: Daily leukocyte trend throughout the admission in the hospital.

TABLE 1: Infectious and immunologic work-up performed during the admission.

Test	Result	Comments
Chest X-ray	Normal examination	
CT chest, abdomen, and pelvis	Unremarkable	Simple cysts in the left kidney.
Blood cultures	Negative	Performed on three different days (two sets each)
Stool analysis	C. albicans isolated in the culture	Negative for bacteria, ova, and parasites.
Influenza rapid diagnostic test	Negative	
Rapid strep test	Negative	
Mononucleosis spot test	Negative	IgM heterophile antibody
Urine analysis	Negative for infection	
Blood parasites	Negative	
Viral hepatitis	Negative	Hepatitis A, B, and C.
Cytomegalovirus	Negative	IgG and IgM
Human immunodeficiency virus	Negative	Elisa and PCR
Parvovirus B19	IgG positive	IgM negative
Babesiosis panel	Negative	PCR for B. microti, B. duncani, and B. divergens.
T. pallidum antibodies	Negative	
Respiratory virus culture	Negative	Reported after 14 days of incubation
Fungitell	Negative	
B. burgdorferi	Negative	IgG and IgM
Rheumatoid factor	Negative	
Anti-nuclear antibodies	Negative	
Ferritin	615 ng/mL	Normal values from 18 to 270 ng/mL
Procalcitonin	0.12 μg/mL	Normal values from 0 to 0.26 μg/mL
C3 level	138 IU	Normal values from 88 to 200 IU
C4 level	37.2 IU	Normal values from 16 to 47 IU
C-reactive protein	17.4 mg/dL	Upper limit of normal 0.5 mg/dL

antibiotics and granulocyte-colony stimulating factor were administered to the patient as part of the treatment for neutropenic fever.

The patient continued to be severely neutropenic despite multiple treatments with granulocyte-colony stimulating factor (G-CSF). There are several hypotheses proposed to explain the phenomenon: the first one is an immune-mediated reaction after the patient is exposed to the drug and the second one, the drug itself inducing a toxic microenvironment in the marrow that inhibits the production of new cells [9].

Four days after G-CSF was started, the bone marrow was still not responding and bone marrow biopsy and aspirate was performed. The pathology department reported 40–60% cellularity with marked myeloid hypoplasia. At the same time, skin biopsy was taken as well for further understanding of the rash and reported perivascular and periadnexal lymphoplasmacytic inflammation. Both of these findings are consistent the with drug-related reaction.

We conclude that over the years, amoxicillin-clavulanate has demonstrated to be a safe drug that has been widely used. Despite the two prior reports and ours, prescription must be continued if there is a formal indication in the appropriate patient to avoid harming the patient and reducing antibiotic resistance rates as much as possible.

Authors' Contributions

All authors contributed equally to the development of the manuscript.

References

[1] CDC Centers for Disease Control and Prevention, OutpatientAntibiotic Prescriptions—United States, CDC Centers for Disease Control and Prevention, Atlanta, GA, USA, 2015, https://www.cdc.gov/antibiotic-use/community/pdfs/Annual-Report-2015.pdf.

[2] D. C. Dale and K. Welte, "Neutropenia and neutrophilia," in *Williams Hematology, 9E*, K. Kaushansky, M. A. Lichtman, J. T. Prchal et al., Eds., McGraw-Hill, New York, NY, USA, 2018, http://accessmedicine.mhmedical.com/content.aspx?bookid=1581&sectionid=101238861.

[3] P. E. Newburger and D. C. Dale, "Evaluation and management of patients with isolated neutropenia," *Seminars in Hematology*, vol. 50, no. 3, pp. 198–206, 2013.

[4] B. L. Strom, J. L. Carson, R. Schinnar et al., "Descriptive epidemiology of agranulocytosis," *Archives of Internal Medicine*, vol. 152, no. 7, pp. 1475–1480, 1992.

[5] N. Spetrino, M. Arazzi, G. Di Fulvio et al., "Severe neutropenia during treatment with amoxicillin/clavulanic acid in a patient on regular hemodialysis treatment," *Giornale Italiano di Nefrologia*, vol. 33, no. 6, 2016.

[6] D. W. Kaufman, J. P. Kelly, S. Issaragrisil et al., "Relative incidence of agranulocytosis and aplastic anemia," *American Journal of Hematology*, vol. 81, no. 1, pp. 65–67, 2006.

[7] B. R. Curtis, "Non-chemotherapy drug-induced neutropenia: key points to manage the challenges," *Hematology*, vol. 2017, no. 1, pp. 187–193, 2017.

[8] D. Tesfa, M. Keisu, and J. Palmblad, "Idiosyncratic drug-induced agranulocytosis: possible mechanisms and management," *American Journal of Hematology*, vol. 84, no. 7, pp. 428–434, 2009.

[9] A. Johnston and J. Uetrecht, "Current understanding of the mechanisms of idiosyncratic drug-induced agranulocytosis," *Expert Opinion on Drug Metabolism & Toxicology*, vol. 11, no. 2, pp. 243–257, 2015.

15

Severe Thrombocytosis in a Newborn with Subcutaneous Fat Necrosis and Maternal Chorioamnionitis

Mitali Sahni ,[1] Pooja Patel,[2] and Akila Muthukumar[2]

[1]*Pediatrix Medical Group, Sunrise Children's Hospital, University of Nevada, Las Vegas, NV, USA*
[2]*Department of Pediatrics, University of Texas Medical Branch, Galveston, TX, USA*

Correspondence should be addressed to Mitali Sahni; mitali12@gmail.com

Academic Editor: Pier Paolo Piccaluga

Background. Subcutaneous fat necrosis (SFN) is a form of transient panniculitis that presents commonly in infants with a history of perinatal insult, particularly hypothermia. It is characterized by subcutaneous nodules and plaques that appear over bony prominences on cheeks, shoulders, buttock, and thighs. SFN is usually associated with various complications including hypercalcemia, thrombocytopenia, hypertriglyceridemia, and hyperglycemia. *Case Presentation.* We present a unique case of a female infant with a history of maternal chorioamnionitis who presented with SFN at 11 days of life with thrombocytosis. The platelet count decreased during the hospital stay, and thrombocytosis resolved over the course of the next two weeks. She did not have any other hematological or metabolic abnormalities associated with SFN. *Conclusion.* Infants with perinatal stress are at increased risk of developing SFN during the first month of life. Infants with a diagnosis of SFN should be monitored closely for various hematological and metabolic abnormalities that can have serious consequences.

1. Background

Subcutaneous fat necrosis (SFN) is a form of transient panniculitis that presents in newborns in their first month of life, as multiple erythematous to violaceous, indurated plaques or nodules. It is usually seen over areas of bony prominences and usually resolves with time. It is however associated with various serious metabolic and hematological complications like hypercalcemia, for which the patient should be monitored. The pathogenesis of SFN is not clearly defined in the literature, but it is seen in infants where the blood supply to the fat tissue may be affected due to environmental stress. We present a unique case of SFN who also presented with severe thrombocytosis. SFN has been associated with thrombocytopenia; however, there are no reported cases of SFN with thrombocytosis in the literature.

2. Case Presentation

An eleven-day-old female infant was admitted to the pediatric inpatient floor due to a two-day history of increase in size and number of nodules on the back. She was born at 38 weeks gestational age, to a G1P1 mother via Cesarean section. The perinatal course was complicated by maternal chorioamnionitis; infant underwent a sepsis workup which was negative and received IV antibiotics for 48 hours only. Complete blood count (CBC) done during this period revealed normal CBC indices including a normal total platelet count. She was discharged from the nursery on day of life 5 and was readmitted on day 11 of life for new-onset nodules and increased irritability. On physical examination, there were multiple oval, rubbery, nonmobile, nonfluctuant 1×1 cm nodules, palpable at occiput and nape of the neck. Also, a large 4 cm violaceous plaque was found on her back interspersed with multiple, firm, nonmobile nodules. These lesions looked erythematous in some areas and were tender to touch. Initial evaluation revealed an elevated platelet count of $1104 \times 10^3/\mu L$ with normal leukocyte count, normal C-reactive protein, and normal blood smear. The platelet count continued to decrease over the course of the hospital stay, and thrombocytosis resolved over the next two weeks. Figure 1 shows the progression of

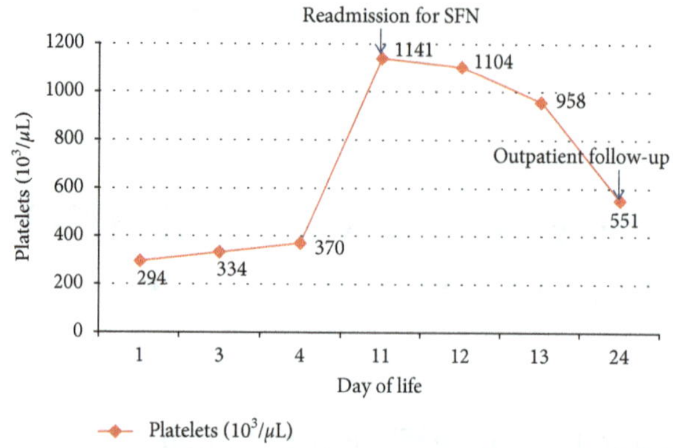

FIGURE 1: Progression of total platelet count-infant with normal platelet count at birth, thrombocytosis noted on the readmission to hospital for SFN and progressive decrease over the next two weeks.

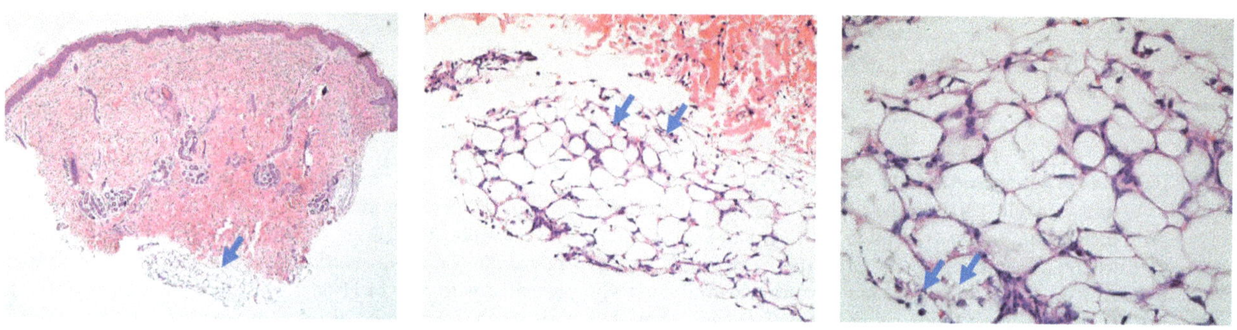

FIGURE 2: Hematoxylin-eosin stained section of the skin biopsy shows in (a) normal epidermis and dermis with underlying lobular panniculitis (blue arrow) and necrosis of the fat globules in the subcutaneous adipose tissue. (b) The panniculitis (blue arrows) comprised of acute (neutrophils) and chronic (lymphocytes) inflammatory cells and histiocytes. (c) shows many fat cells retained their outline but contain fine, eosinophilic cytoplasmic strands and granules, between which are narrow clefts radiating (blue arrow) from a point near the periphery of the cell.

total platelet count from birth until 4 weeks of age. Our initial differential diagnosis included infections like herpes simplex virus, malignancies like neuroblastoma, infantile myofibromatosis and rhabdomyosarcoma, subcutaneous fat necrosis, and skin necrosis due to protein C/S deficiency.

The infant was started on the IV antibiotics ampicillin and gentamicin along with IV acyclovir that were later discontinued after cultures resulted negative. Retroperitoneal ultrasound done to rule out any abdominal mass was reported to be normal. A punch biopsy of the lesion was obtained, and it showed a focus of inflammatory cells in the fat lobule with focal needle-like spaces, consistent with subcutaneous fat necrosis (Figure 2). The nodules remained stable during the hospital stay, and the infant was discharged on DOL 13. Twelve days after discharge, CBC done at the time of outpatient follow-up indicated resolving thrombocytosis ($551 \times 10^3//\mu L$) and stable calcium levels (10.2 mg/dL). Three months after discharge, the large violaceous plaque and skin nodules were mostly resolved.

3. Discussion

SFN is a rare form of benign panniculitis seen in the first four weeks of life in term and postterm infants. It is essential to identify it early, as it has been known to cause many complications including hypercalcemia, which can be fatal. The lesions of SFN are characterized by multiple erythematous to violaceous, indurated plaques or nodules most commonly found on the cheeks, buttocks, posterior trunk, and extremities. Of note, they tend to spare the anterior trunk. Many lesions become calcified or fluctuant with liquefied fat. Mild atrophy of the skin may be noticed after resolution [1].

The cause of SFN is not precisely known; however, there are many risk factors associated with it. A systemic review of 16 patients with SFN performed by Mahé et al. identified newborn failure to thrive (12/16), forceps delivery (7/16), maternal high blood pressure (3/10) and/or diabetes (2/10), macrosomia (7/16), exposure to active (4/10) or passive (3/10) smoking during pregnancy, putative or known maternal/paternal or newborn risk factors for thrombosis (5/10), and dyslipidaemia (2/10) as the possible causes [2]. Another case-series review by Burden and Krafchik described birth asphyxia and meconium aspiration as etiological factors [3]. There have been multiple case reports of SFN developing in patients after receiving therapeutic hypothermia [4, 5] or after application of ice bags for management of supraventricular tachycardia [6]. Given its varied associations, the pathogenesis of this disease remains unclear. However, there is a definite association with infants in distress secondary to the maternal and fetal factors noted above.

Diagnosis of SFN is usually made clinically, but sometimes a biopsy can be helpful for confirmation. The cytology can show a spectrum of changes ranging from fat lobules with opaque cytoplasm to necrotic aspirates containing fat cells with needle-shaped crystals, multinucleated giant cells, foamy macrophages, lymphocytes, and neutrophils. We did a skin biopsy, which showed inflammatory cells in the fat lobule with focal needle-like spaces, consistent with the diagnosis of SFN [7].

Most SFN lesions spontaneously resolve in a few months, but many complications may be seen. The most commonly reported complications include thrombocytopenia, hypoglycemia, hypertriglyceridemia, and hypercalcemia (which may sometimes lead to nephrocalcinosis) [1]. In a retrospective study of 30 patients with SFN, authors reported the clinical characteristics and complications in infants with a diagnosis of SFN. The complications seen with SFN in their study cohort included hypercalcemia (19/30), thrombocytopenia (11/30), recurrent disease (4/30), nephrocalcinosis (3/30), hypoglycemia (3/30), calcinosis of the gallbladder (1/30), and hyperlipidemia (1/30) [8]. Hypercalcemia has been attributed to high levels of 1, 25-dihydroxy vitamin D produced by macrophages leading to increased calcium absorption from the gastrointestinal tract and also to calcium release from necrotic adipose tissue [9, 10]. In our case, we did not encounter any of these complications, but we noted a significant thrombocytosis at the time of presentation and which slowly resolved during the hospital stay. To the best of our knowledge, this is the first reported case of SFN where thrombocytosis has been reported. Although thrombocytopenia has been reported in many cases of SFN, the cause of this association is not known. Chen et al. proposed that the thrombocytopenia was due to the local sequestration of platelets in the subcutaneous tissue [11]. We propose that the thrombocytosis can be attributed to the reactive inflammatory response of SFN. However, the increased number of platelets could have led to increased sequestration in the subcutaneous tissue, thereby worsening the adipose tissue necrosis.

Although SFN is a relatively benign condition, it has been associated with many hematological and metabolic abnormalities that require follow-up and at times interventions. Since we do not know the pathogenesis behind this phenomenon, any new association noted can be helpful to understand this disease better. Infants diagnosed with SFN should be monitored for hematological and electrolyte abnormalities periodically. Most lesions resolve spontaneously over time, but monitoring for complications is suggested to avoid adverse outcomes.

Abbreviations

SFN: Subcutaneous fat necrosis
CBC: Complete blood count
DOL: Day of life.

Acknowledgments

The authors thank Dr. Beamon Agarwal, MD, for his assistance and guidance with the pathology slides.

References

[1] J. T. Tran and A. P. Sheth, "Complications of subcutaneous fat necrosis of the newborn: a case report and review of the literature," *Pediatric Dermatology*, vol. 20, no. 3, pp. 257–261, 2003.

[2] E. Mahé, N. Girszyn, S. Hadj-Rabia, C. Bodemer, D. Hamel-Teillac, and Y. De Prost, "Subcutaneous fat necrosis of the newborn: a systematic evaluation of risk factors, clinical manifestations, complications and outcome of 16 children," *British Journal of Dermatology*, vol. 156, no. 4, pp. 709–715, 2007.

[3] A. D. Burden and B. R. Krafchik, "Subcutaneous fat necrosis of the newborn: a review of 11 cases," *Pediatric Dermatology*, vol. 16, no. 5, pp. 384–387, 2002.

[4] M. Hogeling, K. Meddles, D. R. Berk et al., "Extensive subcutaneous fat necrosis of the newborn associated with therapeutic hypothermia," *Pediatric Dermatology*, vol. 29, no. 1, pp. 59–63, 2012.

[5] B. Strohm, A. Hobson, P. Brocklehurst, A. D. Edwards, and D. Azzopardi, "Subcutaneous fat necrosis after moderate therapeutic hypothermia in neonates," *Pediatrics*, vol. 128, no. 2, pp. E450–E452, 2011.

[6] S. Diamantis, T. Bastek, P. Groben, and D. Morrell, "Subcutaneous fat necrosis in a newborn following icebag application for treatment of supraventricular tachycardia," *Journal of Perinatology*, vol. 26, no. 8, pp. 518–520, 2006.

[7] P. T. Schubert, R. Razack, A. Vermaak, and H. Francois Jordaan, "Fine-needle aspiration cytology of subcutaneous fat necrosis of the newborn: the cytology spectrum with review of the literature," *Diagnostic Cytopathology*, vol. 40, no. 3, pp. 245–247, 2012.

[8] B. R. Del Pozzo-Magaña and N. Ho, "Subcutaneous fat necrosis of the newborn: a 20-year retrospective study," *Pediatric Dermatology*, vol. 33, no. 6, pp. e353–e355, 2016.

[9] P. H. Finne, J. Sanderud, L. Aksnes, D. Bratlid, and D. Aarskog, "Hypercalcemia with increased and unregulated 1,25-dihydroxyvitamin D production in a neonate with subcutaneous fat necrosis," *The Journal of Pediatrics*, vol. 112, no. 5, pp. 792–794, 1988.

[10] K. Kruse, U. Irle, and R. Uhlig, "Clinical and laboratory observations—elevated 1,25-dihydroxyvitamin-d serum concentrations in infants with subcutaneous fat necrosis," *The Journal of Pediatrics*, vol. 122, no. 3, pp. 460–463, 1993.

[11] T. H. Chen, S. W. Shewmake, D. D. Hansen, and H. L. Lacey, "Subcutaneous fat necrosis of the newborn. A case report," *Archives of Dermatology*, vol. 117, no. 1, pp. 36-37, 1981.

16

QT Prolongation and Associated Ventricular Tachycardia due to Cardiac Iron Load in a Patient with Thalassemia Major

Derya Demirtas,[1] Abdullah Orhan Demirtas,[2] Hilmi Erdem Sumbul,[1] and Ayse Selcan Koc[3]

[1]*Assistant Professor in Department of Internal Medicine, Adana Health Practice and Research Center, Health Sciences University, Adana, Turkey*
[2]*Assistant Professor in Department of Cardiology, Adana Health Practice and Research Center, Health Sciences University, Adana, Turkey*
[3]*Assistant Professor in Department of Radiology, Adana Health Practice and Research Center, Health Sciences University, Adana, Turkey*

Correspondence should be addressed to Ayse Selcan Koc; drayseselcankoc@gmail.com

Academic Editor: Håkon Reikvam

We report the case of a 23-year-old male with thalassemia major who developed long QT and continuous ventricular tachycardia (VT). Electrocardiography, echocardiography, and cardiac magnetic resonance imaging (MRI) were used for diagnosis and risk stratification. VT causes and treatments are presented and discussed. Ventricular arrhythmia can be treated by normalizing QT interval with high-dose beta-blocker therapy. However, MRI-compatible internal cardiac defibrillator implantation was performed due to the high risk in this patient.

1. Introduction

Excess iron loading occurs in many organs, primarily the heart and liver, and in patients with thalassemia major. In a study using magnetic resonance imaging (MRI) on a large number of patients, serious heart involvement was reported to be 20%, while in 58% of patients, iron deposition was reported to be within normal limits [1]. Malignant ventricular arrhythmias, which can result in sudden cardiac death due to increased cardiac repolarization, can be seen in patients who develop heart failure due to iron deposition [2]. In the following article, we discussed the treatment of the patient with thalassemia major who developed long QT and continuous ventricular tachycardia (VT) due to severe iron deposition.

2. Clinical Case

A 23-year-old male with a previous diagnosis of beta thalassemia major was admitted to the emergency department with complaints about palpitation, dizziness, blurred vision, weakness, and tiredness. His electrocardiography (ECG) showed VT (Figure 1(a)); thus, the patient was taken to the cardiac intensive care unit (CICU). Serum electrolytes were normal in the emergency department (Na: 138 mmol/lt, K: 4.2 mmol/lt, Ca: 9.8 mg/dl, and Mg: 2.4 mg/dl). The VT continued when the patient was admitted to the CICU (Figure 1(b)). Blood pressure was 80/60 mmHg. He had rough breathing. Synchronized, 100 J biphasic cardioversion was performed by sedating the patient who had an ECG compatible with VT under emergency conditions. VT was successfully corrected with cardioversion. The ECG was in the sinus rhythm and had ventricular premature beats (R on T) and QT-QTc interval prolongations (Figure 1(c)). Immediate beta-blocker treatment was initiated. On the 13th day of treatment, QT-QTc intervals were corrected and ventricular premature beats disappeared with maximum tolerable doses of beta-blocker therapy (Figure 1(d)). He was taking deferoxamine methanesulfonate 500 mg daily for blood chelation.

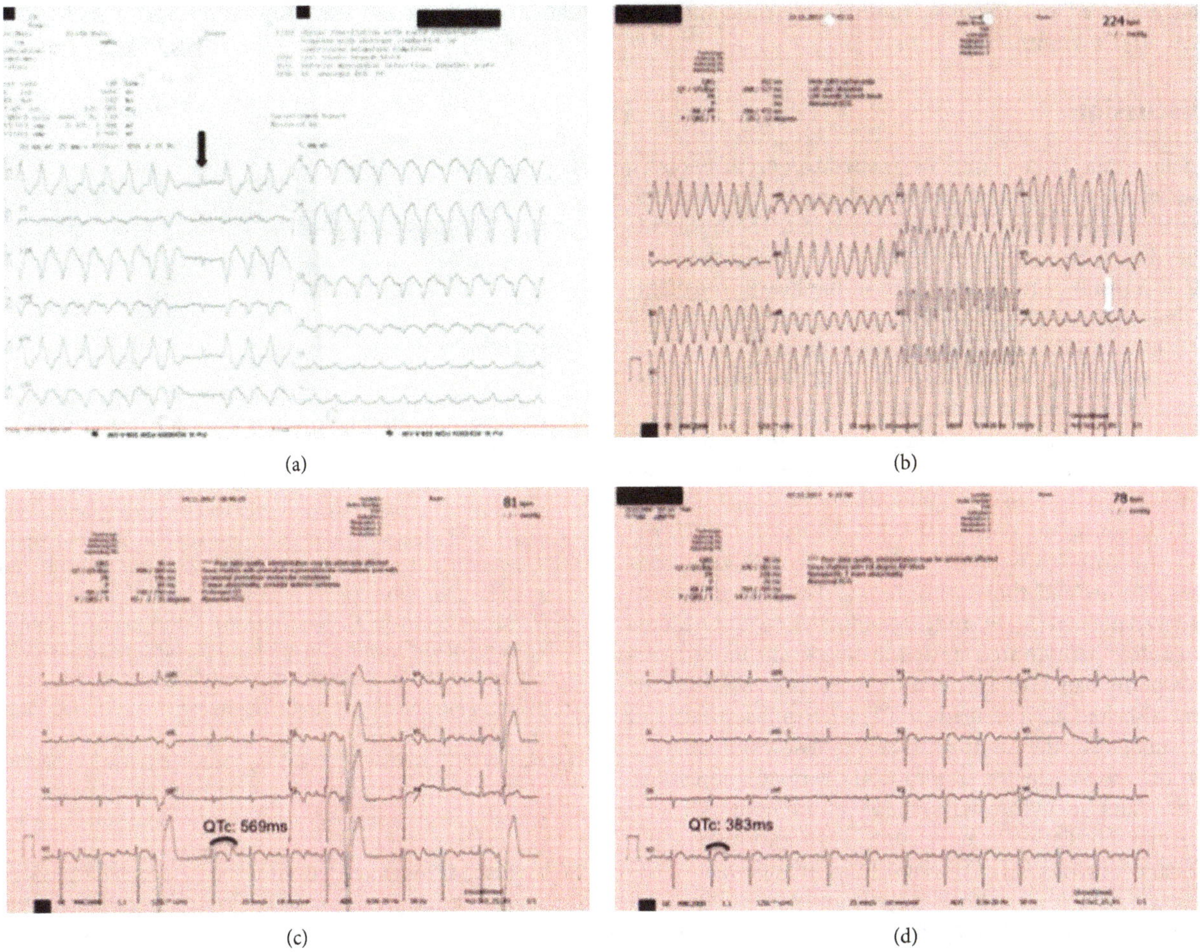

FIGURE 1: Electrocardiographies (ECGs) of patients. (a) Ventricular tachycardia (VT) ECG in emergency department; the capture beat, which is a diagnostic ECG finding for VT, is indicated by the arrow. (b) Another VT ECG in cardiac intensive care unit, another diagnostic ECG finding for VT, and the fusion beat is shown with an arrow. (c) Sinus rhythm ECG after cardioversion (ventricular premature beats (R on T) and long QT/QTc). (d) QT-QTc intervals were corrected and ventricular premature beats disappeared with maximum tolerable doses of beta-blocker therapy.

Hemoglobin value was measured as 8.6 mg/dl in laboratory findings. A unit of blood transfusion was given with the recommendation of the Hematology Clinic. Hemoglobin value after transfusion was 9.6 gr/dl, serum ferritin was >1500 ng/l, and serum iron was 251 pg/dl.

Echocardiography revealed that ejection fraction was 69%, interventricular septum was hypertrophic (1.5 cm), left atrium was dilated (end-diastolic diameter 4.1 cm), and stage III diastolic dysfunction (restrictive filling pattern) was observed. A cardiac MRI was requested to screen the iron deposition in the heart of the patient. On MRI imaging, left ventricle (LV) was diffuse hypertrophic and hypointense (dark) (myocardial T2* value 8.67 milliseconds). However, right ventricle (RV) myocardium was normal, stained with MRI (Figure 2). MRI results were interpreted as deposition of intense iron in the LV myocardium (Figure 2). As a result of the examinations, it was thought that VT might be related to QT prolongation related to iron deposition in the heart. Electrophysiology study was performed when the patient had normal QT interval and tachycardia was not induced in the procedure. Current situation was told to the patient and relatives, secondary internal cardiac defibrillator (ICD) implantation was decided for prophylaxis, and Medtronic brand MRI compatible DDD-ICD implantation was performed. Beta-blocker treatment continued. The patient did

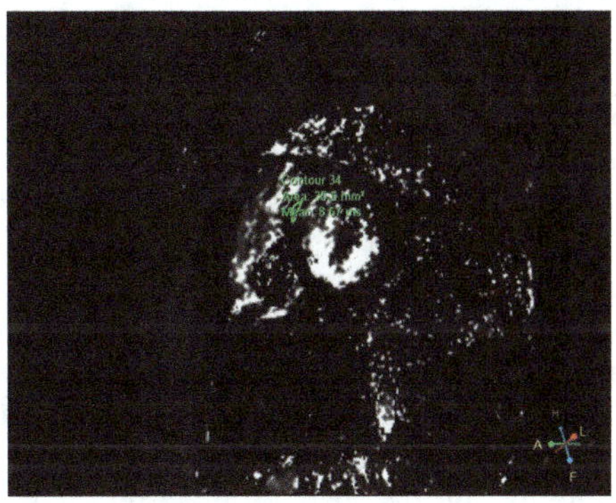

FIGURE 2: Cardiac magnetic resonance imaging (MRI) finding: T2* mapping MRI sagittal midventricular view shows a dark appearance of left ventricle myocardium due to severe iron load (T2* value was 8.67 ms).

not have any VT recordings at routine polyclinic and ICD control after a month.

3. Discussion

In thalassemia major, due to ineffective erythropoiesis, regular blood transfusions are needed and this may lead to excess iron deposition in the liver and heart. These patients are lost due to cardiac failure and cardiac complications that occur as a result of iron deposition in the heart. In patients with thalassemia major, mortality rates reduced significantly due to intravenous and oral chelation therapy [3, 4]. Our patient could have reached the age of 23 because he had received regular chelation therapy.

In patients with thalassemia major, MRI imaging is widely used to detect early onset and general iron overload [1]. In addition, information about RV and LV anatomy and functions can be obtained with MRI. In cardiac MRI, patients with iron loads of T2* <10 milliseconds were considered serious and those with T2* >20 milliseconds were considered normal [5]. In studies conducted, 83% of patients with cardiac arrhythmias and iron-overload-induced cardiomyopathy had MRI T2* levels <20 milliseconds [5]. Our patient also had an iron load of T2* = 8.6 milliseconds and was evaluated in the group with severe iron overload.

In thalassemia major, due to iron overload and cardiac fibrosis, fatal arrhythmias such as continuous VT and ventricular fibrillation may occur [2]. In various studies, parameters such as QT, QTc, and QTp in superficial ECG have been shown to increase significantly in comparison with normal healthy subjects [6]. In our case, QT interval was 490 milliseconds and QTc interval was 569 milliseconds. In our patient, there was also premature ventricular (R on T) beats. Beta-blocker therapy normalized both QT and QTc intervals, and ventricular premature beats disappeared. This suggests that beta-blocker treatment may routinely be initiated in patients with thalassemia major who have ventricular arrhythmia, if not contraindicated.

Because the current guideline [7] considers it as a reversible condition with chelation therapy, it recommends chelation and drug treatment in primer protection and does not recommend ICD in both primary and secondary protection. Information on antiarrhythmic therapy is limited in patients with thalassemia major and accompanying ventricular arrhythmia. The DDD-ICD device was implanted prophylactically on his own request because of the young age of the patient, history of having VT twice, his undergoing iron chelation therapy, and increased risk of sudden cardiac death. Personalized treatment is usually applied in patients with VT due to iron overload. In literature, ICD implantation was performed in two similar cases [4, 8]. In our case, the implantation of DDD-ICD was coordinated with the decision of 3 electrophysiologists.

In conclusion, in patients with thalassemia major, long QT and subsequent VT may occur due to excess iron accumulation. In these patients, ventricular arrhythmia can be treated by normalizing the QT interval with high-dose beta-blocker therapy after acute condition treatment. Beta-blocker therapy must be considered in thalassemia major patients with excess iron deposition and associated ventricular arrhythmia, and ICD therapy should be considered in patients at high risk.

Consent

Written informed consent was obtained from the patient.

References

[1] J.-P. Carpenter, T. He, P. Kirk et al., "On T2* magnetic resonance and cardiac iron," *Circulation*, vol. 123, no. 14, pp. 1519–1528, 2011.

[2] C. A. Obejero-Paz, T. Yang, W.-Q. Dong et al., "Deferoxamine promotes survival and prevents electrocardiographic abnormalities in the gerbil model of iron-overload cardiomyopathy," *Journal of Laboratory and Clinical Medicine*, vol. 141, no. 2, pp. 121–130, 2003.

[3] R. M. Al-Rousan, K. Manzoor, S. Paturi et al., "Long-term efficacy of deferasirox in preventing cardiovascular complications in the iron-overloaded gerbil," *Journal of Cardiovascular Pharmacology and Therapeutics*, vol. 17, no. 1, pp. 117–125, 2012.

[4] N. Bayar, Ş. Arslan, Z. Erkal, and S. Küçükseymen, "Sustained ventricular tachycardia in a patient with thalassemia major," *Annals of Noninvasive Electrocardiology*, vol. 19, no. 2, pp. 193–197, 2014.

[5] P. Kirk, M. Roughton, J. B. Porter et al., "Cardiac T2* magnetic resonance for prediction of cardiac complications in thalassemia major," *Circulation*, vol. 120, no. 20, pp. 1961–1968, 2009.

[6] M. Kayrak, K. Acar, E. E. Gul et al., "The association between myocardial iron load and ventricular repolarization parameters in asymptomatic beta-thalassemia patients," *Advances in Hematology*, vol. 2012, Article ID 170510, 6 pages, 2012.

[7] S. M. Al-Khatib, W. G. Stevenson, M. J. Ackerman et al., "AHA/ACC/HRS guideline for management of patients with ventricular arrhythmias and the prevention of sudden cardiac death: executive summary: a report of the American college of cardiology/American heart association task force on clinical practice guidelines and the heart rhythm society," *Heart Rhythm*, vol. 15, no. 17, pp. e190–e252, 2017.

[8] D. Foo and P. F. Joseph, "Ventricular tachycardia in iron man," *Heart Rhythm Case Reports*, vol. 2, no. 1, pp. 98–100, 2015.

17

"A Dangerous Black Box": Idiopathic Hemophagocytic Lymphohistiocytosis in Adult Patients—A Case Report and Review of the Literature

Nada Agbariah,[1] **Javier Sanz**,[2] **and Alicia Rovó**[1]

[1]*Department of Hematology and Central Hematology Laboratory, Inselspital, Bern University Hospital, University of Bern, Bern, Switzerland*
[2]*Department of Human Genetics, Inselspital University Hospital Bern, Bern, Switzerland*

Correspondence should be addressed to Nada Agbariah; nada.agbariah@gmail.com

Academic Editor: Pier Paolo Piccaluga

Hemophagocytic lymphohistiocytosis (HLH) is a rare potentially life-threatening condition characterized by aberrant inflammation that can be related to genetic or sporadic forms. In both forms, triggering factors may be involved. Early detection of the underlying cause is crucial for therapeutic decision, while early intervention might be associated with better outcomes. The largest descriptions in the literature on HLH refer to pediatric cases. Adolescents and adults may also be affected, but there is scarce evidence regarding their diagnosis and management. We describe here the case of a 68-year-old Swiss woman with HLH, in whom an extensive search for underlying causes was performed, but neither trigger nor pathogenic variant was found. An early intervention first with dexamethasone and later with cyclosporine was performed. The patient showed a favorable response and did not require further hospitalization; however, one year after diagnosis, it was not possible to suspend cyclosporine due to recurrence of laboratory inflammation signs by drug tapering. The occurrence of HLH idiopathic forms represents a challenge; failure to identify the underlying triggering cause generates uncertainty, endless diagnostic investigations, and consequently additional delays in the treatment. This manuscript addresses the difficulties on this issue.

1. Introduction

Hemophagocytic lymphohistiocytosis (HLH) is a rare and potentially life-threatening condition characterized by a cytokine storm that is provoked by aberrant activation of macrophages and T cytotoxic cells [1, 2]. Clinically, HLH patients present with fever, splenomegaly, and a sepsis-like syndrome. The laboratory findings are hyperferritinemia, bicytopenia or pancytopenia, activation of the coagulation cascade, hypertriglyceridemia, often hepatitis, and multi-organ dysfunction [3–5]. Pathophysiology is complex: key factors are the presence of predisposing immunodeficiency and significant immune activation [6]. Although sepsis can trigger HLH, it is important to identify underlying associated HLH as soon as possible, because immunosuppressive therapy is required to suppress the cytokine storm of HLH, a strategy that is not present systematically in sepsis guidelines [7, 8].

The mortality of HLH is highly dependent on provoking conditions and lies between 20% and 88% [9–11]. There are two forms of HLH: the primary/genetic one, more frequent in children, is caused by pathogenic variants in genes involved in lymphocytic cytotoxicity and immune regulation. The secondary form, more frequent in teenagers and adults, is associated with different medical conditions, such as infections with Epstein–Barr virus (EBV) or cytomegalovirus (CMV), malignancy, and rheumatologic diseases and more recent cases reported due to SARS-CoV-2 infection or vaccination or after chimeric antigen receptor T-cell (CART) therapy infusions among others [6, 12–17]. Furthermore, in a variable number of patients, despite extensive investigations,

Table 1: Case series and cohorts of HLH in adult patients. In some studies, more than a possible cause for HLH was identified.

Study	Number of patients	Malignancy	Hematological disease	Primary immunodeficiency	Infection	Autoimmune disease	Post-transplant	Other	Idiopathic	30-day mortality	Overall mortality
Ahn et al., 2010	30	4 (13.3%)	—	—	18 (60%)	1 (3.3)	—	—	7 (23.3%)	14 (46.7%)$^{+}$	NA
Tseng et al., 2010	96	61 (63.5%)	—	—	32 (33.3%)	3 (3.2%)	—	—	—	NA	60 (63%)
Shabbir et al., 2010	18	4 (22%)	1 (6%)	—	5 (28%)	2 (11%)	3 (16%)	—	3 (17%)	5 (27%)	12 (66.7%)
Park et al., 2012	23	Excluded	—	—	17 (74%)	—	—	—	6 (23%)	NA	17 (73.9%)
Kim et al., 2013	14	14 (42.8%)	—	—	14 (14.3%)	14 (14.3%)	—	—	14 (28.6%)	NA	5 (35.7%)
Parikh et al. 2014	62	32 (52%)			21 (34%)	5 (8%)	—	—	4 (6%)	27 (44%)	41 (66%)
Ramos et al., 2014^{++}	2197	1047 (47.66%)	—	—	1108 (50.4%)	276 (12.6%)	—	184 (8.4%)	81 (3.7%)	NA	1109 (41%)
Riviere et al., 2014	162	95 (59.9%)	—	—	40 (24.7%)	5 (3.1%)	—	-	14 (8.6%)	68 (42%)	33 (20%)
Barba et al., 2015	71	21 (30%)	—	—	20 (28%)	13 (13%)	—	—	18 (26%)	40 (41%)	68 (70%)
Li et al., 2015	85	23 (27.1%)	—	—	29 (34.1%)	6 (7.1%)	—	—	27 (31.8%)	NA	39 (65%)$^{+++}$
Schram et al., 2015	68	33 (49%)	—	—	22 (33%)	19 (28%)	—	—	15 (22%)	14 (21%)	46 (69%)
Oto et al., 2015	34	6 (17.6%)	—	—	4 (11.8%)	3 (8.8%)	—	4 (11.7%)	17 (50%)	NA	11 (32.4%)
Li et al., 2016	103	49 (47.6%)	—	—	24 (23.3)	14 (13.6%)	—	—	24 (23.3%)	NA	77 (74.8%)
Lim et al., 2016	264	170 (64.4%)	—	—	48 (18.2%)	15 (23.4%)	—	—	31 (11.7%)	NA	133 (50.37%)
Yuan et al., 2016	45	28 (62.2%)	—	—	10 (22.2%)	—	—	—	—	NA	NA
Zheng et al., 2016	43	31 (72%)	—	—	3 (7%)	3 (7%)	—	—	6 (14%)	NA	31 (72%)
Arslan et al., 2018	26	3 (11.5%)	—	—	9 (34.6%)	4(15.4%)	—	—	10 (38.5%)	NA	13 (50%)
Brito-Zeron et al., 2018	151	48 (31.8%)	—	—	32 (21.2%)	5 (35.1%)	8 (5.3%)	42 (27.8%)	42 (27.8%)	NA	80 (52.9%)
Kapoor et al., 2018	16	2 (13%) $^{+}$infection 5/16 (31%)	—	—	5 (31%)	—	—	—	4 (25%)	6 (37%)	31(81%)
Miao et al., 2018	112	66 (58.9%)	—	—	23 (20.5%)	4 (3.6%)	—	—	19 (17%)	NA	NA
Qiaolei et al., 2018	174	—	92 (52.9%)	—	57 (32%) 33 (18.9%) $^{+}$infection	6 (3.4%)	—	—	24 (13.8%)	NA	102 (58.6%)
Zhou et al., 2018	205	119 (58%)	—	—	83 (40.5%)	14 (6.8%)	—	—	14 (6.8%)	89 (43.3%)	NA
Kumar et al. 2019	12	—	—	—	4 (33.3%)	7 (58.3%)	—	—	1 (8.3%)	NA	NA
Jumic et al., 2019	41	16 (54%)	—	—	22 (41%)	8 (19%)	9 (22%)	—	—	NA	16 (39%)
Birndt et al., 2020	137	48 (35%)	—	—	61 (44.5%)	13 (9.5%)	—		15 (10.9%)	27 (20.6%)	67 (51%)
Diack et al., 2020	26	11 (42.3%)	—	1 (3.8%)	12 (46.1%)	6 (23%)	—	—	2 (7.6%)	NA	19 (73%)
Pandey et al., 2020	41	15 (37%)	—	—	31 (76%)	9 (22%)	—	—	—	NA	22 (54%)
Bichon et al., 2021	260	28 (11%)	205 (79%)	—	—	—	—	—	27 (10%)	NA	147 (75%)

$^{+}$For 2 patients, the outcome is not available; $^{++}$Meta-analysis, 24 studies published between Jan 1, 1974, and Sept 29, 2011, none of them separately listed in our table; $^{+++}$39 deaths among 60 patients followed-up.

Table 2: Laboratory findings.

Parameters (references), units	At admission	After 1 month	After 3 months	After 6 months	After 12 months
Leucocytes (3.00–10.5), g/L	3.97	4.07	4.21	3.35	3.99
Neutrophils (1.60–7.40), g/L	4.70	2.57	2.25	1.89	2.38
Lymphocytes (1.10–3.50), g/L	0.24	0.68	1.44	1.03	1.10
Hemoglobin (121–154), g/L	96	96	91	122	128
Platelet count (150–450), g/L	74	76	337	216	220
Ferritin (20–250), μg/L	33649	49036	77	508*	254
ASAT (<35), U/L	213	175	16	—	31
ALAT (<35), U/L	56	462	30	32	39
Alkaline phosphatase (35–110), U/L	180	211	63	—	121
GGT (<40), U/L	113	504	43	—	48
LDH (<250), U/L	999	838	262	191	158
Triglyceride (<1.70), mmol/L	2.55	—	—	—	—
D-dimer (<500), μg/L	71270	3643	—	<155	—
Fibrinogen (1.80–4.00), g/L	3.12	1.91	3.27	—	3.35

*Iron deficiency was diagnosed one month before, and this value was after iron infusion administration.

Table 3: Saint-Antoine score [23] calculated for this case (https//saintantoine.aphp.fr/score/).

Known underlying immunodepression	No
Maximal temperature (°C)	Strictly greater than 39.4
Hepatomegaly	No
Splenomegaly	Yes
Lower hemoglobin level	Strictly greater than 92 g/L
Lower leukocyte count	Less than or equal to 5 g/L
Lower platelet count	Less than or equal to 110 g/L
Higher ferritin level (ng/ml)	Strictly greater than 6000
Higher triglyceride level (mmol/l)	Between 1.5 and 4
Lower fibrinogen level (g/L)	Strictly greater than 2.5
Higher ASAT/ALAT level (UI/l)	Greater than or equal to 30
Hemophagocytosis features on the bone marrow aspirate	No
	Calculate
HScore	209
Probability of having HS (%)	92.87735027549559

no trigger has been found to explain HLH and they will be considered as idiopathic forms. The latter represents a particular challenge since physicians often might insist on endless diagnosis searches that could lead to an unacceptable delay in the treatment.

HLH is a condition better known in children than in adults [1], although awareness regarding HLH in the adult population is increasing. The incidence of HLH in the pediatric population is 1 in 300.000 [12, 13, 18], whereas the real incidence of HLH in the adult population remains unknown; however, in the last 10 years, the number of cases reported in the literature in the adult population has significantly increased [4, 19, 20]. Diagnostic tools such as HLH-2004 [21] are based on pediatric populations, and despite being applied to adult patients, their interpretation must be performed with caution [22]. In contrast, the HLH-score (HScore), which was published in 2014, is based on an adult population [23] and relies on the summation of points assigned for 9 variables (immunosuppression, fever, organomegaly, triglyceride, ferritin, glutamic oxaloacetic transaminase, fibrinogen, cytopenia, and hemophagocytosis features in bone marrow aspirates), which correlate with the probability of having HLH. The Hscore ranges from 0 to 337, giving a probability of having HLH ranging from <1% to ≥99% [23].

There are recommendations for the treatment of HLH in pediatric patients, and for example, HLH-2004 [24], an established treatment protocol for adult HLH patients, is however missing. Thus, treatment of adult HLH patients follows existing recommendations for pediatric patients with a variety of nonstandard adaptations. It is common practice to start the treatment with glucocorticoids and another immunosuppressive drug, such as cyclosporine. The use of etoposide, as recommended by HLH-2004, despite being frequently used, is still discussed in adult patients. Allogenic stem cell transplantation has rarely been reported in adults with secondary HLH [25].

A literature search was performed in PubMed using MeSH terms (performed on January 23rd, 2022; HLH adult). Among the 1,192 results, 28 cohorts including more than 10 adult patients published from 2010 were identified and evaluated (Table 1).

Table 4: Performed investigations to exclude infections, malignancies, rheumatic conditions, and genetic mutations.

Causes	Investigations	Results
Infections	Blood culture	Sterile
	Lumbar puncture	Sterile
	Transthoracic echocardiography	No vegetations
	QuantiFERON test	Negative
	SARS-CoV-2 PCR, SARS-CoV-2 spike antibodies, influenza PCR	Negative
	Viral serology (EBV, CMV, HIV, HAV, HBV, HCV, HDV, HEV, HHV6, parvovirus B19, *Bartonella*, leptospirosis, toxoplasmosis, *Coxiella*)	Negative
Malignancies	Thorax X-ray, abdominal ultrasound, CT of the thorax, abdomen, and pelvis	No suspected lesions
	Bone marrow biopsy, skin biopsy, liver biopsy	No malignancy
	PET-CT	Metabolic active lesions: 1. Right knee 2. Colon ascendants and sigma
	Right knee MRI	Pigmented villonodular synovitis (PVNS), nonmalignant
	Gastroscopy and colonoscopy	No malignancy
Rheumatic conditions	ANA, Hep2 cytoplasmic, SsA, PR3-ANCA, MPO-ANCA	Negative
	Rheumatic disease symptoms	None
Genetic causes	Genes *PRF1*, *STX11*, *STXBP2*, *UNC13D*	No pathologic variant

Polymerase chain reaction (PCR), Epstein–Barr virus (EBV), cytomegalovirus (CMV), human immunodeficiency virus (HIV), hepatitis A virus (HAV), hepatitis B virus (HBV), hepatitis C virus (HCV), hepatitis B virus (HBV), hepatitis C virus (HCV), hepatitis D virus (HDV), hepatitis E virus (HEV), human herpes virus 6 (HHV6), computed tomography (CT), positron emission tomography-computed tomography (PEC-CT), magnetic resonance imaging (MRI), antinuclear antibodies (ANAs), antineutrophil cytoplasmic antibodies (ANCAs), myeloperoxidase (MPO), perforin 1 (PRF1), syntaxin 11 (STX11), syntaxin binding protein 2 (STXBP2).

2. Case Presentation

We report the case of a 68-year-old Swiss woman who presented to a peripheral hospital in Switzerland after consulting her general doctor about loss of weight (8 kg) in the last month, a maculopapular rash, fatigue, loss of appetite, palpitations, headaches, and cough for 2 weeks. The general doctor assigned her to the peripheral hospital after measuring 39.5°C fever and noticing very high liver parameters in the blood test.

She had a history of pericarditis at the age of 65 years, and paroxysmal atrial fibrillation and depression were also noted.

The family history was negative for hematological diseases.

The laboratory workup at admission showed normocytic, normochromic nonregenerative moderate anemia, mild thrombocytopenia, high D-dimer, slightly lower fibrinogen, liver insufficiency, and high triglycerides. The ferritin level increased (7,069 μg/L, reference value: 10–120 μg/L). An ultrasound scan of the abdomen showed splenomegaly (12.5 cm). The SARS-CoV-2 polymerase chain reaction (PCR) test, chest X-ray, lumbar puncture, blood culture, serology for EBV, CMV, human immunodeficiency virus (HIV), hepatitis A, B, C, and E, *Coxiella*, parvovirus B19, and *Bartonella*, and search for *Mycobacterium tuberculosis* (QuantiFERON test) were negative. After one week of hospitalization, her clinical condition deteriorated, and she was transferred to our center with the suspicion of HLH. At admission, the patient presented with markedly reduced general conditions; she was febrile (38.6°C), hemodynamically compensated, her BMI was 18.5 kg/m^2, and the laboratory tests showed a progressive increase in CRP up to 190 mg/l, hypoosmolar hyponatremia, increased liver values, coagulopathy, and pancytopenia (Table 2). An HScore for reactive HLH was calculated, showing 209/337 points with an estimated probability for HLH of 93% (Table 3). Therefore, therapy with dexamethasone 15 mg/day was immediately started. Additional investigations were performed, including transthoracic echocardiography, computed tomography (CT) of the chest, abdomen, and pelvis, and a biopsy of the liver, skin, and bone marrow; however, none of these examinations contributed to the identification of an underlying trigger for HLH. The bone marrow showed a large number of macrophages but did not show any sign of hemophagocytosis. Furthermore, a rheumatologic disease could be excluded based on negative screening for autoantibodies (antinuclear antibodies, Hep-2, SsA, PR3 antineutrophil cytoplasmic antibodies, and myeloperoxidase antineutrophil cytoplasmic antibodies) and missing related symptoms. After 1 week of treatment, slight clinical and laboratory improvements allowed doctors to start tapering dexamethasone, and the patient was discharged home after 4 weeks of hospitalization.

Four days later, she presented to her scheduled control in the outpatient clinic of hematology with worsened fatigue. The laboratory workup showed an increase of ferritin to 49′036 mcg/L while still being under 5 mg dexamethasone/day. We therefore increased the dexamethasone dose to 16 mg/day and started with cyclosporine, with a trough level goal between 100 and 200 ng/ml. Because up to that point no cause of HLH could be identified, the investigation was completed with positron emission tomography-computed tomography (PEC-CT), which showed intensive metabolic activity behind the right patella and in the ascending and sigmoid colon. Gastroscopy and colonoscopy performed afterward excluded gastrointestinal neoplasia and local inflammatory diseases. Additionally, leg magnetic resonance imaging (MRI) was performed, which suggested pigmented villonodular synovitis (PVNS), a benign entity unlikely to cause HLH, and thus considered an incidental finding.

Only after 3 months from the manifestation of symptoms, the patient reported a significant improvement in her general condition, including regaining appetite and weight.

Furthermore, we performed a genetic analysis searching for variants in genes related to primary HLH (perforin 1 (*PRF1*), syntaxin 11 (*STX11*), syntaxin binding protein 2 (*STXBP2*), and *UNC13D*), revealing no pathogenic variants.

The diagnostic workup is summarized in Table 4.

Vitamins and substrates (folic acid, iron, zinc, and vitamin B12) were administrated to sustain hematopoiesis.

Six months after the diagnosis, the patient was completely back to her routine life with no symptoms and completely normalized laboratory findings (Table 2). Slow tapering to discontinue cyclosporine was performed, but immediately before planned drug withdrawal, laboratory signs of inflammation with increased liver values at a 9-monthfollow-up were observed, and a low dose of cyclosporine was reinstalled. Currently, one year after the diagnosis, the patient is doing well, and tapering of cyclosporine is still ongoing.

3. Discussion/Conclusion

Several causes have been described as possible triggers of HLH in adult patients (Table 4). Nevertheless, the case presented here did not show any underlying trigger despite an exhaustive search.

The most important contribution of bone marrow investigations in HLH is the diagnosis or exclusion of hematological diseases. In the bone marrow cytology and biopsy of the case reported here, there was no evidence of lymphoma or other hematological diseases, which may have triggered HLH, and there was also no evidence of hemophagocytosis. Indeed, hemophagocytosis in the bone marrow is reported in just 25% of HLH cases [26]. It is important to note that finding a hemophagocytosis phenomenon in the bone marrow is neither specific nor sensitive for HLH [27]. Furthermore, in our case, a skin biopsy was performed to rule out Sézary syndrome due to the presence of maculopapular exanthema erythematosus of unknown origin. Likewise, due to the persistence of liver test abnormalities, a liver biopsy was also performed. The results of both biopsies did not show lymphoma or other relevant findings, and in both samples, no hemophagocytosis phenomenon was observed.

Performing PET-CT on HLH patients contributes to the diagnosis of lymphoma and other malignant or inflammatory diseases [28–30].

After excluding a secondary cause of HLH in our patient and despite the low probability due to age, as well as the lack of positive family history, we considered the possibility of primary/genetic HLH. This form is better known in children and often associated with other abnormalities such as immunodeficiency or albinism, such as in Griscelli syndrome [31]. Panel sequencing of HLH-associated genes or exome sequencing have made a great deal of contribution to the diagnosis of congenital forms, particularly in children. In fact, with these investigations, molecular explanation could likely be found in 58% of the studied pediatric patients even in the absence of familial syndromes [32]. The most common pathogenic variants reported in 14% of the cases associated with HLH in adults were identified in *PRF1*, *STXBP2*, and *UNC13D* [33]. In our patient, the analysis of these genes was negative.

With the first suspicion of HLH, despite not knowing the triggering cause, an early intervention first with dexamethasone and later with cyclosporine was performed, as suggested by other authors [1, 5]. The patient initially responded well to glucocorticoid monotherapy, but while tapering at one month (Table 2), she had a relapse. A careful glucocorticoid tapering method combined with another immunosuppressive (cyclosporine) drug was afterward successful in this case.

In the literature review, we found 28 case series or studies published after 2010 based on the adult population [11, 26, 28, 30, 34–57]. Cohorts were collected from different countries and reported on a number of patients, from 12 [46] to 264 [38]. A meta-analysis [11] analyzing 2,197 patients was also included. We found that the most common trigger reported for secondary HLH in adults was malignancy, both solid cancer and hematological diseases, with a weighted average of 50% (from 0% to 72%). The second most common trigger was infection with 39% (from 0% to 76%) and autoimmune diseases with 10% (0% to 58.3%). Idiopathic HLH was reported in 24/28 studies, and the weighted average was 9.4% (0% to 50%). The different observed prevalence of triggers may be explained by the differences in the median age of the studied population. Furthermore, not all centers had the same possibility and easy access to diagnostic tools such as MRI or PET-CT and therefore were not included in publications. This diversification in patients and used diagnostic methods may partially contribute to the variability of the prevalence of idiopathic HLH.

Regarding the mortality, some studies reported just the 30-day mortality, others the mortality during the hospitalization or for the whole follow-up. For this analysis, we focused on the 30-day mortality, which was 38%, and on the overall mortality, which was 53%. In addition, mortality may be influenced by different factors, such as the prevalence of different underlying diseases, comorbidities, and age of the observed population, as well as the experience and resources of the center in diagnosing and treating HLH rapidly.

HLH is a life-threatening condition and requires rapid diagnosis and therapy. Unknown origin of HLH may be frustrating for both physicians and patients. According to our experience, it is very important to perform a complete diagnostic test, including tissue biopsy, different imaging studies, and genetic analysis whenever possible. All possible triggers should be searched because specific treatment of the underlying "trigger" disease may play a key role in management [5]. Every diagnostic and therapeutic step must be explained clearly to the patient to keep high compliance, which is essential in this process that may last several months in some cases. Our patient was very consistent with the prescribed medications and the appointments in our outpatient clinic, and she also had great support from her husband. They understood how dangerous her condition was; nowadays, they are happy with the outcome and the treatment received, and the patient is still under follow-up. A close follow-up is recommended after the first episode of idiopathic HLH to allow early diagnosis of an eventual relapse.

With currently available diagnostic methods, idiopathic forms of HLH still exist. Considering the high reported rate of mortality in many series, it is important to emphasize that in seriously affected patients, the lack of a trigger should not delay the initiation of immunosuppressive treatment, which should be started as soon as possible and should be complemented by the search for underlying causes.

We can conclude that despite the recent contributions of some publications, there is clearly a deficit in the understanding of HLH in adults. Due to the rarity of its presentation, only joint efforts of many centers investigating this disease in a prospective way will better identify its epidemiological, diagnostic, and therapeutic aspects, allowing for tailored management of HLH adults in the future.

Consent

Written informed consent was obtained from the patient for publication of this case report and any accompanying images.

Authors' Contributions

Nada Agbariah and Alicia Rovó contributed to conception and design of the study. Nada Agbariah wrote the first draft of the manuscript. All the authors contributed to manuscript revision, and read and approved the submitted version.

References

[1] P. La Rosée, A. C. Horne, M. Hines et al., "Recommendations for the management of hemophagocytic lymphohistiocytosis in adults," *Blood*, vol. 133, no. 23, pp. 2465–2477, 2019.

[2] L. Zhang, J. Zhou, and L. Sokol, "Hereditary and acquired hemophagocytic lymphohistiocytosis," *Cancer Control*, vol. 21, no. 4, pp. 301–312, 2014.

[3] Z. K. Otrock and C. S. Eby, "Clinical characteristics, prognostic factors, and outcomes of adult patients with hemophagocytic lymphohistiocytosis," *American Journal of Hematology*, vol. 90, no. 3, pp. 220–224, 2015.
[4] A. H. Filipovich and S. Chandrakasan, "Pathogenesis of hemophagocytic lymphohistiocytosis," *Hematology-Oncology Clinics of North America*, vol. 29, no. 5, pp. 895–902, 2015.
[5] K. Bauchmuller, J. J. Manson, R. Tattersall et al., "Journal of the Intensive Care Society," *Haemophagocytic lymphohistiocytosis in adult critical care*, vol. 21, no. 3, pp. 256–268, 2020.
[6] M. B. Jordan, C. E. Allen, S. Weitzman, A. H. Filipovich, and K. L. McClain, "How I treat hemophagocytic lymphohistiocytosis," *Blood*, vol. 118, no. 15, pp. 4041–4052, 2011.
[7] R. Machowicz, G. Janka, and W. Wiktor-Jedrzejczak, "Similar but not the same: Differential diagnosis of HLH and sepsis," *Critical Reviews in Oncology*, vol. 114, pp. 1–12, 2017.
[8] R. Machowicz, G. Janka, and W. Wiktor-Jedrzejczak, "Your critical care patient may have HLH (hemophagocytic lymphohistiocytosis)," *Critical Care*, vol. 20, no. 1, pp. 215–224, 2016.
[9] G. Griffin, S. Shenoi, and G. C. Hughes, "Hemophagocytic lymphohistiocytosis: an update on pathogenesis, diagnosis, and therapy," *Best Practice & Research Clinical Rheumatology*, vol. 34, no. 4, p. 101515, 2020.
[10] M. Arca, L. Fardet, L. Galicier et al., "Prognostic factors of early death in a cohort of 162 adult haemophagocytic syndrome: Impact of triggering disease and early treatment with etoposide," *British Journal of Haematology*, vol. 168, no. 1, pp. 63–68, 2015.
[11] M. Ramos-Casals, P. Brito-Zerón, A. López-Guillermo, M. A. Khamashta, and X. Bosch, "Adult haemophagocytic syndrome," *The Lancet*, vol. 383, no. 9927, pp. 1503–1516, 2014.
[12] R. Q. Cron, S. Davi, F. Minoia, and A. Ravelli, "Clinical features and correct diagnosis of macrophage activation syndrome," *Expert Review of Clinical Immunology*, vol. 11, no. 9, pp. 1043–1053, 2015.
[13] C. E. Allen, X. Yu, C. A. Kozinetz, and K. L. McClain, "Highly elevated ferritin levels and the diagnosis of hemophagocytic lymphohistiocytosis," *Pediatric Blood and Cancer*, vol. 50, no. 6, pp. 1227–1235, 2008.
[14] M. R. Hines, C. Keenan, G. Maron Alfaro et al., "Hemophagocytic lymphohistiocytosis-like Toxicity (carHLH) after CD19-specific CAR T-cell therapy," *British Journal of Haematology*, vol. 194, no. 4, pp. 701–707, 2021.
[15] R. D. Sandler, R. S. Tattersall, H. Schoemans et al., "Diagnosis and management of secondary HLH/MAS following HSCT and CAR-T cell therapy in adults; A review of the literature and a Survey of practice within EBMT Centres on Behalf of the autoimmune diseases working party (ADWP) and transplant complications working party (TCWP)," *Frontiers in Immunology*, vol. 11, p. 524, 2020.
[16] L. V. Tang and Y. Hu, "Hemophagocytic lymphohistiocytosis after COVID-19 vaccination," *Journal of Hematology & Oncology*, vol. 14, no. 1, pp. 87–95, 2021.
[17] A. Prilutskiy, M. Kritselis, A. Shevtsov et al., "SARS-CoV-2 infection-associated hemophagocytic lymphohistiocytosis," *American Journal of Clinical Pathology*, vol. 154, no. 4, pp. 466–474, 2020.
[18] A. M. Schram and N. Berliner, "How I treat hemophagocytic lymphohistiocytosis in the adult patient," *Blood*, vol. 125, no. 19, pp. 2908–2914, 2015.
[19] Y. R. Kim and D. Y. Kim, "Current status of the diagnosis and treatment of hemophagocytic lymphohistiocytosis in adults," *Blood Res*, vol. 56, no. S1, pp. 17–25, 2021;56 April.
[20] J. West, T. R. Card, M. J. Bishton et al., "Incidence and survival of haemophagocytic lymphohistiocytosis: a population-based cohort study from England," *Journal of Internal Medicine*, vol. 291, no. 4, pp. 493–504, 2021.
[21] J.-I. Henter, A. Horne, M. Arico′ et al., "HLH-2004: diagnostic and therapeutic guidelines for hemophagocytic lymphohistiocytosis," *Pediatric Blood and Cancer*, vol. 48, no. 2, pp. 124–131, 2007.
[22] L. Naymagon, "Can we truly diagnose adult secondary hemophagocytic lymphohistiocytosis (HLH)? A critical review of current paradigms," *Pathology, Research & Practice*, vol. 218, no. 2020, Article ID 153321, 2021.
[23] L. Fardet, L. Galicier, O. Lambotte et al., "Development and validation of the hscore, a score for the diagnosis of reactive hemophagocytic syndrome," *Arthritis & Rheumatology*, vol. 66, no. 9, pp. 2613–2620, 2014.
[24] G. E. Janka and K. Lehmberg, "Hemophagocytic syndromes - an update," *Blood Reviews*, vol. 28, no. 4, pp. 135–142, 2014.
[25] A. Hayden, S. Park, D. Giustini, A. Y. Y. Lee, and L. Y. C. Chen, "Hemophagocytic syndromes (HPSs) including hemophagocytic lymphohistiocytosis (HLH) in adults: a systematic scoping review," *Blood Reviews*, vol. 30, no. 6, pp. 411–420, 2016.
[26] S. Rivière, L. Galicier, P. Coppo et al., "Reactive hemophagocytic syndrome in adults: a retrospective analysis of 162 patients," *The American Journal of Medicine*, vol. 127, no. 11, pp. 1118–1125, 2014.
[27] E. Gars, N. Purington, G. Scott et al., "Bone marrow histomorphological criteria can accurately diagnose hemophagocytic lymphohistiocytosis," *Haematologica*, vol. 103, no. 10, pp. 1635–1641, 2018.
[28] L. Yuan, Y. Kan, J. K. Meeks, D. Ma, and J. Yang, "18F-FDG PET/CT for identifying the potential causes and extent of secondary hemophagocytic lymphohistiocytosis," *Diagnostic and interventional radiology*, vol. 22, no. 5, pp. 471–475, 2016.
[29] S. Jacob, B. L. Dunn, Z. P. Qureshi et al., "Ticlopidine-clopidogrel-and prasugrel-associated thrombotic thrombocytopenic purpura: a 20-year review from the southern network on adverse reactions (SONAR)," *Seminars in Thrombosis and Hemostasis*, vol. 38, no. 08, pp. 845–853, 2012.
[30] J. Kim, S. W. Yoo, S. R. Kang, H. S. Bom, H. C. Song, and J. J. Min, "Clinical implication of F-18 FDG PET/CT in patients with secondary hemophagocytic lymphohistiocytosis," *Annals of Hematology*, vol. 93, no. 4, pp. 661–667, 2014.
[31] G. Ménasché, E. Pastural, J. Feldmann et al., "Mutations in RAB27A cause Griscelli syndrome associated with haemophagocytic syndrome," *Nature Genetics*, vol. 25, no. 2, pp. 173–176, 2000.
[32] I. K. Chinn, O. S. Eckstein, E. C. Peckham-Gregory et al., "Genetic and mechanistic diversity in pediatric hemophagocytic lymphohistiocytosis," *Blood*, vol. 132, no. 1, pp. 89–100, 2018.
[33] K. Zhang, M. B. Jordan, R. A. Marsh et al., "Hypomorphic mutations in PRF1, MUNC13-4, and STXBP2 are associated with adult-onset familial HLH," *Blood*, vol. 118, no. 22, pp. 5794–5798, 2011.
[34] F. Li, Y. Yang, F. Jin et al., "Clinical characteristics and prognostic factors of adult hemophagocytic syndrome patients: a retrospective study of increasing awareness of

a disease from a single-center in China," *Orphanet Journal of Rare Diseases*, vol. 10, no. 1, pp. 20–29, 2015.

[35] A. M. Schram, P. Comstock, M. Campo et al., "Haemophagocytic lymphohistiocytosis in adults: a multicentre case series over 7 years," *British Journal of Haematology*, vol. 172, no. 3, pp. 412–419, 2016.

[36] M. Oto, K. Yoshitsugu, S. Uneda, M. Nagamine, and M. Yoshida, "Prognostic factors and outcomes of adult-onset hemophagocytic lymphohistiocytosis: a retrospective analysis of 34 cases," *Hematology Reports*, vol. 7, no. 2, pp. 5841–5851, 2015.

[37] J. Li, Q. Wang, W. Zheng et al., "Hemophagocytic lymphohistiocytosis: clinical analysis of 103 adult patients," *Medicine*, vol. 93, no. 2, pp. 100–105, 2014.

[38] S. H. Lim, S. Park, J. H. Jang et al., "Clinical significance of bone marrow hemophagocytosis in adult patients with malignancy and non-malignancy-induced hemophagocytic lymphohistiocytosis," *Annals of Hematology*, vol. 95, no. 2, pp. 325–335, 2016.

[39] Y. Zheng, G. Hu, Y. Liu et al., "The role of 18F-FDG PET/CT in the management of patients with secondary haemophagocytic lymphohistiocytosis," *Clinical Radiology*, vol. 71, no. 12, pp. 1248–1254, 2016.

[40] F. Arslan, S. Alp, Y. Büyükasık, M. C. Ozkan, F. Şahin, S. Basaran et al., "Hemophagocytic lymphohistiocytosis in adults: low incidence of primary neoplasm as a trigger in a case series from Turkey," *Mediterr J Hematol Infect Dis*, vol. 10, no. 1, pp. e2018047–7, 2018.

[41] P. Brito-Zerón, B. Kostov, P. Moral-Moral et al., "Prognostic factors of death in 151 adults with hemophagocytic syndrome: Etiopathogenically Driven analysis," *Mayo Clinic Proceedings: Innovations, Quality & Outcomes*, vol. 2, no. 3, pp. 267–276, 2018.

[42] S. Kapoor, C. K. Morgan, M. A. Siddique, and K. K. Guntupalli, "Intensive care unit complications and outcomes of adult patients with hemophagocytic lymphohistiocytosis: a retrospective study of 16 cases," *World Journal of Critical Care Medicine*, vol. 7, no. 6, pp. 73–83, 2018.

[43] Y. Miao, H. Y. Zhu, C. Qiao et al., "Pathogenic gene mutations or variants identified by targeted gene sequencing in adults with hemophagocytic lymphohistiocytosis," *Frontiers in Immunology*, vol. 10, no. MAR, p. 395, 2019.

[44] Q. Zhang, L. Li, L. Zhu et al., "Adult onset haemophagocytic lymphohistiocytosis prognosis is affected by underlying disease: analysis of a single-institution series of 174 patients," *Swiss Medical Weekly*, vol. 148, no. 37–38, p. w14641, 2018.

[45] M. Zhou, L. Li, Q. Zhang et al., "Clinical features and outcomes in secondary adult hemophagocytic lymphohistiocytosis," *QJM: International Journal of Medicine*, vol. 111, no. 1, pp. 23–31, 2018.

[46] V. Kumar, B. Sharma, and A. S. Nigam, "Case series of hemophagocytic lymphohistiocytosis from a tertiary care centre: an underdiagnosed entity," *Turk Patoloji Derg*, vol. 35, no. 3, pp. 207–212, 2019.

[47] S. Jumic and S. Nand, "Hemophagocytic lymphohistiocytosis in adults: associated Diagnoses and outcomes , a Ten-year experience at a single institution," *Journal of Hematology*, vol. 8, no. 4, pp. 149–154, 2019.

[48] S. Birndt, T. Schenk, B. Heinevetter et al., "Hemophagocytic lymphohistiocytosis in adults: collaborative analysis of 137 cases of a nationwide German registry," *Journal of Cancer Research and Clinical Oncology*, vol. 146, no. 4, pp. 1065–1077, 2020.

[49] N. D. Diack, B. S. Kane, S. Fall et al., "Adult hemophagocytic lymphohistiocytosis in Sub-Saharan Area: a retrospective study of 26 cases," *Cureus*, vol. 12, no. 3, p. e7258, 2020.

[50] Y. Pandey, D. Atwal, M. Konda et al., "Hemophagocytic lymphohistiocytosis in adults," *Baylor University Medical Center Proceedings*, vol. 33, no. 3, pp. 326–330, 2020.

[51] A. Bichon, J. Bourenne, J. Allardet-servent, L. Papazian, D. Mokart, and M Gainnier, "High Mortality of HLH in ICU," *Regardless Etiology or Treatment*, vol. 8, pp. 1–9, 2021.

[52] J.-S. Ahn, S.-Y. Rew, M.-G. Shin et al., "Clinical significance of clonality and Epstein-Barr virus infection in adult patients with hemophagocytic lymphohistiocytosis," *American Journal of Hematology*, vol. 85, no. 9, pp. 719–722, 2010.

[53] Y. T. Tseng, W. H. Sheng, B. H. Lin et al., "Causes, clinical symptoms, and outcomes of infectious diseases associated with hemophagocytic lymphohistiocytosis in Taiwanese adults," *Journal of Microbiology, Immunology, and Infection*, vol. 44, no. 3, pp. 191–197, 2011.

[54] M. Shabbir, J. Lucas, J. SK. Lazarchick, and K. Shirai, "Secondary hemophagocytic syndrome in adults: a case series of 18 patients in a single institution and a review of literature," *Hematological Oncology*, vol. 29, no. 2, pp. 100–106, 2011.

[55] H. Park, D. Kim, J. Lee, J. Lee, S. Kim, and Y. Park, "Clinical Features of Adult Patients with Secondary Hemophagocytic Lymphohistiocytosis from Causes Other than Lymphoma," *An Analysis of Treatment Outcome and Prognostic Factors*, pp. 897–904, 2012.

[56] S. A. Parikh, P. Kapoor, L. Letendre, S. Kumar, and A. P. Wolanskyj, "Prognostic factors and outcomes of adults with hemophagocytic lymphohistiocytosis," *Mayo Clinic Proceedings*, vol. 89, no. 4, pp. 484–492, 2014.

[57] T. Barba, D. Maucort-Boulch, J. Iwaz et al., "Hemophagocytic lymphohistiocytosis in intensive care Unit: a 71-caseStrobe-Compliant retrospective study," *Medicine*, vol. 94, no. 51, pp. 23188–e2327, 2015.

18

Secondary Squamous Cell Carcinoma of the Tongue Complicated with Bronchiolitis Obliterans as a Manifestation of Graft-versus-Host Disease following Peripheral Blood Stem Cell Transplantation

Kengo Hashimoto,[1] Toru Nagao,[1] Shin Koie,[2] Satoru Miyabe,[1] and Terumi Saito[2]

[1]*Department of Oral and Maxillofacial Surgery, Aichi-Gakuin University School of Dentistry, Nagoya, Japan*
[2]*Department of Oral and Maxillofacial Surgery, Okazaki City Hospital, Okazaki, Japan*

Correspondence should be addressed to Toru Nagao; tnagao@dpc.agu.ac.jp

Academic Editor: Vincent Ribrag

Peripheral blood stem cell transplantation (PBSCT) has increasingly been used for hematologic cancer therapy, resulting in improved survival rates. However, risks include graft-versus-host disease (GVHD) and secondary solid tumors. Here, we describe a case of tongue squamous cell carcinoma (SCC) complicated by bronchiolitis obliterans (BO) following PBSCT. A 42-year-old man with a history of acute lymphocytic leukemia treated with PBSCT presented with multiple white lesions and erosions on the tongue and buccal mucosa that are compatible with oral chronic GVHD (NIH criteria: score 2). The lesions were presented for 8 years. The patient had a history of BO manifested as GVHD. During follow-up, an exophytic mass was rapidly developed on the left dorsum of the tongue. Biopsy of this lesion confirmed SCC (cT2N0M0). Pulmonary function testing for general anesthesia was almost normal. Hemiglossectomy, supraomohyoid neck dissection, and tongue reconstruction were performed. Thirteen months after surgery, the patient showed neither recurrence of tumor nor progression of oral GVHD. However, the patient died of respiratory failure due to repeated pneumothoraxes and deterioration of BO.

1. Introduction

In recent years, peripheral blood stem cell transplantation (PBSCT) has increasingly been used to treat hematologic malignancies, resulting in improved survival rates [1]. However, PSBCT generally has a higher risk of graft-versus-host disease (GVHD) and secondary solid tumor development than bone marrow transplantation [1]. In addition, bronchiolitis obliterans (BO) has been reported in patients undergoing PBSCT [2]. BO is an important respiratory complication which may lead to late morbidity and decreased survival after transplantation. Here, we describe a case of oral squamous cell carcinoma (OSCC) of the tongue complicated by bronchiolitis obliterans (BO) due to GVHD following PBSCT.

2. Case Presentation

In March 2012, a 42-year-old man was referred to our department for evaluation of whitish and erosive lesions that involved the tongue, buccal mucosa, palate, and lip. The patient previously received PBSCT for treatment of acute lymphocytic leukemia (ALL) in December 2005; his sister was the related donor, and she matched for HLA antigens. PBSCT was carried out after induction by combined chemotherapy and total body irradiation (TBI). The patient's ALL went into remission without evidence of acute GVHD. Cyclosporine A (100 mg) and prednisolone (10 mg) were utilized for posttransplantation GVHD prophylaxis. However, chronic GVHD (cGVHD) of the skin and eyes were developed 3 months after PBSCT. One month later, airflow obstruction developed, which was considered as evidence of BO. Later, white spots and erosions of the oral mucosa were noted, which persisted without significant change during follow-up until the first visit of our department. In August 2008, he became aware of respiratory discomfort due to pneumothorax of the right lung. The pneumothorax was successfully treated with a thoracic cavity drainage.

Intraoral examination revealed lichenoid changes and atrophic mucosa located on the buccal mucosa, tongue, and lip, compatible with oral cGVHD (Figure 1(a)). The patient was received plaque control instruction to improve poor oral hygiene associated with severe xerostomia. A lip biopsy for confirmation of oral cGVHD was performed on June 7, 2012. The biopsy specimen demonstrated a lichenoid infiltration compatible with cGVHD (NIH criteria: score 2).

In January 2013, 8 years after PBSCT, a raised mucosal lesion appeared on the left dorsal surface of the tongue base, with a background of lichenoid mucositis. This lesion decreased in size by 50% over the next month. However, the lesion then enlarged over the following 3 months and appeared as an exophytic mass (20 × 15 mm) (Figure 1(b)). The lesion was then biopsied; histopathologic examination showed well-differentiated OSCC (T2N0M0: stage II). After preoperative examination, we determined that the patient had adequate cardiorespiratory function to undergo an invasive operation under general anesthesia. In July 2013, hemiglossectomy and left supraomohyoid neck dissection and reconstruction with a rectus abdominis musculocutaneous flap were performed after cessation of immunosuppressants. Histopathologically, the excised specimen revealed a well-keratinized OSCC with negative tumor margins; regional lymph nodes were negative for metastasis. On the 7th day after the operation, the patient's respiratory status was suddenly deteriorated. Bilateral infiltrations were noted on plain chest radiography (Figure 2(a)), and significant ground-glass abnormalities were seen on a chest computed tomography (Figure 2(b)), indicating acute respiratory distress syndrome (ARDS). Subsequently, mechanical ventilation, intravenous antibiotics and sivelestat sodium, and control of body fluids were administered. The ARDS improved over two weeks. Adjuvant therapy for OSCC was not considered, given the patient's status. Although the surgical site remained clinically stable, approximately 2 months later, recurrent pneumothorax developed on the right. In October 2013, the patient was discharged after the pneumothorax improved. Thirteen months after surgery, the patient showed neither recurrence of tumor nor progression of oral GVHD. However, the patient died of respiratory failure due to repeated pneumothorax and deterioration of BO.

3. Discussion

The incidence of oral cancer as a secondary malignancy in patients with previous hematopoietic stem cell transplantation (HSCT) is 4 to 7 times that of the general population [3]. The risk for developing a malignant neoplasm after PBSCT is 3.5% at 10 years and 11.5% at 15 years; the overall incidence of malignant tumors is approximately 5 folds greater after adjusting for age and sex [3]. SCC of the skin and mouth accounts for one-third of all solid second malignancies. OSCC represents 50% of these cases [4]. Kruse and Gratz [3] reported that the most OSCC appear 5 to 9 years after HSCT. Several risk factors for the development of solid tumors after HSCT have been previously discussed, including TBI, chemotherapy, male gender, viral infection, young age, cGVHD, and immunosuppressive therapy [3–5]. Of these, cGVHD has been considered to be a significant risk factor for the development of any solid tumor, particularly oral and esophageal cancer. Oral lesions are common in patients with cGVHD and occur in 45%–83% of patients within 3 years after HSCT [6]. Any oral site may be involved, with the buccal mucosa and tongue among most commonly affected [6]. Moreover, Curtis et al. [1] reported that cGVHD may be more intense and more frequent in general after PBSCT, which may alter the risk for subsequent SCC.

Oral manifestations of cGVHD can be characterized as mucosal or salivary sclerotic in nature and resemble several autoimmune conditions, including Sjogren's syndrome, oral lichen planus, and scleroderma in both clinical features and histological appearance [7]. Oral cGVHD is characterized by lesions clinically similarly to lichen planus, a relatively common disorder of the oral cavity with a malignant potential. Long-term immunologic damage to the mucosa by T cells has been implicated in predisposing this tissue to malignant transformation. Imanguli et al. [6] noted that multiple factors must be considered when treating a patient with oral GVHD. Even though oral GVHD may have serious health consequences, GVHD of the liver or lungs is life-threatening. Therefore, therapeutic decisions must include consideration of the patient's medical regimen for nonoral GVHD conditions; cooperation between treating physicians and dentists is required. Systemic immunosuppressive therapy is generally used for treatment of cGVHD. Its primary limitation is the increased risk for opportunistic infections, a leading cause of mortality in HSCT patients [6]. Moreover, chronic inflammation induced by systemic immunosuppressive therapy has also been identified as a potential risk factor for secondary oral cancer [4]. The interactions between chronic inflammation and therapy-induced immunosuppression are not fully understood, but immunosuppression in the context of chronic inflammation, as in cGVHD, may interfere with tissue repair, thereby promoting the risk for tumor development [8]. In our case, long-term immunosuppression and chronic inflammation associated with cGVHD and poor oral hygiene were potential risk factors, which are considered to play a pivotal role in carcinogenesis after PBSCT. The differential diagnosis for OSCC in patients with cGVHD includes hyperplastic candidiasis, papilloma virus-induced verrucae, herpetic mucositis, and benign tongue nodule.

The occurrence of tongue OSCC located on the dorsum is rare, even in the Japanese population, accounting for only 3%–5% of cases [9]. OSCC of the dorsum of the tongue is characterized by the existence of predisposing conditions such as long-standing lichen planus, median rhomboid glossitis, Fanconi's anemia, and cGVHD of the oral mucosa [9]. Moreover, OSCC after HSCT has been reported to be

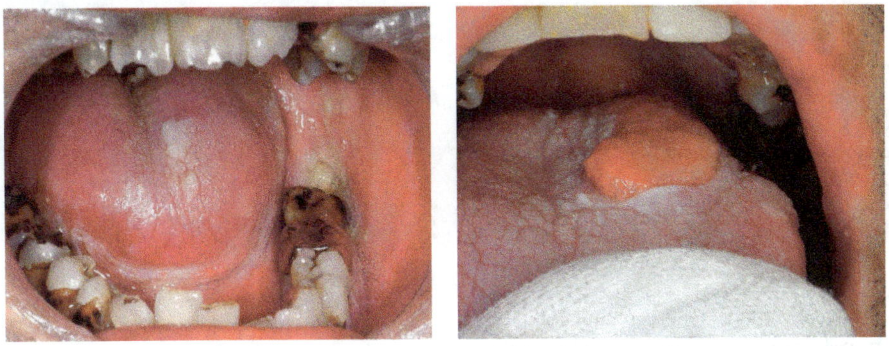

(a) (b)

FIGURE 1: (a) A 42-year-old man presenting with lichenoid changes and atrophic mucosa located on the buccal mucosa, tongue, and lip, compatible with oral chronic graft-versus-host disease. Multiple dental caries is present due to poor oral hygiene associated with xerostomia. (b) An exophytic mass (20×15 mm) with induration on the left dorsum of the tongue base with a background of lichenoid mucositis.

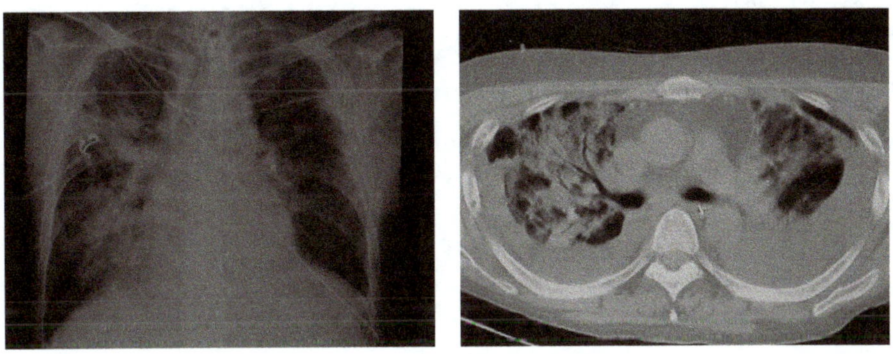

(a) (b)

FIGURE 2: (a) Plain chest radiography showing bilateral infiltrations on the 7th day after surgery. (b) Chest computed tomography imaging showing a significant ground-glass pattern, compatible with acute respiratory distress syndrome.

more aggressive than in non-HSCT patients [4]. In our case, the reconstructive surgery was required due to the aggressiveness of the tumor and its location on the dorsum and nearby tongue base, which can greatly influence the ingestion and swallowing function. As a result, this invasive treatment was considered to be a possible cause of the patient's postoperative severe pulmonary complications.

Pulmonary complications are a major cause of morbidity and mortality in transplant recipients, occurring in 40%–60% of patients [2]. Though relatively uncommon, BO may result in late morbidity and decreased survival after HSCT [2, 9]. Previously described risk factors are existence of GVHD, PBSCT, a long interval from diagnosis to transplant, female donor to male recipient, and a prior episode of interstitial pneumonitis [2, 9]. To date, there are no definitive criteria or guidelines regarding appropriateness of general anesthesia for BO patients. Surgical decision-making should consider pulmonary function and respiratory symptoms. We determined that the patient's pulmonary function could enough tolerate an operation under general anesthesia. However, postoperative management required strict control of respiratory function and body fluids due to the development of ARDS. Invasive surgery and the load of general anesthesia may have triggered the development of repeated pneumothoraxes and deterioration of BO. The mechanism of pneumothorax associated with BO is thought to occur from the rupture of subpleural blebs [10].

In conclusion, transplant recipients should be followed closely to detect early OSCC or precursor lesions. However, the difficulty in discriminating malignant changes from oral GVHD lesions must be recognized because of atypical clinical tumor features and the wide distribution of oral GVHD lesions throughout the oral cavity. Moreover, Elad et al. [11] noted an increased risk for recurrence of OSCC in patients after HSCT. From comparison of their cases, our case might be at high risk for recurrence. The surveillance should be frequent in patients with OSCC post-HSCT, and repeated biopsies should be considered whenever recurrence is suspected.

Acknowledgments

The authors would like to thank Enago for the English language review.

References

[1] R. E. Curtis, C. Metayer, J. D. Rizzo et al., "Impact of chronic GVHD therapy on the development of squamous-cell cancers after hematopoietic stem-cell transplantation: an international case-control study," *Blood*, vol. 105, no. 10, pp. 3802–3811, 2005.

[2] L. H. S. Tomas, F. R. Loberiza, J. P. Klein et al., "Risk factors for bronchiolitis obliterans in allogeneic hematopoietic stem-cell transplantation for leukemia," *Chest*, vol. 128, no. 1, pp. 153–161, 2005.

[3] A. L. D. Kruse and K. W. Gratz, "Oral carcinoma after hematopoietic stem cell transplamtation-anew classification based on a literature review over 30 years," *Head & Neck Oncology*, vol. 1, no. 1, pp. 29–35, 2009.

[4] H. Mawardi, S. Elad, M. E. Correa et al., "Oral epithelial dysplasia and squamous cell carcinoma following allogeneic hematopoietic stem cell transplantation: clinical presentation and treatment outcomes," *Bone Marrow Transplantation*, vol. 46, no. 6, pp. 884–891, 2011.

[5] Y. Atsuta, R. Suzuki, T. Yamashita et al., "Continuing increased risk of oral/esophageal cancer after allogeneic hematopoietic stem cell transplantation in adults in association with chronic graft-versus-host disease," *Annals of Oncology*, vol. 25, no. 2, pp. 435–441, 2014.

[6] M. Imanguli, I. Alevizos, R. Brown, S. Pavletic, and J. Atkinson, "Oral graft-versus-host disease," *Oral Diseases*, vol. 14, no. 5, pp. 396–412, 2008.

[7] C. W. Bassim, H. Fassil, J. W. Mays et al., "Validation of the national institutes of health chronic GVHD oral mucosal score using component-specific measures," *Bone Marrow Transplantation*, vol. 49, no. 1, pp. 116–121, 2014.

[8] L. Montebugboli, D. B. Gissi, C. Marchetti, and M. P. Foschini, "Multiple squamous cell carcinomas of the oral cavity in a young patient with graft-versus-host disease following allogenic bone marrow transplantation," *International Journal of Oral and Maxillofacial Surgery*, vol. 40, no. 5, pp. 556–558, 2011.

[9] A. O. Soubani, K. B. Miller, and P. M. Hassoun, "Pulmonary complications of bone marrow transplantation," *Chest*, vol. 109, no. 4, pp. 1066–1077, 1996.

[10] S. Rahmanian and K. L. Wood, "Bronchiolitis obliterans and the risk of pneumothorax after transbronchial biopsy," *Respiratory Medicine CME*, vol. 3, no. 2, pp. 87–89, 2010.

[11] S. Elad, Y. Zadik, I. Zeevi, A. Miyazaki, M. A. Z. de Figueiredo, and R. Or, "Oral cancer in patients after hematopoietic stem-cell transplantation: long-term follow-up suggests an increased risk for recurrence," *Transplantation*, vol. 90, no. 11, pp. 1243-1244, 2010.

19

Efficacy of CRISPR-Based Gene Editing in a Sickle Cell Disease Patient as Measured through the Eye

Alexander Pinhas[1] **Davis B. Zhou**[1,2] **Oscar Otero-Marquez**[1] **Maria V. Castanos Toral**[1] **Justin V. Migacz**[1] **Jeffrey Glassberg**[3] **Richard B. Rosen**[1,2] **and Toco Y. P. Chui**[1,2]

[1]*Department of Ophthalmology, New York Eye and Ear Infirmary of Mount Sinai, New York, NY, USA*
[2]*Department of Ophthalmology, Icahn School of Medicine at Mount Sinai, New York, NY, USA*
[3]*Departments of Emergency Medicine,Hematology and Medical Oncology, Icahn School of Medicine at Mount Sinai, New York, NY, USA*

Correspondence should be addressed to Toco Y. P. Chui; ychui@nyee.edu

Academic Editor: Kostas Konstantopoulos

Sickle cell disease (SCD) exists on a phenotypic spectrum with variable genetic expressivity, making it difficult to assess an individual patient's risk of complications at any particular point in time. Current and emerging SCD treatments, including CRISPR-based gene editing, result in a variable proportion of affected red blood cells (RBCs) still vulnerable to sickling. Clinical serological indicators of disease such as hemoglobin, indirect bilirubin, and reticulocyte count and clinical metrics including number of emergency department visits and hospitalizations over time often fall short in their ability to objectively quantify ischemic disease activity and efficacy of treatments. Clearly, better clinical biomarkers are needed. The rapidly developing field of oculomics leverages the transparent nature of the ocular tissue to directly study the retinal microvasculature in order to characterize the status of systemic diseases. In this case report, we demonstrate the ability of optical coherence tomography angiography (OCT-A) to detect and measure micro-occlusive events within the retinal capillary bed before and after RBC exchange transfusion and following CRISPR-based gene editing, as an indicator of systemic ischemic disease activity and measure of treatment efficacy. The implications of these findings are discussed.

1. Introduction

Sickle cell disease (SCD) is the most common inherited blood disorder in the world and causes significant body pains, morbidity secondary to ischemic end-organ damage, and mortality at a relatively young age [1]. Evidence suggests that SCD exists on a phenotypic spectrum with variable genetic expressivity, making it difficult to stratify risk of complications for a given individual [2]. Even with current and emerging SCD treatments, including CRISPR-based gene editing of bone-marrow-derived hematopoietic stem cells, studies have shown that a variable degree of phenotypic mosaicism persists, with a variable proportion of red blood cells (RBCs) still able to sickle and cause disease [3].

Current indicators of disease severity and treatment response used in clinic and in clinical drug trials include serological biomarkers of hemolytic anemia and number of vaso-occlusive crises (VOCs), emergency room visits, and hospitalizations over time [4]. These clinical indicators lack the ability to immediately and objectively measure ischemic disease activity in SCD patients before or after treatment, which limits their ability to stratify patients according to prognosis and risk [5]. Improved biomarkers are clinically needed to help assess disease activity and response to therapy [6].

Oculomics, a rapidly developing field dedicated to identifying ocular biomarkers for systemic disease, is gaining attention for several cardiovascular and neurological applications [7]. A variety of retinal microvasculature features have become recognizable for their associations with systemic disease states [8]. Optical coherence tomography angiography (OCT-A) has emerged as a powerful clinical tool to image the retinal capillary bed, as it provides higher transverse and axial resolution than conventional color fundus photography or intravenous fluorescein angiography [9,10].

OCT-A allows direct visualization of dynamic occlusive events of the microvasculature secondary to SCD within the macula. Quantitative biomarkers using sequential OCT-A scans, measuring macular capillary density and intermittent perfusion indices, provide an indication of systemic SCD activity and treatment response [11]. Recently, adaptive optics scanning light ophthalmoscopy (AO-SLO) has been used for *in vivo* study of intermittent perfusion events detected by OCT-A and has revealed the role of sickled RBCs in promoting intravascular thrombus formations [12].

The purpose of this case report was to demonstrate the use of OCT-A in an SCD patient in assessing disease activity and the impact of treatment with RBC exchange transfusion therapy versus CRISPR-based gene editing. BCL11A has been identified as a potent repressor of γ-globin expression and hemoglobin F (HbF) production in adult erythrocytes [13]. The patient in this case report underwent CRISPR-based gene editing targeting the *BCL11A* gene with the purpose of disease modification through HbF elevation.

1.1. Case Description. A 23-year-old male had severe HbSS disease diagnosed at birth with an extensive history of complications. His sickle cell anemia required chronic monthly RBC transfusions and multiple RBC exchange transfusions (approximately 100 transfusions over his lifetime), resulting in hemochromatosis necessitating oral iron chelation therapy. Other SCD complications included frequent VOCs with hypoxia and fevers, multiple episodes of acute chest syndrome (ACS; intubated once at age 9), two episodes of pneumonia, one episode of hyperhemolytic crisis, recurrent cellulitis from oxacillin-susceptible *Staphylococcus aureus*, nocturnal enuresis, avascular necrosis of both hips and left shoulder, history of priapism, and a history of cholecystitis status post cholecystectomy at age 15. His history was negative for clinical stroke. The patient averaged 6–8 emergency room visits per year over the 2 years leading up to gene editing, for which he was usually admitted. Occasionally, he would receive intravenous pain medications in the clinic as well.

The patient's past ocular history was significant for high myopia (OD -6.0D and OS -6.75D), dry eye disease, and nonproliferative sickle cell retinopathy of both eyes. His family history was significant for both parents with sickle cell trait and a brother with HbSS disease.

The patient's medications included L-glutamine 15 g two times a day, folic acid 1 mg daily, and deferasirox 1.8 g daily. The patient required an occasional albuterol but did not meet the clinical criteria for asthma. His pain control medications included gabapentin 100 mg three times a day, ibuprofen 600 mg every 6 hours as needed for pain, dilaudid 4 mg every 4 hours as needed for pain, and oxycodone-acetaminophen 10–325 mg every 4 hours as needed for pain. The patient required 15–30 tablets of dilaudid per month and 20–30 tablets of oxycodone-acetaminophen per month for pain control.

The patient had a history of treatment with hydroxyurea 2 g/2.5 g, alternating every other day, starting from age 13. The patient tolerated hydroxyurea well and maintained a good serological response to it, as evidenced by his average % HbF of 20% while on hydroxyurea. However, clinically, the patient's severe cycles of VOCs and hemolytic anemia continued, and the decision was made to pursue further investigational treatment with gene editing. Thus, in preparation for gene editing, the patient's hydroxyurea was discontinued and the patient underwent gene editing approximately 1 year later.

During a hematology clinic visit a few days prior to his first OCT-A imaging visit, the patient described continued limitation in his physical abilities, complaining of shortness of breath and hip pain with moderate physical exertion, such as climbing a few flights of stairs. He denied brain fog or limitations in his mental capacity. His vital signs included a blood pressure of 109/65 mmHg, a heart rate of 91 beats per minute, a temperature of 37.3°C (99.1°F) (oral), respirations of 17 breaths per minute, a blood oxygen saturation of 94% on room air, a weight of 79.1 kg (174 lb 6.4 oz), a height of 5′9″, and a body mass index of 25.02 kg/m^2. On physical exam, he had tenderness over his hip joints and limited range of motion with pain in both hips. Relevant serological values within 1 year before gene editing (range of values from when patient was not taking hydroxyurea and was awaiting gene editing) and at 5 months after gene editing (single time point) are shown in Table 1.

His eye exam on the day of his first OCT-A imaging showed a best-corrected visual acuity with corrective spectacles of 20/20 in both eyes and intraocular pressures of 15 and 14 mm Hg in the right and left eye, respectively. His anterior segment exam was significant for decreased tear breakup time and scleral pallor, and was otherwise unremarkable. Dilated fundus examination and ultrawide-field fluorescein angiography revealed temporal peripheral nonperfusion without evidence of neovascularization (Optos California icg, Optos PLC, Dunfermline, United Kingdom). OCT macula showed mild temporal macular thinning (Heidelberg Spectralis HRA + OCT, Heidelberg Engineering Inc, Heidelberg, Germany).

Three months prior to and in preparation for gene editing, the patient's frequent RBC transfusions were replaced with RBC exchange transfusions. The patient was imaged longitudinally with OCT-A during 3 serial visits using the protocol described below. His first imaging visit took place 2 months after receiving his initial exchange transfusion. His second imaging visit occurred 1 month later, which was 2 weeks after his second exchange transfusion. The patient underwent a CRISPR-based gene editing procedure 1 month after his second imaging visit. His third imaging visit was 7 months after his second and approximately 6 months after his gene editing.

At a hematology clinic visit 5 months following gene editing, the patient reported that he was no longer

TABLE 1: Serologies before and after gene editing.

Serology	Before gene editing	After gene editing	Normal range
Hb	7.7–9.6 g/dL	13.3 g/dL	13.9–16.3 g/dL
% Hb A	45%	0.00%	N/A
% Hb S	70–80%	50%	N/A
% Hb F	1.9%	45%	N/A
Hct	23–27.5%	36%	42.0–52.0%
MCV	88.7–109.2 FL	95.7 FL	80.0–98.0 FL
RDW	22.9–24.1%	15%	11.5–15.0%
Indirect bilirubin	2.7–8.1 mg/dL	3.3 mg/dL	0.2–0.8 mg/dL
Reticulocytes	7.0–10.2%	4.70%	0.7–2.8%

Hb, hemoglobin; %, percent; Hct, hematocrit; MCV, mean corpuscular volume; RDW, red blood cell distribution width; g, grams; dL, deciliter; N/A, nonapplicable; FL, femtoliter; mg, milligram.

experiencing shortness of breath with physical exertion; however, he reported persistent hip pains. His vital signs at that visit were a blood pressure of 116/77 mm Hg, a heart rate of 94 beats per minute, a temperature of 36.1°C (97°F) (tympanic), respirations of 19 breaths per minute, a blood oxygen saturation of 96% on room air, a weight of 77.1 kg (170 lb), a height of 5′9″, and a body mass index of 25.1 kg/m^2.

The patient had no SCD complications in the 6 months following gene editing. Due to persistent hip pains from avascular necrosis, the patient was scheduled for hip replacement. He was less reliant on his pain control medications following gene editing but they were continued mainly for his hip pain and included gabapentin 100 mg three times a day, ibuprofen 600 mg every 6 hours as needed for pain, and oxycodone-acetaminophen 10–325 mg every 4 hours as needed for pain. The patient was continued on L-glutamine 15 g two times a day, folic acid 1 mg daily, and deferasirox 1.8 g daily.

2. Methods

Prior to gene editing, the patient was recruited to participate in the imaging research study using OCT-A to quantify systemic SCD severity and treatment efficacy. The study was conducted at the New York Eye and Ear Infirmary of Mount Sinai. It followed the tenets of the Declaration of Helsinki and was HIPAA compliant and was approved by the Institutional Review Board of New York Eye and Ear Infirmary of Mount Sinai. Written informed consent was obtained from the patient after an explanation of the nature and risks of the study. The left eye was randomly chosen as the eye of interest in this patient.

2.1. OCT-A Image Acquisition. Mydriasis and cycloplegia of the left eye were induced at the beginning of each imaging visit, with 1 drop each of 2.5% phenylephrine hydrochloride ophthalmic solution (Bausch & Lomb Inc., Tampa, FL) and 1% tropicamide ophthalmic solution (Akorn Inc., Lake Forest, IL).

The OCT-A imaging protocol was performed at each of the three imaging visits as previously described [11, 14], using a commercial SD-OCT system with the illumination source centered at 840 nm, a bandwidth of 45 nm, an axial resolution of 5 μm, and an acquisition rate of 70,000 A-scans per second (Avanti RTVue-XR; AngioAnalytics software version 2017.1.0; Optovue, Fremont, California, USA). Each imaging visit consisted of 2 sessions, 1 hour apart. During both sessions of each imaging visit, 10 sequential 3×3 mm en face OCT-A scans centered on the fovea were acquired.

2.2. OCT-A Image Processing. The OCT-A scans were segmented to include the full vascular slab, extending from the inner limiting membrane to 9 μm below the posterior boundary of the outer plexiform layer, in order to include the superficial, intermediate, and deep capillary plexuses. Each set of 10 sequential OCT-A scans was registered and averaged using ImageJ (ImageJ, US National Institutes of Health, Bethesda MD, USA) [15]. Thus, each of the three imaging visits resulted in two averaged images, one from the first session and one from the second session 1 hour later. The foveal avascular zone (FAZ) and noncapillary vessel areas were then removed by thresholding from each averaged OCT-A (Adobe Photoshop CS6, Adobe Systems, Inc., San Jose, CA, USA; MATLAB 2018b; MathWorks, Natick, MA).

For each visit, between-session pixel intensity differences were calculated by subtracting the first session averaged OCT-A from that of the second session. Pixels at which the difference in pixel intensity was outside the normal range (0.01st–99.99th percentile) of between-session pixel intensity variations were defined as regions with significant intermittent perfusion. Capillaries that were perfused in the averaged OCT-A from the first imaging session that then lost perfusion at the 1-hour follow-up imaging session were labeled nonperfused. Conversely, capillaries not visible during the first imaging session which appeared in the 1-hour follow-up session were labeled reperfused. The between-session intermittent perfusion index (IPI) was defined as the percent of the entire OCT-A scan (minus FAZ and noncapillary vessel area) demonstrating either nonperfusion or reperfusion.

Intermittent perfusion maps were created to highlight nonperfused and reperfused capillary segments. Segments demonstrating subsequent nonperfusion were highlighted in red, and those exhibiting subsequent reperfusion were highlighted in cyan.

3. Results and Discussion

At the first OCT-A imaging visit, the patient was 2 months after his first of the two exchange transfusions in preparation for gene editing. OCT-A showed a relatively high disease activity, with an IPI of 2.83%, a nonperfusion area of 1.69%, and a reperfusion area of 1.14% (Figure 1, Column 1). These results suggested that the effects of the initial exchange transfusion were wearing off. One month later, 2 weeks after the second exchange transfusion, the second imaging session

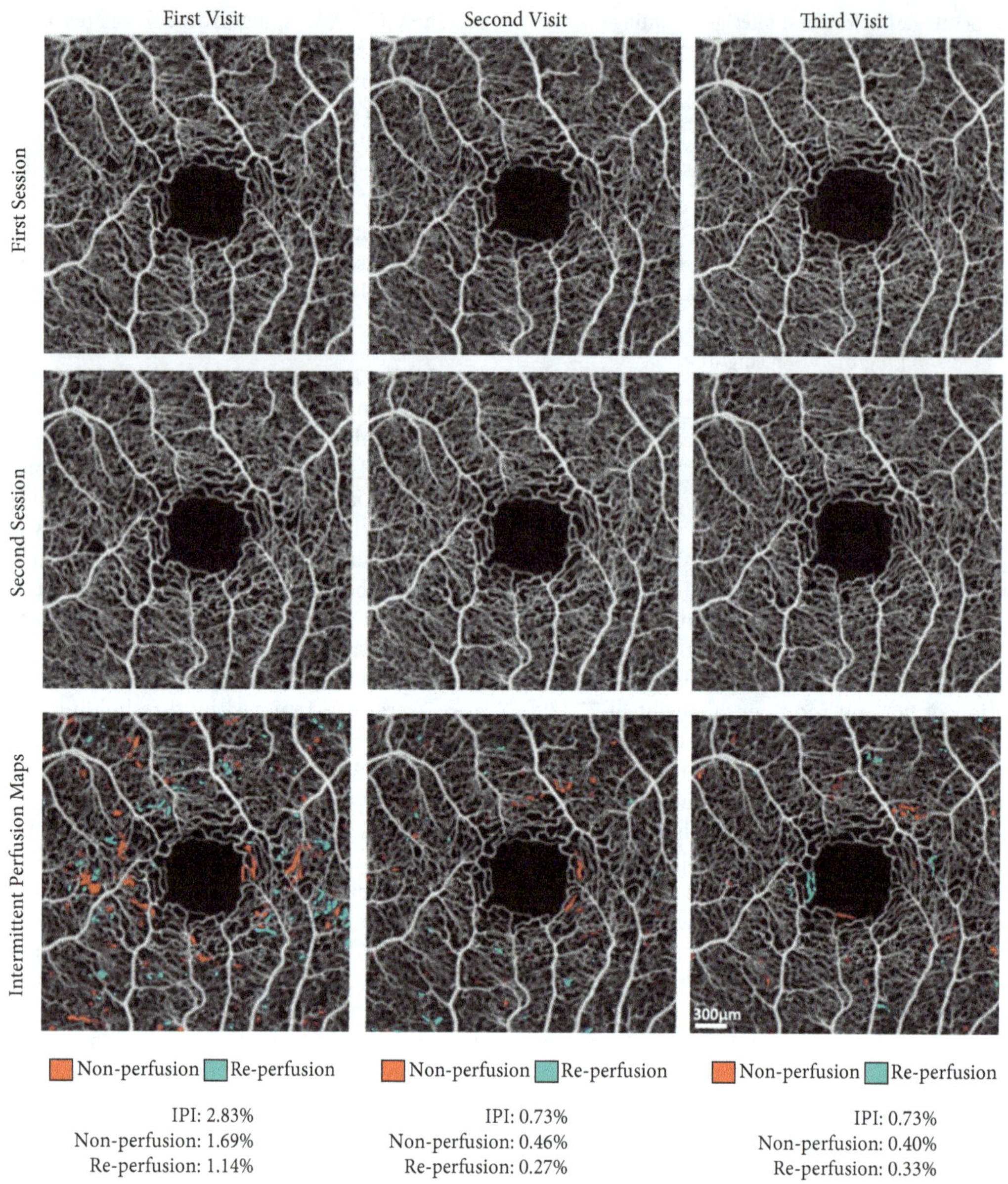

FIGURE 1: OCT-A images of the left eye of the HbSS patient, imaged across 3 imaging visits. The left column shows averaged OCT-A images from the first visit, the middle column from the second visit, and the right column from the third visit. The first and second rows show the averaged OCT-A images from the first and second sessions, respectively, taken 1 hour apart during each visit. The third row of images represents the computed intermittent perfusion maps. Nonperfusion between sessions is highlighted in red, and reperfusion between sessions is highlighted in cyan. The sum of the nonperfusion and reperfusion percent densities equals the intermittent perfusion index (IPI).

showed that IPI had improved substantially to 0.73%, with a nonperfusion area of 0.46% and a reperfusion area of 0.27% (Figure 1, Column 2). This substantial improvement in IPI reflected the expectation that most of the circulating blood 2 weeks after exchange transfusion was healthy donor blood.

The patient underwent CRISPR-based gene editing 1 month after his second imaging visit. The patient did not undergo any repeat blood transfusions after undergoing gene editing. OCT-A images from the third imaging visit, approximately 6 months after gene editing and 7 months after the second imaging visit, showed an IPI of 0.73%, with a nonperfusion area of 0.40% and a reperfusion area of 0.33% (Figure 1, Panel 3). Thus, CRISPR-based gene editing achieved a reduction in microvascular occlusive events that was comparable to exchange transfusion, but without the need to continually repeat therapy. Fundus photography and OCT repeated at all 3 visits did not show appreciable change.

Our case report demonstrates how OCT-A can be used to measure systemic SCD disease activity and response to treatment noninvasively through the visualization and measurement of dynamic vaso-occlusive episodes in the retinal capillary bed. This is the first report documenting macular OCT-A before and after gene editing in SCD. Our results are consistent with the prior paper by Zhou et al. establishing this imaging methodology [11]. In that paper, the IPI of all SCD patients ($n = 13$; including 1 sickle cell trait patient without treatment, 1 HbSC patient without treatment, 3 HbSS patients without treatment, 4 HbSS patients on hydroxyurea, and 1 HbSS patient after gene editing) was 0.36 ± 0.72% (median ± interquartile range). Subgroup analysis showed that IPI was 2.59 ± 1.00% for the HbSS patients without treatment and 0.52 ± 0.39% for the HbSS patients on hydroxyurea. Zhou et al. also reported an IPI of 3.0% in a treatment-naïve HbSS patient, which was reduced to 0.5% following two months of oral hydroxyurea therapy. For comparison, the IPI of unaffected controls was found to be 0.01 ± 0.03%. Since oral hydroxyurea therapy and gene editing targeting the *BCL11A* gene are both disease-modifying treatments based on HbF induction, it is interesting to compare the similar IPI values between the HbSS patients on hydroxyurea from the previous publication and our patient after gene editing (0.52% ± 0.39% versus 0.73%, respectively). Of note, the HbSS patient after gene editing from the previous publication had a reported IPI of 0.16%, although the baseline IPI prior to gene editing was unknown. It is thus difficult to draw conclusions on the relative effectiveness of treatments from these results given the multiple limitations, including limited sample sizes and lack of detail on patients' serologies and disease courses in the prior publication. Future studies combining traditional biomarkers with OCT-A need to elucidate the relative effects of various treatments and combinations of treatments in SCD, including hydroxyurea, blood transfusions, and gene editing.

SCD is a complex and multifactorial disease process that begins with polymerization of HbS and deformation of sickled RBCs, initiating rheological, inflammatory, and cellular events leading to cycles of vaso-occlusion and hemolytic anemia [5]. Conventional biomarkers of disease fall short in objectively measuring immediate ischemic disease activity in SCD. Serological biomarkers of hemolytic anemia, such as hemoglobin, hematocrit, indirect bilirubin, and reticulocyte count, correlate to episodes of VOCs; however, they record their hemolytic aftermath and not the VOCs themselves. The number of VOCs and hospitalizations over time attempt to estimate ischemic disease burden over months to years but lack the granularity to measure the severity and dynamics of vaso-occlusions occurring at any particular point in time.

In our patient, prior to gene editing, serologies indicated significant hemolytic anemia (Hgb 7.7–9.6 g/dL, indirect bilirubin 2.7–8.1 mg/dL, and reticulocyte count 7.0–10.2%). There was evidence of significant ischemic disease burden, as he averaged 6–8 emergency room visits per year for VOCs and ACSs and was dependent on opiate medications for pain control. Five months following gene editing, hemolytic anemia was significantly improved (Hgb 13.3 g/dL, indirect bilirubin 3.3 mg/dL, and reticulocyte count 4.7%). It was difficult to measure the degree of ongoing subclinical ischemic burden since the patient was no longer exhibiting clinical phenomena of VOCs or ACS and was using opiate medications for pain control for his avascular necrosis of the hip.

The severity of SCD micro-occlusive activity, as measured by OCT-A at the first and third imaging visits, was in concordance with the severity of ongoing hemolytic anemia evident on serologies before and after gene editing. OCT-A provided a more sensitive tool for measuring the subclinical vaso-occlusive events than measures dependent on clinically evident VOC and ACS.

This case confirms that CRISPR-based gene editing in SCD, while substantially effective, may not completely eliminate vaso-occlusive activity. This is consistent with prior reports that show that the success of gene editing varies between individuals and gene editing results in a phenotypic spectrum [3]. What was unclear in our case, since % HbS after gene editing was 50%, is whether the continued vaso-occlusive events in our patient were due to residual circulating sickled RBCs, persistent dysfunction of the endothelium and coagulation cascade, or a combination of both. Future studies using AO-SLO along with OCT-A may help answer this question. The clinical significance of residual vaso-occlusive episodes measured on OCT-A following gene editing in SCD also remains unclear and will need to be studied prospectively.

Noninvasive ocular biomarkers such as IPI have the potential to allow hematologists to be less reliant on blood draws and measures such as number of VOCs and hospitalizations over time to grade ischemic disease activity, measure disease progression, prognosticate risk of systemic and ophthalmic complications, and measure treatment response objectively and quantitatively. OCT-A may be useful for minimizing time to decision making to maintain or alter therapy, including identifying candidates for adjunctive oral therapy following gene editing, which can decrease patient morbidity and mortality while reducing healthcare expenditures.

Disclosure

Alexander Pinhas M.D. is a paid employee of Tesseract Health.Richard B. Rosen M.D. is a paid consultant to OptoVue, Boehringer-Ingelheim, Ocusciences, CellView, Topcon, and has personal financial interest in Opticology and Guardion. Jeffrey Glassberg M.D. is a paid consultant to Global Blood Therapeutics and performs contracted research for Pfizer. The remaining authors have no disclosures to make. The sponsors and funding organizations had no role in the design or conduct of this research. The content is solely the responsibility of the authors and does not necessarily represent the official views of the National Institutes of Health.

Acknowledgments

This study was supported by the National Institutes of Health under award numbers R01EY027301 and R01HL159116. Additional funding for this research was provided by the New York Eye and Ear Infirmary Foundation Grant, the Marrus Family Foundation, a Challenge Grant, departmental awards from Research to Prevent Blindness, and the Jorge N. Buxton Microsurgical Foundation.

References

[1] G. J. Kato, F. B. Piel, C. D. Reid et al., "Sickle cell disease," *Nature Reviews Disease Primers*, vol. 4, no. 1, Article ID 18010, 2018.

[2] A. Habara and M. H. Steinberg, "Minireview: genetic basis of heterogeneity and severity in sickle cell disease," *Experimental Biology and Medicine*, vol. 241, no. 7, pp. 689–696, 2016.

[3] T. O. Rosanwo and D. E. Bauer, "Editing outside the body: ex vivo gene-modification for beta-hemoglobinopathy cellular therapy," *Molecular Therapy*, vol. 29, no. 11, pp. 3163–3178, 2021.

[4] P. Houston-Yu, S. R. Rana, B. Beyer, and O. Castro, "Frequent and prolonged hospitalizations: a risk factor for early mortality in sickle cell disease patients," *American Journal of Hematology*, vol. 72, no. 3, pp. 201–203, 2003.

[5] R. Kalpatthi and E. M. Novelli, "Measuring success: utility of biomarkers in sickle cell disease clinical trials and care," *Hematology*, vol. 2018, no. 1, pp. 482–492, 2018.

[6] A. T. Farrell, J. Panepinto, C. P. Carroll et al., "End points for sickle cell disease clinical trials: patient-reported outcomes, pain, and the brain," *Blood Advances*, vol. 3, no. 23, pp. 3982–4001, 2019.

[7] S. K. Wagner, D. J. Fu, L. Faes et al., "Insights into systemic disease through retinal imaging-based oculomics," *Translational Vision Science & Technology*, vol. 9, no. 2, p. 6, 2020.

[8] T. M. Ranchod, "Systemic retinal biomarkers," *Current Opinion in Ophthalmology*, vol. 32, no. 5, pp. 439–444, 2021.

[9] Y. Jia, O. Tan, J. Tokayer et al., "Split-spectrum amplitude-decorrelation angiography with optical coherence tomography," *Optics Express*, vol. 20, no. 4, pp. 4710–4725, 2012.

[10] R. F. Spaide, J. G. Fujimoto, N. K. Waheed, S. R. Sadda, and G. Staurenghi, "Optical coherence tomography angiography," *Progress in Retinal and Eye Research*, vol. 64, pp. 1–55, 2018.

[11] D. B. Zhou, M. V. Castanos, A. Pinhas et al., "Quantification of intermittent retinal capillary perfusion in sickle cell disease," *Biomedical Optics Express*, vol. 12, no. 5, pp. 2825–2840, 2021.

[12] A. Pinhas, D. B. Zhou, M. V. Castanos et al., "Insights into sickle cell disease through the retinal microvasculature: AOSLO correlates to clinical OCT angiography," *Ophthalmology Science*, 2022.

[13] E. B. Esrick, L. E. Lehmann, A. Biffi et al., "Post-transcriptional genetic silencing of BCL11A to treat sickle cell disease," *New England Journal of Medicine*, vol. 384, no. 3, pp. 205–215, 2021.

[14] G. Lynch, J. S. A. Romo, R. Linderman et al., "Within-subject assessment of foveal avascular zone enlargement in different stages of diabetic retinopathy using en face OCT reflectance and OCT angiography," *Biomedical Optics Express*, vol. 9, no. 12, pp. 5982–5996, 2018.

[15] C. A. Schneider, W. S. Rasband, and K. W. Eliceiri, "NIH Image to ImageJ: 25 years of image analysis," *Nature Methods*, vol. 9, no. 7, pp. 671–675, 2012.

20

Severe Hemolysis in a COVID-19 Patient with Paroxysmal Nocturnal Hemoglobinuria

Steve Biko Otieno,[1,2,3] **Alaa Altahan**,[1,2,3] **Fnu Kaweeta**,[1] **Saradasri Karri**,[1,2,3] **Fnu Alnoor**,[2,4] **and Robert Johnson**[3]

[1]*The University of Tennessee Health Science Center, Department of Hematology and Oncology, 19 S. Manassas, Memphis, TN 38103, USA*
[2]*The Veterans Affairs Medical Center, 1030 Jefferson Ave, Memphis, TN 38104, USA*
[3]*The West Cancer and Research Institute, 7945 Wolf River Blvd, Germantown, TN 38138, USA*
[4]*The University of Tennessee Health Science Center, Department of Pathology, 930 Madison Ave, Memphis, TN 38103, USA*

Correspondence should be addressed to Steve Biko Otieno; sotieno@uthsc.edu

Academic Editor: Tatsuharu Ohno

Severe acute respiratory syndrome coronavirus 2 (SARS-CoV-2), the virus that causes coronavirus disease 2019 (COVID-19), has been demonstrated to be able to activate complement, making patients with deficiency in negative complement regulation, such as paroxysmal nocturnal hemoglobinuria (PNH), particularly vulnerable to complement-mediated cell damage. We report a case of a patient who presented with fatigue, facial swelling, and upper respiratory infection (URI) symptoms and was found to have COVID-19 with laboratory tests showing severe hemolysis and pancytopenia secondary to PNH.

1. Background

Severe acute respiratory syndrome coronavirus 2 (SARS-CoV-2) has infected more than 150 million worldwide and caused over 3 million deaths since December 2019, and these numbers continue to rise. It was declared a pandemic by the World Health Organization (WHO) on March 11, 2020. SARS-CoV-2 has been shown to be able to activate complement, making patients with a deficiency in negative complement regulation, such as paroxysmal nocturnal hemoglobinuria (PNH), particularly vulnerable to complement-mediated cell damage [1, 2] Patients with PNH have a mutation in the *PIG-A* gene which controls a key step in the biosynthesis of cell surface linker glycosyl-phosphatidyl-inositol (GPI) which tethers the negative complement regulators CD55 and CD59 to cell surfaces. The lack of the GPI linker results in the absence of these two key negative complement regulators [3]. On erythrocytes, the absence of the GPI linker results in complement-mediated hemolysis which is a common presentation of PNH. We report a case of a patient with COVID-19 who was diagnosed with PNH after she presented with fatigue, facial swelling, and URI symptoms with laboratories showing severe hemolysis and pancytopenia.

2. Case Presentation

The patient is a 19-year-old female with no significant past medical history who presented to the Emergency Department (ED) with left-sided facial swelling. 3 weeks prior to presentation, she developed cough, subjective fever, severe fatigue, and swelling of the gums of her left teeth. The gum swelling got worse, and she started having facial swelling. She underwent a COVID-19 test in the community prior to presentation but had not received the results at the time of presentation. The jaw swelling worsened and started draining pus despite taking amoxicillin prescribed by her dentist. She presented to the ED for further evaluation. On review of systems, she denied any history of recurrent infections, anemia, bleeding, rashes, jaundice, or thrombosis.

Her only medication was amoxicillin. She denied smoking, alcohol, or illicit drug use. Family history was notable for a cousin, aunt, and grandmother with leukemia.

On exam, her temperature was 37.3°C, blood pressure was 114/75, heart rate was 130, and oxygen saturation was 99% on room air. She was noted to have left face and neck swelling. Lungs were clear to auscultation bilaterally. She had no bruises, petechiae, or lymphadenopathy. The rest of her exam was unremarkable. A maxillofacial computed tomographic scan (CT) showed diffuse soft tissue edema throughout the left face without drainable fluid collection to suggest an abscess. Initial labs showed pancytopenia with a white blood cell count of 2.6×10^3 per microliter (reference range 4.2×10^3 to 10.2×10^3), an absolute neutrophil count of 1.8×10^3 per microliter (reference range 1.8×10^3 to 7.1×10^3), a hemoglobin of 2.7 grams per deciliter (reference range 11.5 to 14.8), and a platelet count of 30×10^3 per microliter (reference range 150×10^3 to 400×10^3). Other notable laboratory results were a total bilirubin level of 1.3 milligrams per deciliter (reference range 0.2 to 1.0), haptoglobin of 22 milligrams per deciliter (reference range 30–200), lactate dehydrogenase (LDH) of 2218 U per liter (reference range 84 to 246), reticulocyte count of 55.3×10^3 per microliter (reference range 30–90), prothrombin time of 20.3 seconds (reference range 23.2 to 34.1), international normalized ratio of 1.3 (reference range 0.8 to 1), partial thromboplastin time of 15.5 seconds (reference range 11.7 to 14.5), and fibrinogen of 514 milligrams per deciliter (reference range 208 to 475). A direct Coombs test was negative. Parvovirus B19 IgG was positive with a titer of 7.4 (reference range <0.9), but the IgM was negative. The results of the rest of her initial tests are shown in Table 1. She received four units of packed red blood cells (pRBCs) and was started on broad-spectrum antibiotics.

The patient developed a fever with a maximum temperature of 38.5°C after admission. Her COVID-19 test result returned as positive. Since the initial labs were consistent with hemolysis in the context of pancytopenia, a peripheral smear was ordered as well as flow cytometry on peripheral blood and flow cytometry for PNH. A bone marrow aspiration and core biopsy were performed. A CT chest, abdomen, and pelvis did not reveal any adenopathy and was negative for pulmonary embolism.

Flow cytometry was positive for PNH (Figure 1). The peripheral blood smear showed leukopenia with absolute neutropenia and thrombocytopenia. The observed neutrophils and lymphocytes were mature without significant morphological abnormality. Schistocytes were not present (Figure 2(a)). Bone marrow biopsy showed large areas of the marrow that were less than 10% cellular (Figure 2(b)); however, focally, the marrow is 40–50% cellular with erythroid predominant trilineage hematopoiesis (Figure 2(c)). Megakaryocytes were present but markedly decreased without any significant dysplasia. Few mature neutrophils were present. Blasts were not increased. Immunohistochemical stains performed with appropriate controls demonstrated numerous E-cadherin-positive erythroid precursors (Figure 2(d)). There were rare CD34-positive blasts and few scattered CD3-positive T cells and CD20-positive B cells. Terminal deoxynucleotidyl transferase (TdT) stain was negative. Bone marrow aspirate showed small hypocellular spicules with erythroid predominance. Some of these erythroid precursors were binucleated and had nuclear budding or irregular nuclear contours. Neutrophil precursors were present but infrequent. Blasts were not increased. A cytogenetics study revealed normal female karyotype (46XX). No mutations were detected by targeted next-generation sequencing.

The patient was treated with 2 doses of 600 milligrams of the C5 complement inhibitor eculizumab as inpatient with improvement in counts. She was seen in clinic after discharge, and she received 2700 mg of the longer acting C5 complement inhibitor ravulizumab a week after the last dose of eculizumab and a 3300 mg dose 2 weeks later. Her last blood counts showed a white blood cell count of 4×10^3 per microliter, absolute neutrophil count of 2.2×10^3 per microliter, hemoglobin level of 7.8 grams deciliter, and platelet count of 50×10^3 per microliter. Haptoglobin was 30, and LDH was normal. In the subsequent visits, the patient's pancytopenia persisted, and she was referred to a transplant center for evaluation.

3. Discussion

The patient in this case presented with a tooth infection, severe fatigue, and upper respiratory infection symptoms with work-up revealing severe hemolysis in the setting of COVID-19. Flow cytometry analysis of peripheral blood revealed a PNH clone. PNH is characterized by severe fatigue, smooth muscle dystonias, hemolysis, and thrombosis [3]. The patient did not have a history of hemolysis or thrombosis. Iron studies were not consistent with a chronic blood loss process as the patient had a normal mean corpuscular volume (MCV). The underlying pathophysiology of PNH is the absence of the negative complement regulatory proteins CD55 and CD59 on the surface of erythrocytes (Figure 3). Processes that activate the complement pathway make these erythrocytes vulnerable to complement-mediated hemolysis. SARS-CoV-2 has been implicated in overactivation of the complement system. Gao et al. reported that SARS-CoV-2 can activate the lectin complement pathway [1]. In another study, Yu et al. demonstrated that the SARS-CoV-2 spike proteins can activate the alternative complement pathway and also showed that disrupting interaction of the spike proteins and factor D or C5 inhibited this immunopathology [2]. The COVID-19 of this patient activated complement, resulting in the diagnosis of PNH in this previously asymptomatic patient. A complement-mediated thrombotic microangiopathy (TMA) has also been described in COVID-19 [4]. This type of TMA is usually characterized by hemolytic anemia, thrombocytopenia, and end-organ damage [4]. While the patient in this case had hemolytic anemia and thrombocytopenia, she did not have any end-organ damage suggesting that her pathophysiology was not driven by a TMA. In addition, TMAs usually have schistocytes on the peripheral blood smear. No schistocytes were observed on the peripheral blood smear for the patient in this case report.

TABLE 1: Laboratory values.

	Reference ranges	Initial labs	Before starting eculizumab	After 2 doses of eculizumab
White cells (thou/mcL)	4.2–10.20	2.6	3.2	5.4
Hemoglobin (g/dL)	11.5–14.8	2.7	9.0	8.2
Hematocrit (%)	34.6–43.8	8.5	26.6	24.9
Platelets (thou/mcL)	150–400	30	14	45
Absolute neutrophil count (thou/mcL)	1.8–7.1	1.8	0.2	3.0
Retic count (%)	0.5–2.0	2.57	1.73	5.63
Iron (mcg/dL)	50–170	58	152	
Ferritin (ng/mL)	8.0–252.0	246		517
Transferrin (mg/dL)	200–360	250	176	
Vitamin B12 (pg/mL)	211–911	345	552	
Lactate dehydrogenase (unit/L)	84–246	2218	566	189
Haptoglobin (mg/dL)	30–200	22	27	13
Fibrinogen (mg/dL)	208–475	514	391	
Partial thrombin time (sec)	11.7–14.5	20.3	24.1	29.4
International normalized ratio	0.8–1.0	1.3	1.0	1.0
Direct antiglobulin test	Negative	Negative	Negative	
Sodium (mmol/L)	136–145	139	141	140
Potassium (mmol/L)	3.5–5.1	3.6	3.5	3.8
Chloride (mmol/L)	98–107	108	106	109
Carbon dioxide (mmol/L)	22–32	19	29	24
Urea nitrogen (mg/dL)	7–18	19	14	5
Creatinine (mg/dL)	0.52–1.21	1.15	0.43	0.58
Alkaline phosphatase (unit/L)	45–117	82	92	197
Aspartate aminotransferase (unit/L)	15–37	75	26	22
Alanine aminotransferase (unit/L)	13–56	28	76	21
Total bilirubin (mg/dL)	0.2–1.0	1.3	0.7	0.6

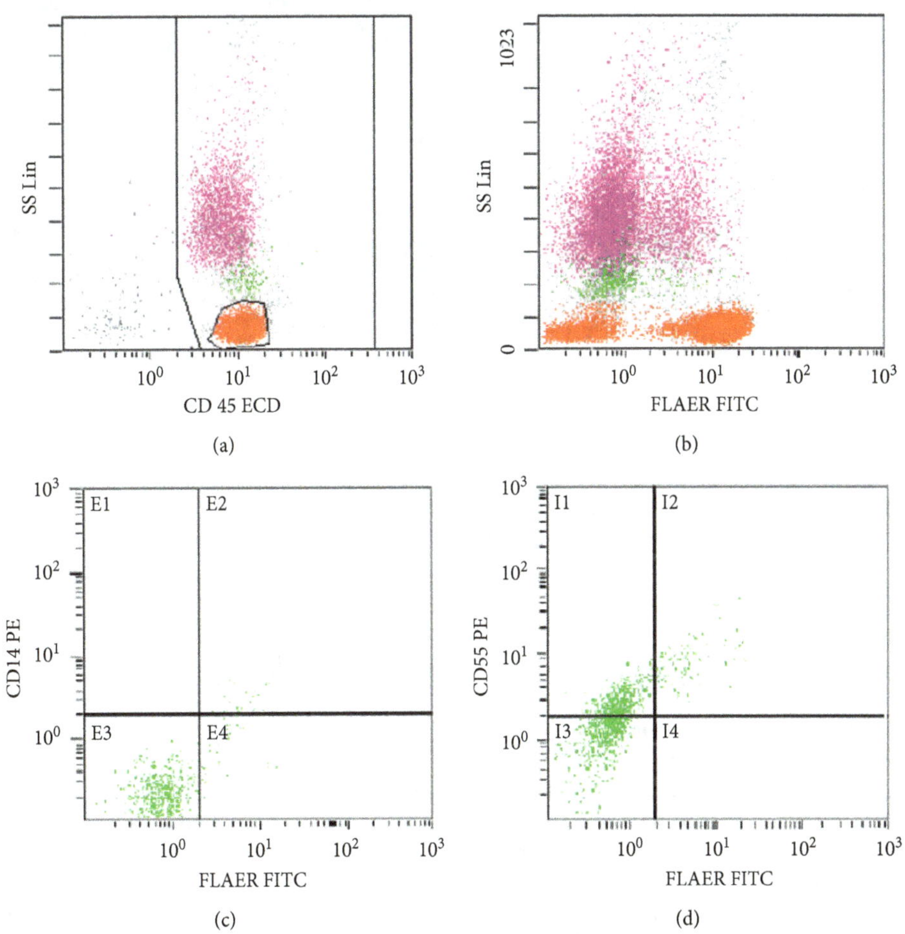

FIGURE 1: Continued.

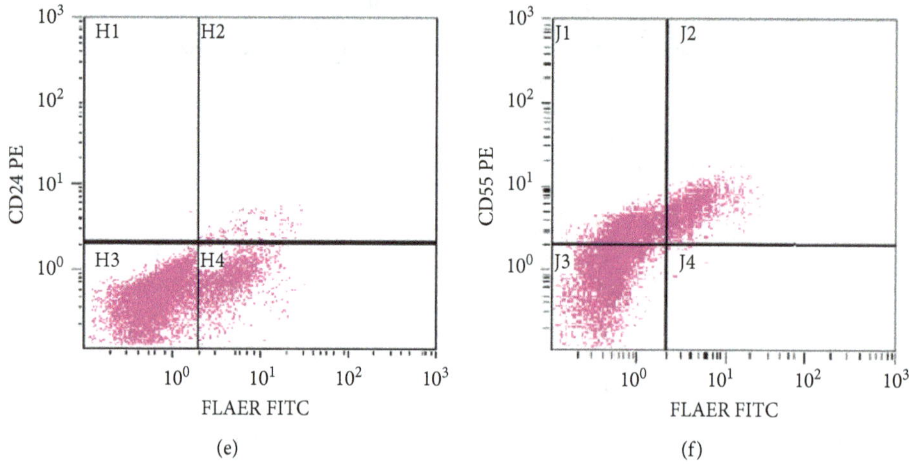

FIGURE 1: PNH flow cytometry. Lymphocytes (red), monocytes (green), and granulocytes (pink) were displayed on the CD 45 side scattered (SS) plot (a). The SS plot demonstrating fluorescein-labeled-proaerolysin- (FLAER-) negative different cell populations (b). 51% of monocytes and 52% of granulocytes had PNH immunophenotype; FLAER-/CD14-/CD55 and FLAER-/CD24-/CD55, respectively ((c)–(f)).

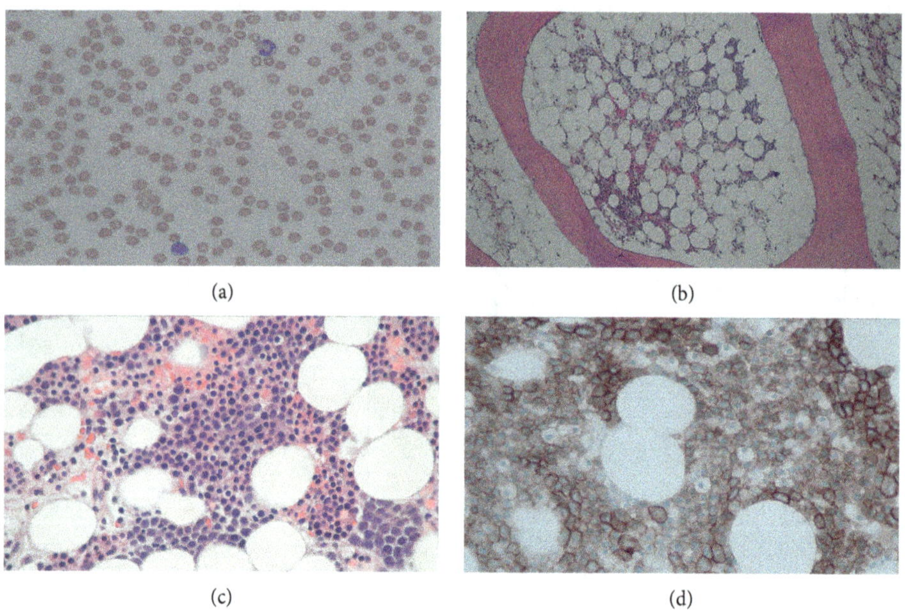

FIGURE 2: Peripheral blood and bone marrow biopsy. The peripheral blood smear showed leukopenia with absolute neutropenia and thrombocytopenia. The observed neutrophils and lymphocytes were mature without significant morphological abnormality. Schistocytes were not present (a). Bone marrow biopsy showed large areas of the marrow that are less than 10% cellular (b); however, focally, the marrow is 40–50% cellular with erythroid predominant trilineage hematopoiesis (c). Immunohistochemical stains performed with appropriate controls demonstrated numerous E-cadherin-positive erythroid precursors (d).

PNH is classified into 3 groups: (1) subclinical PNH which usually has few PNH clones but no clinical or laboratory manifestation of hemolysis or thrombosis; (2) classical PNH, which has clinical and laboratory manifestations of hemolysis and thrombosis; and (3) PNH in the setting of other marrow failure syndromes such as aplastic anemia or myelodysplastic syndrome [5]. It is important to note that a bone marrow biopsy in cases on PNH typically reveals a normal to increased cellularity with erythroid predominance [3]. The patient in this case had a hypocellular marrow suggesting a secondary process. She had likely had a concomitant severe aplastic anemia. Since the predominant clinical presentation of this patient was complement-mediated hemolysis, the goal of primary treatment was to control the hemolysis through complement inhibition.

The use of complement inhibitors such as eculizumab or ravulizumab is well established in treating PNH. Both drugs are monoclonal antibodies against the C5 component of complement preventing its cleavage into to C5a and C5b. This prevents the terminal complement cascade and the formation of the membrane attack complex (MAC), as shown in Figure 3. Pike et al. reported an institutional

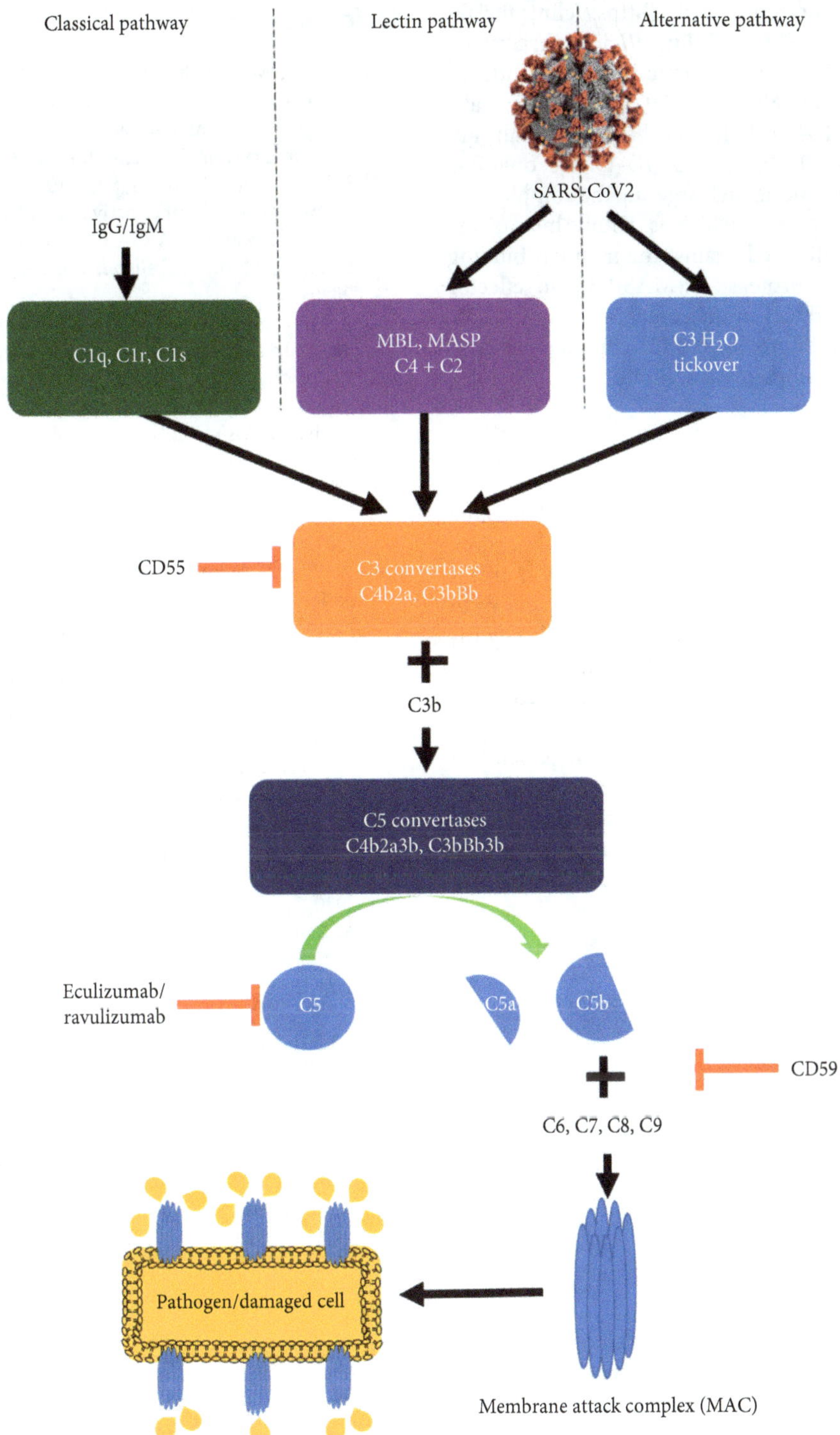

FIGURE 3: The complement system and its inhibitors. SARS-CoV-2 activates complement through the lectin and alternative pathways. CD55 negatively regulates the activity of C3 convertase and CD59 negatively regulates the formation of the membrane attack complex. Eculizumab and ravulizumab prevent the cleavage of C5 and prevent formation of the membrane attack complex. MBL: mannose-binding lectin; MASP: MBL-associated serine protease.

experience of 4 patients with COVID-19 who had a history of PNH and were on complement inhibitors [6]. Kulasekararaj et al. also reported an institutional experience of another 4 patients with COVID-19 and a history of PNH [7]. Two of these patients were treatment naïve, and two were established on complement inhibitor therapy [7]. The results of a small study of 80 patients suggested that eculizumab may improve survival and reduce hypoxia in patients with severe COVID-19 [8]. However, there is no approved indication yet for use in COVID-19 patients. Clinical trials investigating the use of eculizumab (https://clinicaltrials.gov/ct2/show/NCT04288713 and https://clinicaltrials.gov/ct2/show/NCT04346797) and ravulizumab (https://clinicaltrials.gov/ct2/show/NCT04570397, https://clinicaltrials.gov/ct2/show/NCT04390464, and https://clinicaltrials.gov/ct2/show/NCT04369469) in COVID-19 are ongoing. Other potential therapeutic agents targeting the complement pathway include narsoplimab which is a fully human Ig4 monoclonal antibody directed against the mannan-binding lectin-associated serine protease-2 (MASP-2), an effector enzyme of the lectin pathway of the complement system [9], AMY-101, a peptide inhibitor of the C3 complement [10], and Zilucoplan, a C5 complement inhibitor [11].

4. Conclusions

This 19-year-old female with undiagnosed PNH became symptomatic in the context of a SARS-COV-2 infection. Management of PNH in the setting of SARS-CoV-2 infection poses a great challenge. SARS-CoV-2 has been shown to activate complement, and patients with PNH lack key inhibitors of complement regulation, CD55 and CD59, and are, therefore, predisposed to complement-mediated damage. This case raises a great concern for patients who, at baseline, have clinically evident PNH. In such patients, a SARS-CoV-2 infection would potentially cause significant morbidity and mortality. In this patient population, it may be prudent to consider anticomplement therapy, for patients not on this therapy, to mitigate potentially catastrophic SARS-CoV-2-mediated complement activation. This case shows that complement inhibitors may potentially be effective in controlling SARS-CoV-2-mediated complement-activation-dependent hemolysis in PNH patients.

Consent

No written consent has been obtained from the patient as there are no patient identifiable data included in the case report.

Authors' Contributions

Steve Biko Otieno, MD, PhD, Alaa Altahan, MD, Fnu Kaweeta, MD, and Saradasri Karri, MD, wrote and edited the article Fnu Alnoor, MD, wrote and edited the section on pathology. Robert Johnson, MD, reviewed the article and provided comments.

Acknowledgments

The authors would like to acknowledge the Centers of Disease Control (https://www.cdc.gov/media/subtopic/images.htm) for making publicly available images of the SARS-CoV-2 virus used in making Figure 3.

References

[1] T. Gao, M. Hu, X. Zhang et al., "Highly pathogenic coronavirus N protein aggravates lung injury by MASP-2-mediated complement over-activation," *medRxiv*, 2020, https://www.medrxiv.org/content/10.1101/2020.03.29.20041962v3.

[2] J. Yu, X. Yuan, H. Chen, S Chaturvedi, E. M Braunstein, and R. A Brodsky, "Direct activation of the alternative complement pathway by SARS-CoV-2 spike proteins is blocked by factor D inhibition," *Blood*, vol. 136, no. 18, pp. 2080–2089, 2020.

[3] R. A. Brodsky, "How I treat paroxysmal nocturnal hemoglobinuria," *Blood*, vol. 113, no. 26, pp. 6522–6527, 2009.

[4] E. Gavriilaki and R. A. Brodsky, "Severe COVID-19 infection and thrombotic microangiopathy: success does not come easily," *British Journal of Haematology*, vol. 189, no. 6, pp. e227–e230, 2020.

[5] C. J. Parker, "Update on the diagnosis and management of paroxysmal nocturnal hemoglobinuria," *Hematology*, vol. 2016, no. 1, pp. 208–216, 2016.

[6] A. Pike, P. Muus, T. Munir et al., "COVID-19 infection in patients on anti-complement therapy: the Leeds National Paroxysmal Nocturnal Haemoglobinuria service experience," *British Journal of Haematology*, vol. 191, no. 1, pp. e1–e4, 2020.

[7] A. G. Kulasekararaj, I. Lazana, J. Large et al., "Terminal complement inhibition dampens the inflammation during COVID-19," *British Journal of Haematology*, vol. 190, no. 3, pp. e141–e143, 2020.

[8] D. Annane, N. Heming, L. Grimaldi-Bensouda et al., "Eculizumab as an emergency treatment for adult patients with severe COVID-19 in the intensive care unit: a proof-of-concept study," *EClinicalMedicine*, vol. 28, Article ID 100590, 2020.

[9] A. Rambaldi, G. Gritti, M. C. Micò et al., "Endothelial injury and thrombotic microangiopathy in COVID-19: treatment with the lectin-pathway inhibitor narsoplimab," *Immunobiology*, vol. 225, no. 6, Article ID 152001, 2020.

[10] S. Mastaglio, A. Ruggeri, A. M. Risitano et al., "The first case of COVID-19 treated with the complement C3 inhibitor AMY-101," *Clinical Immunology*, vol. 215, Article ID 108450, 2020.

[11] J. Declercq, C. Bosteels, K. Van Damme et al., "Zilucoplan in patients with acute hypoxic respiratory failure due to COVID-19 (ZILU-COV): a structured summary of a study protocol for a randomised controlled trial," *Trials*, vol. 21, no. 1, pp. 934–2020, 2020.

21

Acute Myeloid Leukemia with Concomitant BCR-ABL and NPM1 Mutations

Benedetta Mariotti,[1] **Federico Meconi**,[1] **Raffaele Palmieri**,[1] **Eleonora De Bellis**,[1] **Serena Lavorgna**,[1] **Tiziana Ottone**,[1] **Vincenza Martini**,[2] **Francesco Lo-Coco**,[1] **and Laura Cicconi**[1]

[1]*Department of Biomedicine and Prevention, University Tor Vergata, Rome, Italy*
[2]*UOC Ematologia, Ospedale "Fabrizio Spaziani", Frosinone, Italy*

Correspondence should be addressed to Benedetta Mariotti; benedetta_mariotti@hotmail.it

Academic Editor: Stephen Langabeer

We present a case report of a patient with acute myeloid leukemia (AML) characterized by the simultaneous presence of nucleophosmin 1 (NPM1) mutation and the breakpoint cluster region-Abelson (BCR-ABL) fusion oncogene. Our findings emphasize the importance of routinely including BCR-ABL in the diagnostic workup of AML in order to offer to the patients the most appropriate risk category and treatment options.

1. Introduction

Mutations in the *NPM1* gene are the most frequent genetic abnormalities occurring in AML and are highly specific for *de novo* AML [1]. The BCR-ABL fusion gene is the genetic hallmark of chronic myeloid leukemia (CML) but can also be found in approximately 30% of acute lymphoblastic leukemia (ALL) and rarely in AML (0.3–2% of newly diagnosed cases). In the updated WHO classification published in 2016, AML with BCR-ABL has been introduced as a provisional new entity [2, 3]. In BCR-ABL-positive AML, molecular and cytogenetic profile may help to distinguish *de novo* AML cases from CML-blastic phase (CML-BP).

To the best of our knowledge, the co-occurrence of *BCR-ABL* fusion gene and *NPM1* mutations in *de novo* AML has been reported in only few cases [4]. Herein, we report a 74-year-old patient diagnosed with AML harboring a complex three-way translocation t(9;22;12)(q34;q13;q11) encoding for two isoforms of BCR-ABL transcript (b3a2;b2a2) and a concomitant type A mutation in the *NPM1* gene.

2. Case Report

A 74-year-old male, with a history of type II diabetes and previous ischemic heart disease, was admitted on September 2014 to the emergency room of the hospital complaining severe asthenia and nasal bleeding. There was no previous history of hematological disorders. Blood cell count disclosed Hb 6.4 gr/dL (12.0–16.0 g/dL), Plts 35×10^9/L ($150–450 \times 10^9$/L), a WBC of 62×10^9 ($4.30–10.80 \times 10^9$/L), basophils <2% (0–1.5%), and with 50% of blasts. The coagulation profile showed INR 1.5 (0.8–1.2), fibrinogen 69 mg/dL (200–400 mg/dL), ATIII 77% (75–128%), and D-dimer 10757 ng/mL (0–500 ng/mL), suggesting a disseminated intravascular coagulopathy (DIC). Bone marrow aspirate showed infiltration by 89% of hypergranular leukemic blasts (Figures 1 and 2).

Immunophenotyping of the leukemic population showed positivity for CD45, CD33, CD117, and MPO and negativity for CD34, HLA-DR, CD13, and CD56, compatible with a diagnosis of AML. Clinical examination showed mild

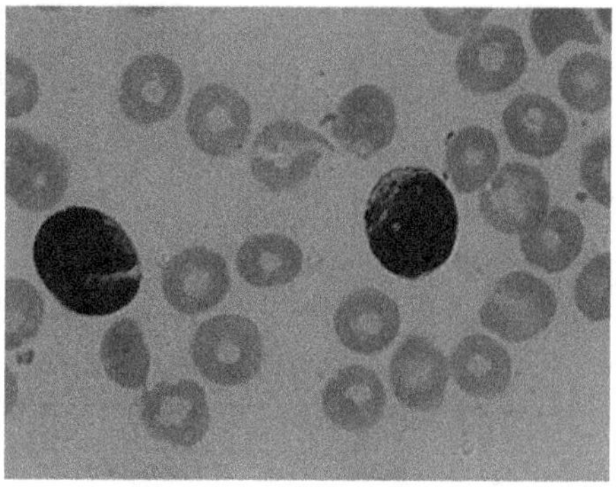

Figure 1

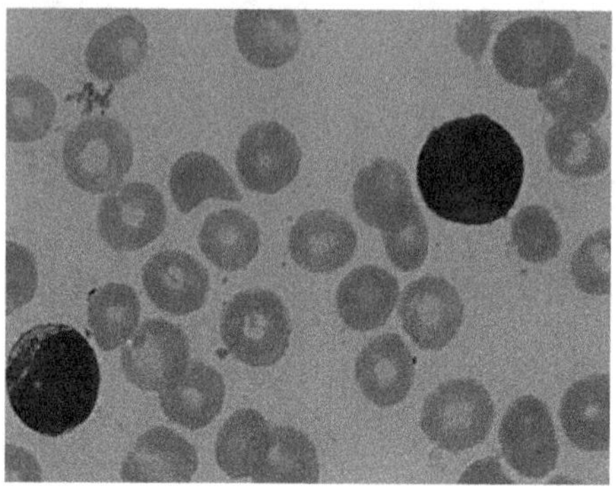

Figure 2

splenomegaly (14 cm) and multiple thick and erythematous skin lesions localized on the back. A biopsy of one such lesion followed by histologic examination was consistent with extramedullary localization of AML.

Conventional karyotyping (Figure 3) and FISH (Figure 4) showed the presence of a three-way translocation t(9; 12;22)(q34;q13;q11) on 15/15 metaphases.

The p210 BCR-ABL fusion transcript was detected by standard RT-PCR, which allowed to identify both b3a2 and b2a2 transcript isoforms [5]. Nowadays, no data are available regarding prognostic value of these transcripts in AML; however, studies regarding CML have shown that in some cases transcript, b2a2 has slower molecular and inferior response rates to TKI and a poorer long-term outcome [6]. In addition, molecular screening allowed to detect the presence of a type A mutation in the *NPM1* gene [7] and the absence of BCR/ABL p190, RUNX1/RUNXT1, CBFbeta/MYH11, DEK/CAN, FLT3-ITD, and PML/RARalpha rearrangements. Quantitative RQ-PCR showed IS 36% of BCR-ABL, with a copy number of BCR-ABL p210 of $7{,}152 \cdot 10^4$/ABL [8] and NPM1 copies of $101{,}160 \cdot 10^4$/ABL [7].

The CT scan showed hepatic lesions suggestive for extramedullary involvement and disseminated venous thrombosis localized in the sovrahepatic veins and the right frontal sinus. Lumbar puncture showed no central nervous system involvement. The patient was started on initial cytoreductive treatment with hydroxyurea for ten days and was subsequently treated with second-generation tyrosine kinase inhibitor (TKI) dasatinib 140 mg PO daily. Dasatinib was preferred over imatinib, a first generation TKI, due to high risk of the central nervous system involvement, extramedullary localization [9, 10] and, as proven for CML, it gives deeper and longer molecular responses [11].

In December 2014, due to trilineage pancytopenia, research for point mutations in BCR/ABL fusion gene was detected and showed, unfortunately after patient died, T315I mutation.

In January 2015, three months after the start of dasatinib, he was hospitalized for neutropenic fever and was diagnosed with pneumonia. He died of sepsis few days later.

3. Discussion

To the best of our knowledge, only few cases of AML with concomitant *BCR-ABL* rearrangement and *NPM1* mutation have been reported so far [4]. In clinical practice, the distinction between *de novo* BCR-ABL +ve AML and CML-BP is still challenging [12, 13]. In the present case, patient clinical features (no history of previous hematologic disorders, lack of basophilia, mild splenomegaly, and a lower bone marrow myeloid/erythroid ratio [14]) and molecular abnormalities (concomitant presence of *NPM1* mutation) were more suggestive of a *de novo* AML rather than of CML-BP. In previous reports of simultaneous *NPM1* mutation and *BCR-ABL* rearrangement, the p210 and p190 transcripts were detected in 2 and 4 cases, respectively. However, the concomitant presence of b3a2 and b2a2 BCR-ABL p210 isoforms combined to simultaneous NPM1 mutation, as observed in the present report, has been reported to date in only one case [12]. An additional peculiarity detected in leukemic cells of our patient is the presence of a complex three-way translocation involving chromosomes 9, 22, and 12 a karyotypic aberration previously unreported in either AML or CML.

BCR-ABL seems to cooperate with several AML-specific aberrations, including *CBFB-MYH11* and *NPM1*, although the precise molecular interaction among the altered proteins remains poorly understood [15].

In our case, RQ-PCR analysis of NPM1 and BCR-ABL detected in both instances a high transcript copy number. Together with the elevated number of metaphases harboring the Philadelphia chromosome (15/15), these findings suggest that the two molecular aberrations were present within the same leukemic clone rather than occurring in two separate clones. However, in recently reported patients with Ph-positive AML, targeted treatment with TKIs was able to abrogate the BCR-ABL +ve clone but did not lead to complete hematologic response, indicating that the *BCR-ABL* lesion was present at the subclonal level [16]. This highlights the more complex clonal architecture of Ph-positive AMLs as compared to CML. In addition, BCR-ABL has been described only occasionally as a minor subclone arising during AML

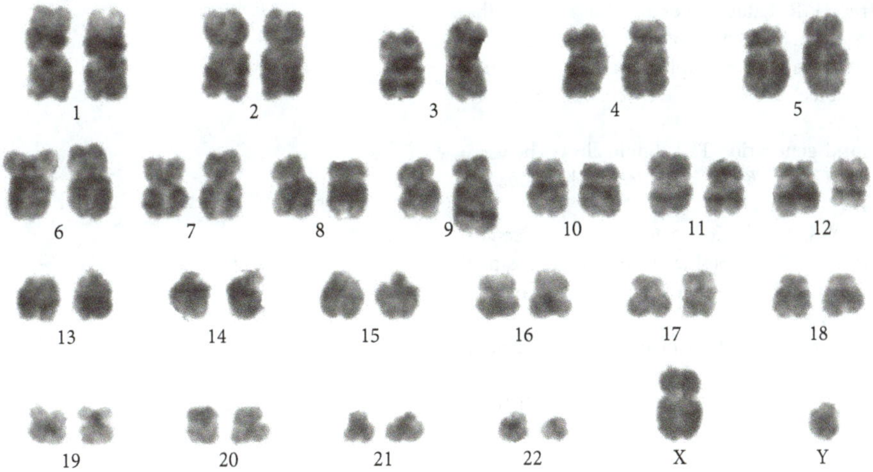

FIGURE 3: G-banding karyotype from a bone marrow blood metaphase.

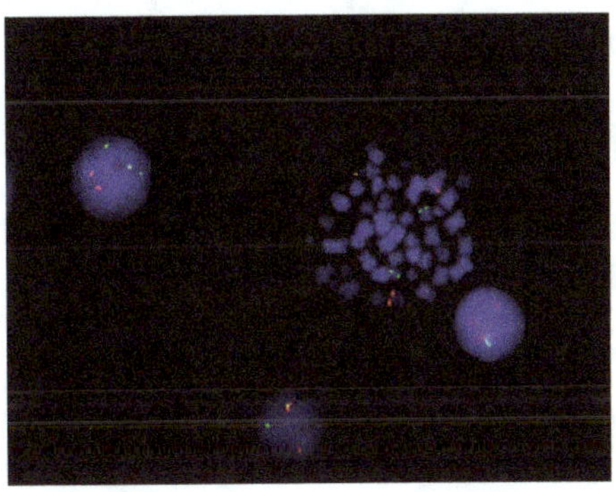

FIGURE 4: FISH BCR/ABL dual color dual fusion probe.

progression. Unfortunately, due to early death of our patients, we were not able to assess the cytogenetic/molecular response to TKI therapy.

At the moment, there is no standardized treatment for patients with Ph-positive AML although few case reports suggested a favorable response to TKIs [17]. In light of the new ELN classification [2], our findings further highlight the need of including BCR-ABL screening in routine diagnostic workup of AML. *BCR-ABL* and *NPM1* mutation are considered distinct entities in the WHO classification of AML with recurrent genetic abnormalities. According to the updated ELN criteria, the presence of *BCR-ABL* fusion gene classifies AML in the adverse risk category while *NPM1* mutation is generally regarded as a favorable prognostic in absence of the *FLT3*-ITD aberration. This case report highlights the possibility to concomitantly detect these two alterations in rare cases of AML and emphasizes the importance of including BCR-ABL screening in routine AML diagnostic panel in order to better assign the patient to the correct risk category and targeted treatment.

Acknowledgments

The authors thank Associazione Italiana Ricerca sul Cancro (AIRC Grant no. 21267).

References

[1] E. Papaemmanuil, M. Gerstung, L. Bullinger et al., "Genomic classification and prognosis in acute myeloid leukemia," *New England Journal of Medicine*, vol. 374, no. 23, pp. 2209–2221, 2016.

[2] H. Döhner, E. Estey, D. Grimwade et al., "Diagnosis and management of AML in adults: 2017 ELN recommendations from an international expert panel," *Blood*, vol. 129, no. 4, pp. 424–447, 2017.

[3] D. A. Arber, A. Orazi, R. Hasserjian et al., "The 2016 revision to the World Health Organization classification of myeloid neoplasms and acute leukemia," *Blood*, vol. 127, no. 20, pp. 2391–2405, 2016.

[4] N. R. Neuendorff, T. Burmeister, B. Dörken, and J. Westermann, "BCR-ABL-positive acute myeloid leukemia: a new entity? Analysis of clinical and molecular features," *Annals of Hematology*, vol. 95, no. 8, pp. 1211–1221, 2016.

[5] J. J. M. van Dongen, E. A. Macintyre, J. A. Gabert et al., "Standardized RT-PCR analysis of fusion gene transcripts from chromosome aberrations in acute leukemia for detection of minimal residual disease," *Leukemia*, vol. 13, no. 12, pp. 1901–1928, 1999.

[6] F. Castagnetti, G. Gugliotta, M. Breccia et al., "The BCR-ABL1 transcript type influences response and outcome in Philadelphia chromosome-positive chronic myeloid leukemia patients treated frontline with imatinib," *American Journal of Hematology*, vol. 92, no. 8, pp. 797–805, 2017.

[7] P. Gorello, G. Cazzaniga, F. Alberti et al., "Quantitative assessment of minimal residual disease in acute myeloid leukemia carrying nucleophosmin (NPM1) gene mutations," *Leukemia*, vol. 20, no. 6, pp. 1103–1108, 2006.

[8] J. Gabert, E. Beillard, V. H. J. van der Velden et al., "Standardization and quality control studies of "real-time" quantitative reverse transcriptase polymerase chain reaction of fusion gene transcripts for residual disease detection in leukemia—a Europe against cancer program," *Leukemia*, vol. 17, no. 12, pp. 2318–2357, 2003.

[9] Y. Isobe, K. Sugimoto, A. Masuda, Y. Hamano, and K. Oshimi, "Central nervous system is a sanctuary site for chronic myelogenous leukaemia treated with imatinib mesylate," *Internal Medicine Journal*, vol. 39, no. 6, pp. 408–411, 2009.

[10] G. Alimena, M. Breccia, R. Latagliata et al., "Dasatinib in the management of lymphoid blast crisis of Philadelphia-positive chronic myeloid leukemia with multiple extra-medullary and intracranial localizations," *Leukemia Research*, vol. 33, no. 8, pp. e134–e136, 2009.
[11] J. E. Cortes, "A second-generation TKI should always be used as initial therapy for CML," *Blood Advances*, vol. 2, no. 24, pp. 3653–3655, 2018.
[12] S. Konoplev, C. C. Yin, S. M. Kornblau et al., "Molecular characterization ofde novoPhiladelphia chromosome-positive acute myeloid leukemia," *Leukemia & Lymphoma*, vol. 54, no. 1, pp. 138–144, 2013.
[13] C. P. Soupir, J. A. Vergilio, P. Dal Cin et al., "Philadelphia chromosome-positive acute myeloid leukemia: a rare aggressive leukemia with clinicopathologic features distinct from chronic myeloid leukemia in myeloid blast crisis," *American Journal of Clinical Pathology*, vol. 127, no. 4, pp. 642–650, 2007.
[14] E. P. Nacheva, C. D. Grace, D. Brazma et al., "DoesBCR/ABL1positive acute myeloid leukaemia exist?," *British Journal of Haematology*, vol. 161, no. 4, pp. 541–550, 2013.
[15] E. Han, H. Lee, M. Kim et al., "Characteristics of hematologic malignancies with coexisting t(9;22) and inv(16) chromosomal abnormalities," *Blood Research*, vol. 49, no. 1, p. 22, 2014.
[16] J. Aoki, K. Kakihana, T. Kobayashi et al., "Tyrosine kinase inhibitor therapy for acute myeloid leukemia with late-appearing Philadelphia chromosome," *Leukemia Research*, vol. 36, no. 1, pp. e41–e42, 2012.
[17] K. Ueda, S. Horiike, K. Zen, S. Misawa, and M. Taniwaki, "Complete cytogenetic and molecular response to treatment with imatinib mesylate for philadelphia chromosome positive acute myeloid leukemia with multilineage dysplasia," *Leukemia & Lymphoma*, vol. 47, no. 9, pp. 1967–1969, 2006.

Familial Hemophagocytic Lymphohistiocytosis Secondary to *PRF1* Mutation

Albaraa T. Alfaraidi,[1] Abdulaziz A. Alqarni,[1] Mohammed T. Aqeel,[1] Turki A. Albalawi,[1] and Ahmed S. Hejazi[2]

[1]*College of Medicine, King Saud Bin Abdulaziz University for Health Sciences, King Abdullah International Medical Research Centre, King Abdulaziz Medical City, Ministry of the National Guard-Health Affairs, Jeddah, Saudi Arabia*
[2]*Department of Oncology, King Abdulaziz Medical City, Ministry of the National Guard-Health Affairs, Jeddah, Saudi Arabia*

Correspondence should be addressed to Ahmed S. Hejazi; drashejazi@yahoo.com

Academic Editor: Pier Paolo Piccaluga

Hemophagocytic lymphohistiocytosis (HLH) is a life-threatening hyperinflammatory syndrome that causes systemic inflammation which can progress to multiorgan failure and death. Symptoms and signs commonly seen in HLH include high fever, hepatosplenomegaly, pancytopenia, and hypertriglyceridemia. This report describes the 8-month clinical course of a 17-year-old male with G6PD deficiency who presented with intermittent high fever of unknown origin for 8 months accompanied by pancytopenia and bilateral lower limb weakness. A pathogenic homozygous missense mutation (c.1081A > T p.(Arg361Trp)) in the *PRF1* gene was detected by whole exome sequencing (WES). The brain and the whole spine MRI showed leptomeningeal enhancement at different levels involving both the brain and the spine. Therefore, a diagnosis of familial HLH type 2 with CNS involvement was confirmed. Accordingly, treatment with dexamethasone, cyclosporin, and etoposide in addition to intrathecal methotrexate and hydrocortisone was given. The patient showed a dramatic response with significant neurological improvement of the bilateral lower limb weakness. Genetic analysis has helped the patient's family with appropriate genetic counselling. This case highlights the importance of immediate treatment with immunosuppressants and the high clinical suspicion of physicians regarding HLH in areas where consanguinity is common.

1. Introduction

Hemophagocytic lymphohistiocytosis (HLH) is a life-threatening hyperinflammatory syndrome characterized by hypercytokinemia and lymphohistiocytic proliferation. In patients with HLH, dysregulated hyper-reactive immune cells cause systemic inflammation that can progress to multiorgan failure and death. The altered interaction between natural killer (NK) cells, CD 8+ cytotoxic T cells, and their antigens leads to a vicious cycle of inflammation which recruits more cytotoxic cells. This results in hypercytokinemia that causes widespread activation of macrophages and hemophagocytosis [1–4]. With mortality rates between 42% and 88%, due to the nature of the disease, prompt initiation of immunosuppressants is essential as soon as a diagnosis is confirmed [5]. HLH is common in infancy; however, it has been reported among all age groups [6]. The inflammatory syndrome has been grouped into two types: familial and acquired HLH. Familial HLH is an autosomal recessive condition in which consanguineous marriage plays an important role in inheriting the disease-causing mutation. It occurs due to a mutation in the genes responsible for normal natural killer (NK) cell activity and the cytotoxic function of T lymphocytes. The acquired form of HLH has been associated with infectious, autoinflammatory, autoimmune, and metabolic diseases [7]. Patients with HLH may present with nonspecific signs of inflammation such as fever, malaise, and fatigue. HLH is characterized by edema, hepatosplenomegaly, and liver dysfunction. Laboratory studies may show pancytopenia, coagulation abnormalities, hypofibrinogenemia, and hypertriglyceridemia [2]. We report this case of a 17-year-old male diagnosed with familial HLH due to a mutation in the *PRF1* gene with a literature review of the current treatment options and an emphasis on the importance of genetic counselling in families affected by HLH.

2. Case Presentation

A 17-year-old male, known to have glucose-6-phosphate dehydrogenase (G6PD) deficiency, was admitted to our hospital due to pancytopenia accompanied by a high-grade intermittent fever of unknown origin for the last eight months which was not relieved by antipyretics. The patient had significant weight loss accompanied by generalized weakness and myalgia. On physical examination, the patient looked sick, pale, and cachectic. Abdominal examination was remarkable for hepatosplenomegaly. On neurological examination, the patient had bilateral lower limb weakness with a power of 4 out of 5 in both limbs. Blood laboratory studies showed pancytopenia, hypertriglyceridemia (3.13 mmol/L), and hyperferritinemia (1912 μg/L). Other laboratory studies showed increased liver enzymes, low fibrinogen (1.4), and increased cerebrospinal fluid (CSF) total protein concentration (1.37, reference range: 0.15–0.45 g/L) (Table 1). In our patient, the soluble interleukin-2 receptor (sIL-2R) level was significantly elevated (15900 U/mL). The viral workup which included CMV and hepatitis A, B, and C serological markers was negative. A bone marrow biopsy was performed which revealed a hypercellular bone marrow with prominent hemophagocytic activity and an increased number of histiocytic cells. The proband is an offspring of first-cousin parents with no previously documented genetic disease in the family (Figure 1). The brain and the whole spine MRI showed leptomeningeal enhancement at different levels involving both the brain and the spine.

The patient was assumed to be a case of HLH with CNS involvement as he met the diagnostic criteria of HLH-2004. Accordingly, treatment with dexamethasone, cyclosporin, and etoposide in addition to intrathecal methotrexate and hydrocortisone was started. The first two doses of etoposide treatment were reduced to 50% due to high bilirubin levels (Table 1). The patient showed a dramatic response after starting treatment and had an uneventful treatment course. Symptomatically, the patient became afebrile and vitally stable. On day 20 of treatment, ferritin levels improved to 881 μg/L, and hemoglobin, platelets, WBC, and LFTs had improved (Table 1). After completion of the first two months of treatment, the patient showed a significant neurological improvement in terms of his bilateral lower limb weakness. Postinduction MRI of the brain and the whole spine showed a partial improvement of the previously seen leptomeningeal enhancement.

To determine whether our patient is a case of familial HLH, genomic DNA was extracted from peripheral blood and was sent for whole exome sequencing (WES). WES identified that our patient had a homozygous missense mutation (NM_001083116.3 (PRF1): c.1081A > T, p.Arg361Trp) in the *PRF1* gene, which is classified as pathogenic and has been previously described in the literature in a family with HLH (PMIDs: 14757862, 23592409, 32542393, 27577878, and 15755897). Considering the homozygous pathogenic variant in *PRF1* and the supportive phenotype of the patient, a genetic diagnosis of familial HLH type 2 was confirmed (OMIM: 603553). Parental samples for which WES was equally performed revealed that parents were heterozygous for the identified mutation. Therefore, an autosomal recessive pattern of inheritance was confirmed in the family. Given the confirmed diagnosis of familial HLH disease with CNS involvement, the patient was a candidate for an allogeneic bone marrow transplant and HLA typing, and a search for a compatible stem cell donor was carried out. Screening of all siblings by WES revealed an 8-year-old HLA-matched sister who had a negative WES for the relevant mutations. Accordingly, the patient was offered an allogeneic bone marrow transplant.

3. Discussion

Familial HLH are a group of autosomal recessive diseases that occur frequently in consanguineous families [8]. Pathological variants in *PRF1*, *UNC13D*, *STX1*, and *STXBP2* have been linked to cause different forms of familial HLH (familial HLH2-HLH5). Familial HLH type 2 is the most common in this group and accounts for 20–40% of all familial HLH cases [9]. These forms of familial HLH lead to a defect in lymphocyte granule-mediated cytotoxicity [10]. Perforin gene mutations were the first genetic causes of familial HLH which were discovered in 1999 [11]. About half of the primary HLH cases were attributed to *PRF1* mutations [2, 12]. *PRF1* variants have been described in the literature in other diseases such as multiple sclerosis, non-Hodgkin's lymphoma, and leukemia [13–15]. The reported incidence of *PRF1* mutations that cause FHLH-2 varies between different ethnic groups [12].

In our patient, whole exome sequencing (WES) found that our patient had a homozygous missense mutation (NM_001083116.3 (PRF1): c.1081 A > T, p.Arg361Trp) in the *PRF1* gene. The *PRF1* gene is located on chromosome 10q22.1 and codes for the perforin protein which is responsible for lymphocyte granule-mediated cytotoxicity [10]. In patients with perforin deficiency, the immune system is unable to kill the target cells as the released contents of the cytotoxic granules cannot penetrate these cells. Mutations in *UNC13D*, *STX11*, and *STXBP2* genes cause familial HLH types 3 to 5, respectively, and lead to defective lymphocyte granule-mediated cytotoxicity [10].

According to the revised diagnostic criteria of the HLH-2004 protocol, HLH is assumed if a genetic defect consistent

TABLE 1: An overview of relevant laboratory parameters during the clinical course of the patient.

Parameters	Reference range	Admission Day 0	Day 5	Day 1 of HLH-04 protocol	Day 5 of HLH-04 protocol	Day 10 of HLH-04 protocol	Day 15 of HLH-04 protocol	Day 20 of HLH-04 protocol	Day of discharge
Hemoglobin (g/-dL)	13.0–18.0	8.7	7.8	10.8	10.2	9.7	8.2	8.5	9.5
Neutrophils (10^9xL)	2.0–7.5	0.8	0.99	0.75	0.92	1.02	0.79	0.42	3.44
Lymphocytes (10^9/L)	1.5–4.0	1.61	1.07	1.44	2.3	0.48	0.41	0.84	2.16
Platelet count (10^9/L)	150–450	63	54	41	87	68	69	221	273
Ferritin (μg/L)	11–172	1420	1912	948	1821	1612	976	881	371
Fibrinogen (g/L)	2.0–4.0	—	1.5	1.6	0.9	1.2	1.4	1.6	1.9
Triglyceride (mmol/L)	0.5–2.20	3.13	—	—	—	—	—	—	—
Direct bilirubin (μmol/L)	1.7–6.7	20	80	—	—	—	—	—	34
ALT (IU/L)	9–24	502	707	611	323	303	257	274	128
AST (IU/L)	14–35	354	608	390	189	113	79	89	63
ALP (IU/L)	59–164	994	885	967	631	413	305	309	253
GGT (IU/L)	7–21	250	219	569	424	535	647	782	1025
sIL-2r (U/ml)	158–623	—	—	—	15900	—	—	—	—

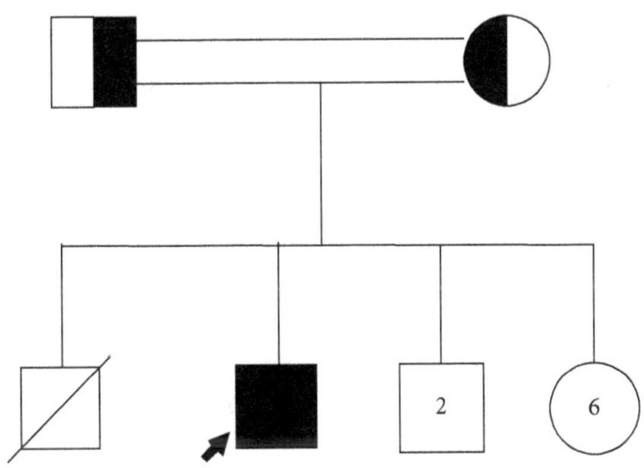

FIGURE 1: Pedigree chart of the proband.

with HLH has been found or clinical and laboratory criteria are met. Etoposide, steroids, and cyclosporin A with or without intrathecal methotrexate are considered first-line therapy for patients with HLH [16]. CNS involvement in HLH has been associated with poorer prognosis and long-term neurological sequelae [17]. The frequency of CNS involvement varies widely in the literature and ranges from 10% to 73% of patients [17, 18]. Histopathological changes may range from minimal infiltration of leptomeninges by macrophages and lymphocytes to advanced infiltration of the parenchyma and tissue necrosis. The most important finding is the presence of hemophagocytosis, which is frequently observed in leptomeninges [19].

Currently, the only long-term curative treatment for primary HLH is allogeneic bone marrow transplantation. The HLH steering committee of the Histiocyte Society urgently recommends consulting a stem cell transplant expert about the treatment options offered since these patients carry a high risk of reactivation even after the acute episode has subsided [20].

4. Conclusion

The diagnosis of HLH remains challenging as patients present with nonspecific symptoms. Without a bone marrow transplant, patients with HLH have a lifelong risk of relapse. The lack of a gold standard confirmatory test for HLH makes it difficult to diagnose HLH in an emergency setting. High clinical suspicion of physicians is essential in areas where consanguinity is common if a patient presents with a fever of unknown origin accompanied by clinical features and laboratory studies that are suggestive of HLH. Immediate treatment with immunosuppressants can be lifesaving and should be provided once a diagnosis has been reached. If indicated, a prenatal analysis may be offered to the family of the patient. Testing for HLH mutations in siblings and family members should be performed before being considered as donors. Genetic counselling regarding future children is recommended to be offered to consanguineous parents with a family history of individuals affected by familial HLH.

Abbreviations

HLH: Hemophagocytic lymphohistiocytosis
PRF1: Perforin 1
FHL: Familial hemophagocytic lymphohistiocytosis
WES: Whole exome sequencing
G6PD: Glucose-6-phosphate dehydrogenase
ALT: Alanine transaminase
AST: Aspartate transaminase
ALP: Alkaline phosphatase
GGT: Gamma-glutamyl transferase
PT: Prothrombin time
TG: Triglycerides
LDH: Lactate dehydrogenase
RBCs: Red blood cells
CMV: Cytomegalovirus
MRI: Magnetic resonance imaging
PIDs: Primary immunodeficiencies
IUIS: International Union of Immunological Societies
sIL-2r: Soluble interleukin-2 receptor
HLA: Human leukocyte antigen
HSCT: Hematopoietic stem cell transplantation.

Consent

Informed written consent was obtained from the patient for the publication of this case report.

Authors' Contributions

AA, AA, MA, and TA collected, assembled, and clinically evaluated the patient's interpreted data and wrote the manuscript. AH critically revised the manuscript and is the corresponding author for all article-related questions. All authors approved the final manuscript and the order of authors.

Acknowledgments

The authors would like to thank the patient and his family for their approval and cooperation.

References

[1] H. Al-Samkari and N. Berliner, "Hemophagocytic lymphohistiocytosis," *Annual Review of Pathology: Mechanisms of Disease*, vol. 13, no. 1, pp. 27–49, 2018.
[2] A. Morimoto, Y. Nakazawa, and E. Ishii, "Hemophagocytic lymphohistiocytosis: pathogenesis, diagnosis, and management," *Pediatrics International*, vol. 58, no. 9, pp. 817–825, 2016.
[3] G. E. Janka, "Familial hemophagocytic lymphohistiocytosis," *European Journal of Pediatrics*, vol. 140, no. 3, pp. 221–230, 1983.
[4] A. M. Schram, P. Comstock, M. Campo et al., "Haemophagocytic lymphohistiocytosis in adults: a multicentre case series over 7 years," *British Journal of Haematology*, vol. 172, no. 3, pp. 412–419, 2016.
[5] G. Griffin, S. Shenoi, and G. C. Hughes, "Hemophagocytic lymphohistiocytosis: an update on pathogenesis, diagnosis, and therapy," *Best Practice & Research Clinical Rheumatology*, vol. 34, no. 4, Article ID 101515, 2020.
[6] G. Elyamany, A. Alzahrani, H. Elfaraidi et al., "Hemophagocytic lymphohistiocytosis: single-center series of 12 cases from Saudi Arabia," *Clinical Medicine Insights: Pediatrics*, vol. 106 pages, 2016.
[7] Y. M. Esteban, J. L. O. de Jong, and M. S. Tesher, "An overview of hemophagocytic lymphohistiocytosis," *Pediatric Annals*, vol. 46, no. 8, pp. e309–e313, 2017.
[8] K. Göransdotter Ericson, B. Fadeel, S. Nilsson-Ardnor et al., "Spectrum of perforin gene mutations in familial hemophagocytic lymphohistiocytosis," *The American Journal of Human Genetics*, vol. 68, no. 3, pp. 590–597, 2001.
[9] M. Madkaikar, S. Shabrish, and M. Desai, "Current updates on classification, diagnosis and treatment of hemophagocytic lymphohistiocytosis (HLH)," *Indian Journal of Pediatrics*, vol. 83, no. 5, pp. 434–443, 2016.
[10] S. W. Canna and R. A. Marsh, "Pediatric hemophagocytic lymphohistiocytosis," *Blood*, vol. 135, no. 16, pp. 1332–1343, 2020.
[11] S. E. Stepp, R. Dufourcq-Lagelouse, F. L. Deist et al., "Perforin gene defects in familial hemophagocytic lymphohistiocytosis," *Science*, vol. 286, no. 5446, pp. 1957–1959, 1999.
[12] C. Gholam, S. Grigoriadou, K. C. Gilmour, and H. B. Gaspar, "Familial haemophagocytic lymphohistiocytosis: advances in the genetic basis, diagnosis and management," *Clinical and Experimental Immunology*, vol. 163, no. 3, pp. 271–283, 2011.
[13] M. Camiña-Tato, C. Morcillo-Suárez, M. F. Bustamante et al., "Gender-associated differences of perforin polymorphisms in the susceptibility to multiple sclerosis," *The Journal of Immunology*, vol. 185, no. 9, pp. 5392–5404, 2010.
[14] S. Mhatre, M. Madkaikar, F. Jijina, and K. Ghosh, "Unusual clinical presentations of familial hemophagocytic lymphohistiocytosis type-2," *Journal of pediatric hematology/oncology*, vol. 36, no. 8, pp. e524–e527, 2014.
[15] S. Mhatre, M. Madkaikar, M. Desai, and K. Ghosh, "Spectrum of perforin gene mutations in familial hemophagocytic lymphohistiocytosis (FHL) patients in India," *Blood Cells, Molecules, and Diseases*, vol. 54, no. 3, pp. 250–257, 2015.
[16] P. Collins, M. Watts, M. Brocklesby, B. Gerritsen, and P. Veys, "Successful engraftment of haploidentical stem cell transplant for familial haemophagocytic lymphohistiocytosis using both bone marrow and peripheral blood stem cells," *British Journal of Haematology*, vol. 96, no. 3, pp. 644–646, 1997.
[17] H. W. Goo and Y. C. Weon, "A spectrum of neuroradiological findings in children with haemophagocytic lymphohistiocytosis," *Pediatric Radiology*, vol. 37, no. 11, pp. 1110–1117, 2007.
[18] I. H. Solomon, H. Li, L. A. Benson et al., "Histopathologic correlates of familial hemophagocytic lymphohistiocytosis isolated to the central nervous system," *Journal of Neuropathology & Experimental Neurology*, vol. 77, no. 12, pp. 1079–1084, 2018.
[19] J.-I. Henter and I. Nennesmo, "Neuropathologic findings and neurologic symptoms in twenty-three children with hemophagocytic lymphohistiocytosis," *The Journal of Pediatrics*, vol. 130, no. 3, pp. 358–365, 1997.

[20] S. Ehl, I. Astigarraga, T. von Bahr Greenwood et al., "Recommendations for the use of etoposide-based therapy and bone marrow transplantation for the treatment of HLH: consensus statements by the HLH Steering Committee of the Histiocyte Society," *Journal of Allergy and Clinical Immunology: In Practice*, vol. 6, no. 5, pp. 1508–1517, 2018.

23

SARS-CoV-2 Infection-Associated Aortic Thrombosis Treated with Oral Factor Xa Inhibition

Alena Strýčková,[1,2] Jakub Benko,[2] Martin Jozef Péč,[2] Monika Péčová,[1] Jana Žolková,[1] Monika Brunclíková,[1] Tomáš Bolek,[2] Ján Staško,[1] Matej Samoš,[2] and Marián Mokáň[2]

[1]*National Centre of Hemostasis and Thrombosis, Department of Hematology and Blood Transfusion, Jessenius Faculty of Medicine in Martin, Comenius University in Bratislava, Martin, Slovakia*
[2]*Department of Internal Medicine I, Jessenius Faculty of Medicine in Martin, Comenius University in Bratislava, Martin, Slovakia*

Correspondence should be addressed to Matej Samoš; matej.samos@gmail.com

Academic Editor: Kostas Konstantopoulos

Coronavirus disease 2019 (COVID-19) is an acute complex systemic disorder caused by the severe acute respiratory syndrome coronavirus 2 (SARS-CoV-2).While SARS-CoV-2 is known to cause significant pulmonary disease, various extrapulmonary manifestations of COVID-19 have also been reported. Growing evidence suggests that COVID-19 is associated with coagulopathy leading to micro and macrovascular complications. Although in patients with COVID-19, venous thromboembolic events are more frequent, arterial thrombosis also occurs at an increased rate. These often lead to acute life-threatening ischemia, which requires urgent diagnosis and treatment. We present case reports of two patients with an abnormal thrombus formation in the thoracic aorta who recently overcame COVID-19, which led to systemic embolism and splenic infarction. Ambulatory oral factor Xa inhibitor therapy led to aortic thrombosis resolution in both patients.

1. Introduction

Coronavirus disease 2019 (COVID-19), an acute complex systemic disorder, is caused by the severe acute respiratory syndrome coronavirus 2 (SARS-CoV-2). COVID-19 causes a spectrum of disorders, with various clinical manifestations. Patient condition might vary from asymptomatic or mildly symptomatic respiratory infection to severe interstitial pneumonia progressing to acute respiratory distress syndrome (ARDS), sepsis, and multiorgan failure [1, 2]. Some patients develop a severe proinflammatory state associated with a unique coagulopathy and procoagulant endothelial phenotype. Several changes in hemostasis, such as prolongation of prothrombin time, elevated levels of D-dimer, fibrinogen, factor VIII and von Willebrand factor, and low platelet count, have been previously reported in patients with COVID-19 [2, 3]. In addition, the disease was repeatedly associated with higher risk of venous thromboembolism (VTE) in hospitalized patients [3]. Several studies reported a VTE incidence of 2–5% [4]. Nevertheless, patients with COVID-19 could be at increased risk for arterial thrombosis due to suggested COVID-19-associated endothelial damage, usually manifesting in individuals without significant preexisting atherosclerosis [2, 5, 6]. We present a case series of patients with acute aortic thrombosis manifesting with systemic embolism associated with recent COVID-19 infection. Ambulatory oral factor Xa inhibition (FXaI) was used for the treatment of thromboembolic events.

2. Case Reports

2.1. Case No. 1. A 58-year-old male patient was admitted to our department for left subcostal pain. The patient had a history of symptomatic COVID-19 disease one month prior the hospitalization, leading symptoms were an elevated body temperature of up to 38°C lasting three days and weakness. The patient had a history of arterial hypertension and was treated with perindopril, amlodipine, and indapamide. Laboratory tests showed an elevated C-reactive protein (CRP) levels, creatinine levels, elevated concentration of D-dimer (3.86 g/mL), and fibrinogen (12.06 g/L). Leukocytosis with neutrophilia was present in the blood count. Other coagulation parameters were normal. Microbiological examinations were negative. A computed tomography pulmonary angiogram (CTPA) was performed without signs of pulmonary embolism. An accessory finding of a mural thrombus on the posterior wall of the descending aorta just behind the subclavian artery was found (Figure 1), together with a finding of a splenic infarction. A regular clinical examination for malignancy was performed, but no signs of cancer were found. No other risk factors for arterial or venous thrombosis were found. We examined antiphospholipid and anticardiolipin antibodies to exclude antiphospholipid syndrome with negative results. We started anticoagulation therapy immediately (nadroparin dosed 9500 IU twice daily subcutaneously for initial 5 days, then apixaban dosed 5 mg twice daily). Blood cultures were negative; thoracic and transesophageal echocardiography was performed, and no cardiac source of embolism was found. The further course of hospitalization went uncomplicated. The patient was discharged home on oral apixaban with an outpatient follow-up. Two months after the discharge, a control CT angiography of the aorta was performed. There was no residual thrombosis in the descending aorta. During this follow-up period, the white blood cells count restored to normal values. Based on these results, anticoagulation was subsequently terminated.

2.2. Case No. 2. A 62-year-old female patient with a history of arterial hypertension, gastroesophageal reflux disease, autoimmune thyroiditis, and recent COVID-19 infection presented with sudden pain and paresthesia in the left lower extremity. Laboratory tests showed slightly elevated CRP (21.6 mg/L) and elevated concentration of D-dimer (1.2 g/mL) and fibrinogen (4.45 g/L). Other coagulation parameters were normal. Antiphospholipid and anticardiolipin antibodies were negative. The patient overcame COVID-19 infection a month before, with bilateral pneumonia requiring hospitalization and oxygen supplementation. CT angiography was performed showing a fluttering thrombus in the descending aorta (Figure 2) and a closure of the left popliteal artery. The patient had no history of arterial or venous thrombosis, and evaluation for malignancy was also negative. The popliteal artery thrombotic closure was confirmed by digital subtraction angiography (DSA), and local thrombolysis was administrated, followed by intravenous body weight-adjusted heparin administration. Control DSA showed successful recanalization of the occluded popliteal artery. The patient was discharged home on oral rivaroxaban (20 mg daily) and aspirin (100 mg daily). A month later, a control CTA of the thoracic and abdominal aorta was performed with no signs of thrombosis.

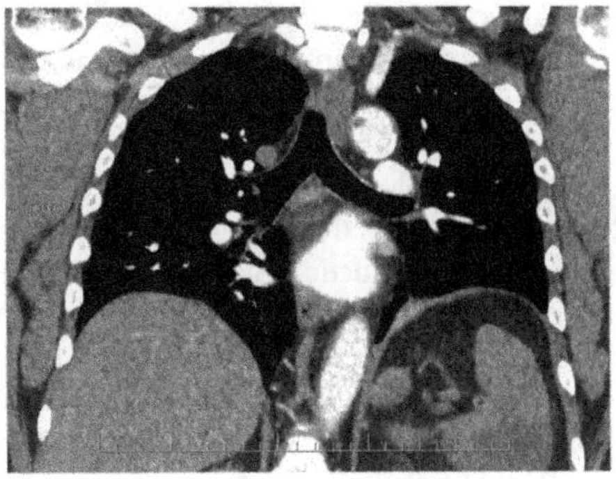

Figure 1: CT angiography showing aortic thrombosis (case no. 1).

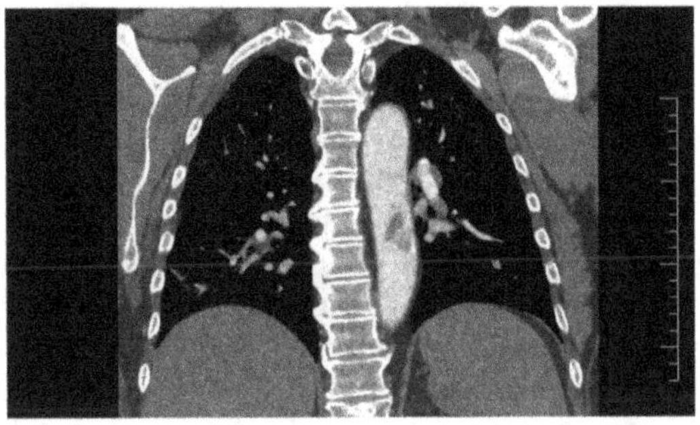

Figure 2: Fluttering aortic thrombosis on CT angiography (case no. 2).

3. Discussion

COVID-19 may predispose patients to an increased risk of thrombotic complications through various pathophysiological mechanisms [7]. Although venous thrombotic events in COVID-19 patients have been well described, there is limited evidence about arterial thrombosis in patients with COVID-19 [8]. According to the study of Cheruiyot et al., the anatomical distribution of arterial thrombotic events occurred in limb arteries (39%), cerebral arteries (24%), great vessels (aorta, common iliac artery, common carotid artery, and brachiocephalic trunk; 19%), coronary arteries (9%), and superior mesenteric artery (8%) [8]. In our cases, patients with initial abnormal thrombus formation in thoracic aorta manifested with secondary systemic embolism (with splenic infarction and acute limb ischemia). Therefore, CT-aortography should be probably included in the diagnostic approaches when searching for "cardiac source" of systemic embolism in patients with COVID-19. In both patients, COVID-19 was confirmed by a reverse transcription-polymerase chain reaction (PCR). Both patients overcame COVID-19 approximately one month before the diagnosis of aortic thrombosis. Whereas one patient had a mild course of the disease, the second patient had a moderate course of the disease with the need for hospitalization and oxygen administration. This indicates that there is no direct relationship between the risk of COVID-19-associated arterial thrombosis and COVID-19 clinical severity.

Another, yet not answered, question is how to treat COVID-19-related arterial thrombosis and systemic embolism. Therapeutic anticoagulation is being traditionally administrated in acute phase, preferring parenteral heparin or low-molecular-weight heparin (LMWH) administration in COVID-19 patients. Systemic thrombolysis could be an option in severe cases with life-threatening acute ischemia [9]; however, systemic thrombolysis is connected with high risk of serious bleeding. Thus, local thrombolysis could be a favorable approach, allowing the reduction of drug doses and reducing the risk of hemorrhage [10]. In our best knowledge, one of our cases is just the second one reporting the successful use of local (catheter-derived) thrombolysis in patient with COVID-19-related acute limb ischemia. Going further, LMWH anticoagulation is traditionally preferred in individuals with COVID-19. However, long-term LMWH therapy is unpleasant, connected with local complications, which reduce the compliance and possibly lead to increased risk of therapy failure. Oral direct FXaI could be a useful alternative therapeutic option, as it demonstrates the therapeutic effect in both arterial and venous thrombosis [11]. Nevertheless, the real-world experiences with this therapy in patients with COVID-19-related arterial thrombosis/systemic embolism are very limited. In our best knowledge, this is the first report about successful use of ambulatory oral FXaI inhibition for the treatment of COVID-19-related aortic thrombosis and systemic embolism. Furthermore, it is not entirely clear whether to coadminister antiplatelet therapy in these patients or not. Searching the relevant medical literature, there is no study dealing with this problem. Right now, the issue remains unexplained, and it is probably necessary to use a "patient-tailored" approach and assess the risk of future atherosclerosis-related vascular events. Concluding, the issue of optimal antithrombotic therapy for arterial thrombosis and systemic requires further research.

Consent

The patient agreed to participate in the research and signed informed consent for research participation.

Acknowledgments

This study was supported by project APVV 16-0020 (Slovakia Research and Development Agency), by Project of Research Agency of Slovakia Ministry of Education, Science and Sports ((VEGA) 1/0090/20), and by research project of Comenius University in Bratislava (UK/183/2021).

References

[1] A. Hajra, S. V. Mathai, S. Ball et al., "Management of thrombotic complications in COVID-19: an update," *Drugs*, vol. 80, no. 15, pp. 1553–1562, 2020.

[2] G. D. Wool and J. L. Miller, "The impact of COVID-19 disease on platelets and coagulation," *Pathobiology*, vol. 88, no. 1, pp. 15–27, 2021.

[3] N. C. Chan and J. I. Weitz, "COVID-19 coagulopathy, thrombosis, and bleeding," *Blood*, vol. 136, no. 4, pp. 381–383, 2020.

[4] Y. Sandoval, J. L. Januzzi Jr, and A. S. Jaffe, "Cardiac troponin for assessment of myocardial injury in COVID-19: JACC review topic of the week," *Journal of the American College of Cardiology*, vol. 76, no. 10, pp. 1244–1258, 2020.

[5] G. T. Gerotziafas, M. Catalano, M. P. Colgan et al., "Guidance for the management of patients with vascular disease or cardiovascular risk factors and COVID-19: position paper from VAS-European independent foundation in angiology/vascular medicine," *Thrombosis & Haemostasis*, vol. 120, no. 12, pp. 1597–1628, 2020.

[6] F. Moroni and L. Baldetti, "COVID-19 and arterial thrombosis: a potentially fatal combination," *International Journal of Cardiology*, vol. 322, pp. 286–290, 2021.

[7] L. Ortega-Paz, D. Capodanno, G. Montalescot, and D. J. Angiolillo, "Coronavirus disease 2019-associated thrombosis and coagulopathy: review of the pathophysiological characteristics and implications for antithrombotic management," *Journal of American Heart Association*, vol. 10, no. 3, Article ID e019650, 2021.

[8] I. Cheruiyot, V. Kipkorir, B. Ngure, M. Misiani, J. Munguti, and J. Ogeng'o, "Arterial thrombosis in Coronavirus disease 2019 patients: a rapid systematic review," *Annals of Vascular Surgery*, vol. 70, pp. 273–281, 2021.

[9] P. Patel, Y. Yu, S. Zia, F. Padberg, M. Curi, and J. Huang, "Systemic thrombolysis as initial treatment of COVID-19 associated acute aortoiliac and lower extremity arterial thrombosis," *Annals of Vascular Surgery*, vol. 70, pp. 297–301, 2021.

[10] K. Muhammad, T. G. Tantawy, R. R. Makar, and O. Olojugba, "Successful catheter-directed thrombolysis for acute lower limb ischemia secondary to COVID-19 infection," *Annals of Vascular Surgery*, vol. 71, pp. 103–111, 2021.

[11] A. Polzin, L. Dannenberg, M. Thienel et al., "Noncanonical effects of oral thrombin and factor Xa inhibitors in platelet activation and arterial thrombosis," *Thrombosis & Haemostasis*, vol. 121, no. 02, pp. 122–130, 2021.

24

A Rare Case of Extensive Cerebral Venous Sinus Thrombosis Complicated by Heparin-Induced Thrombocytopenia

Noman Ahmed Jang Khan, Ashar Farooqi, and Mohamed Alsharedi

Joan C. Edwards School of Medicine at Marshall University, Huntington, WV 25701, USA

Correspondence should be addressed to Noman Ahmed Jang Khan; khanno@marshall.edu

Academic Editor: Gergely Feher

Cerebral venous sinus thrombosis (CVST) is a rare but potentially life-threatening cause of stroke. Several risk factors have been identified including hypercoagulable state, malignancy, use of oral contraceptives, pregnancy, head injury, infection, and prothrombotic states such as heparin-induced thrombocytopenia (HIT). HIT is a prothrombotic state leading to thrombosis in several distinct locations including CVST requiring prompt discontinuation of heparin and initiation of nonheparin anticoagulation to prevent catastrophic consequences. Very rarely, HIT can complicate the ongoing CVST leading to worsening thrombosis and clinical deterioration. We here report an exceedingly rare case of CVST complicated by HIT in a 22-year-old female patient who showed remarkable clinical improvement after discontinuation of heparin and initiation of argatroban.

1. Introduction

Cerebral venous sinus thrombosis (CVST) is a rare but life-threatening cause of cerebrovascular events [1]. Anticoagulation remains the mainstay treatment for CVST even in cases with associated intracerebral hemorrhage [2]. Heparin is one of the most used anticoagulation agents used in the treatment of CSVT. In rare instances, heparin can cause heparin-induced thrombocytopenia (HIT) which can lead to worsening of ongoing thrombosis. We here report a case of a genetically predisposed patient who developed extensive CVST due to use of vaginal estradiol ring, in whom heparin treatment was complicated by HIT. Very few similar cases have been reported in the literature [3].

2. Case Presentation

A 22-year-old right-handed female was brought to the hospital with generalized tonic clonic seizures and reduced level of consciousness. Her initial vitals were temperature 98 F, blood pressure 110/67, pulse 105 bpm, and respiratory rate 20 breaths/min. Initial laboratory workup including complete blood count, electrolytes, creatinine, and liver function panel were unremarkable. During the initial neurological exam, the patient was stuporous and minimally responsive to verbal and tactile stimulation. On motor and sensory testing, she grimaced and appropriately withdrew to noxious stimuli in all four extremities. No nuchal rigidity or other signs of meningism were noted. No prior history of central nervous system abnormalities was reported. The patient had an etonogestrel/ethinyl estradiol vaginal ring for the past few months, and family history was also significant for unprovoked deep vein thrombosis (DVT) at an early age in a maternal uncle. Initial magnetic resonance imaging (MRI) brain with and without contrast demonstrated extensive thrombosis and complete occlusion of the superior, straight, left transverse, and sigmoid sinuses extending into the left cortical draining veins proximally and into the left internal jugular vein distally (Figure 1). FLAIR sequence also showed cortical edema in left posterior parietal region correlated with an area of diffusion restriction on DWI sequence which raised concern for venous infarction (Figure 2). Due to the extensive CVST, the patient was started on unfractionated heparin therapy with frequent/interval monitoring of activated partial thromboplastin time (aPTT) and the vaginal ring was removed. Mannitol was started for

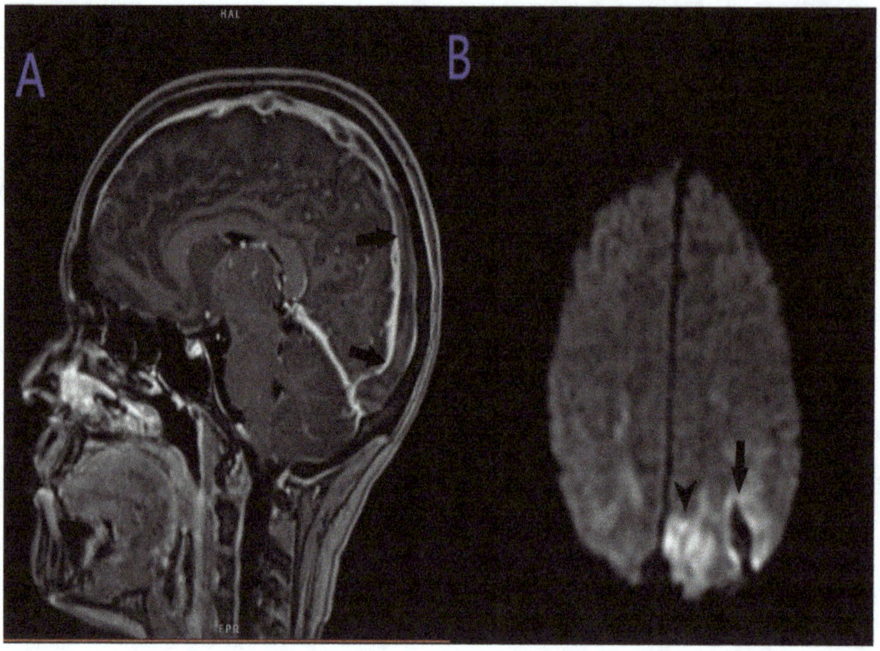

FIGURE 1: Magnetic resonance imaging (MRI) of the brain with contrast. (a) Postcontrast sagittal view showing extensive filling defect in the superior sagittal sinus consistent with thrombosis. (b) Diffusion weighted imaging (DWI) coronal view demonstrating left parietal lobe infarct (arrow) and hemorrhage (arrowhead).

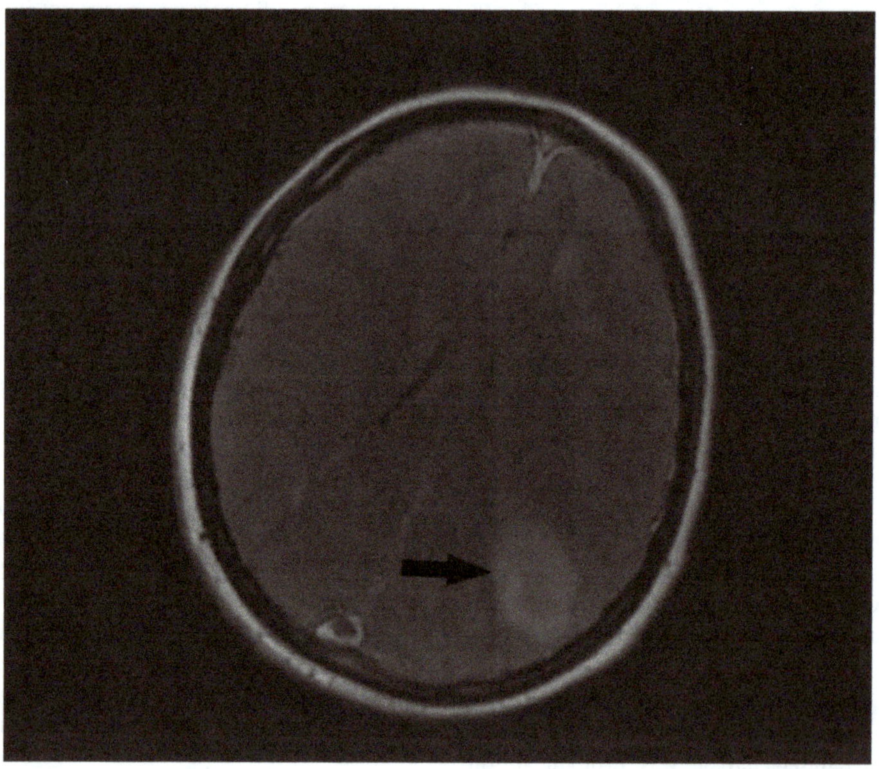

FIGURE 2: Magnetic resonance imaging (MRI) of the brain with contrast, T2 flair showing left parietal lobe hemorrhagic infarct (arrow).

persistently elevated intracranial pressure (ICP). Video electroencephalogram (vEEG) findings were suggestive of encephalopathy with a potential epileptic focus in the left temporal region. No clinical electrographic seizure was noted, and the patient was kept on levetiracetam for seizure prophylaxis. Subsequently, hypercoagulability workup showed positive Factor V Leiden heterozygous mutation. Despite treatment with anticoagulation (AC) and hyperosmolar therapies, no improvement was appreciated in the patient's overall condition. Cerebral angiography with

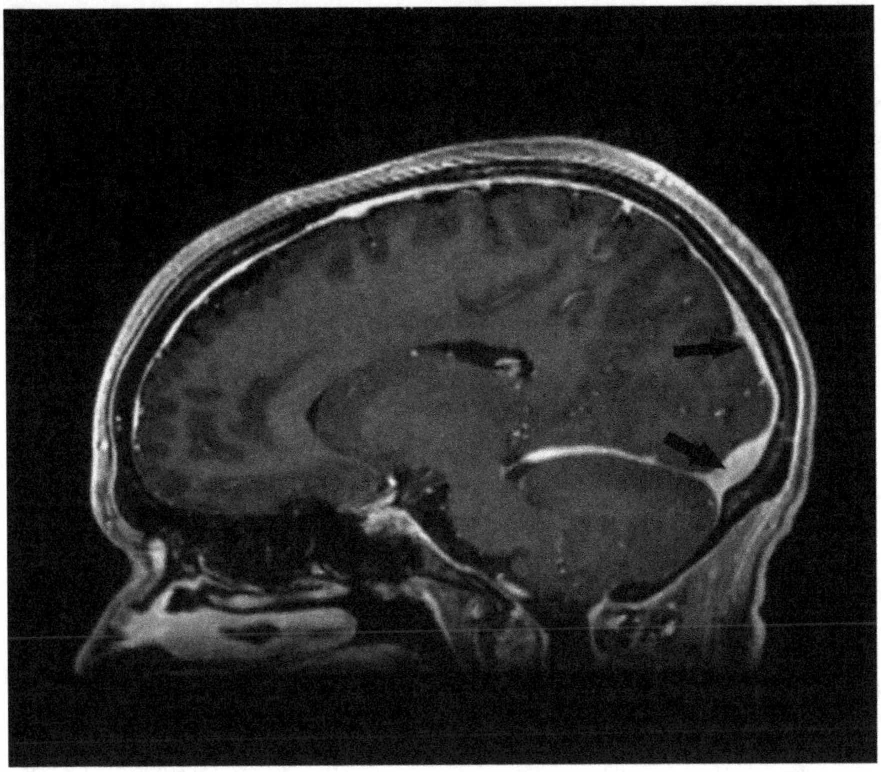

FIGURE 3: Magnetic resonance imaging (MRI) of the brain with contrast, postcontrast sagittal view showing marked improvement in the previously seen filling defect in the superior sagittal sinus (arrows).

endovascular thrombolysis was attempted twice to recanalize but were not successful in relieving the clot burden. After 6 days of continuous heparin administration, there was a sudden drop in platelet counts, i.e., from 217,000 to 117,000 per microliter of blood. The 4T score was 5, indicative of intermediate probability HIT. Heparin was immediately stopped for a presumptive diagnosis of HIT. Repeat MRI brain with and without contrast showed persistent thrombosis and infarct (Figure 2). Due to extensive thrombosis and ongoing need for AC, the patient was started on parenteral argatroban and a HIT panel was sent. The platelet factor 4 (PF-4) assay came back elevated at 1.211 OD (optical density) which was later confirmed with a strongly positive serotonin release assay (SRA). Patient's clinical condition markedly improved and became more awake and responsive in the next few days. Repeat MRI brain demonstrated improvement in clot burden and markedly reduced density of thrombosis with much improved intraluminal contrast flow (Figure 3). Her platelets rebounded on argatroban, and a decision was made to switch to direct oral AC such as apixiban. She was eventually discharged in a stable condition.

3. Discussion

CVST is a life-threatening venous thrombosis which accounts for approximately 0.5 to 1% of all strokes [1]. Several risk factors have been identified, including hypercoagulable states, malignancy, use of oral contraceptives, pregnancy, head injury, infection, and rarely prothrombotic states such as HIT [4]. Very rarely, CVST can be complicated by HIT, leading to worsening of thrombosis and clinical deterioration [3]. HIT is a transient prothrombotic state triggered by exposure to heparin products, predominantly with unfractionated heparin and less likely with low molecular weight heparin (LMWH). The incidence of HIT is approximately 0.5–1% of patients who received therapeutic doses of heparin [3]. In a large analysis by Dhakal et al. where HIT coding was used for the diagnosis of HIT in the National Inpatient Sample (NIS), it was found that 0.065% or 1/1500 of inpatients had HIT [5]. Older age, female gender, higher versus lower doses of heparin, cardiovascular procedures, and UFH versus LMWH are some of the reported risk factors for HIT [6, 7].

The mechanism of HIT is complex. It is an immune-mediated prothrombotic state caused by the formation of antibodies against platelet factor 4 (PF-4) and heparin complex. It then leads to the initiation of a severe procoagulant response by vascular endothelial cells, generating platelets, microparticles, monocytes, and neutrophil extracellular traps, causing thrombocytopenia and thrombosis [8]. Thrombocytopenia is the hallmark of HIT, while thromboembolic complications were found in approximately one third of patients [5].

The most common presentation is a drop in platelet count, occurring at least 4 to 5 days and up to 15 days after exposure to heparin. Rarely, thrombosis can precede the manifestation of thrombocytopenia, making the diagnosis challenging [3]. In patients with CVST and underlying HIT, the most common symptom was headache (60%), followed by altered mental status, visual disturbances, and seizures

[9]. HIT should be suspected in patients with a 30–50% decrease in platelet count and recent heparin exposure. In our patient, the workup for HIT was promptly pursued when platelets dropped from 217,000 to 117,000.

The 4T score is the most widely used pretest clinical score for HIT validated by the American Society of Hematology [10]. The score includes thrombocytopenia, the presence of thrombosis, the timing relative to heparin exposure, and other causes of thrombocytopenia. The HIT Expert Probability (HEP) score is another validated pretest clinical test based on the consensus of 26 HIT experts and was found to be equally effective in several studies [11]. In patients with CVST, intracranial hemorrhage (ICH) was the most dreaded complication and was primarily due to occluded cerebral sinus. This highlights the importance of early diagnosis and discontinuation of heparin in cases where HIT is suspected, as it can lead to further worsening of the thrombosis and higher mortality [9].

The diagnosis of HIT is well established. Two types of assays are well described in the guidelines: functional and immunoassays. Immunoassays are easily available screening tests with a high negative predictive value (NPV) but lack specificity, requiring confirmatory testing in positive cases [12]. However, in a large meta-analysis of approximately 15,000 patients, several immunoassays such as polyspecific enzyme-linked immunosorbent assay (ELISA) with an intermediate threshold, polyspecific chemiluminescent immunoassay (CLIA) with a high threshold, lateral flow immunoassay, and immunoglobulin G (IgG)-specific CLIA with a low threshold were found to be associated with sensitivity and specificity of >95% [13]. The serotonin release assay (SRA) is the most widely accepted functional assay for the diagnosis of HIT and detects platelet activation by identifying the serotonin release in the presence of the patient's serum and heparin [14]. It is considered the gold standard test for the diagnosis of HIT with a sensitivity and specificity of >95%.

The first step in the management of HIT with CVST is the discontinuation of all sorts of heparin products, including UFH, LMWH, and heparin flushes. Due to the highly prothrombotic state, anticoagulation with a nonheparin agent is essential [15]. The association of CVST with ICH makes it extremely challenging but requires continued anticoagulation despite the hemorrhage, as discontinuation of the anticoagulation will lead to drastic worsening of thrombosis and hemorrhage [9]. Our patient suffered worsening clinical deterioration despite being on therapeutic dose heparin and showed remarkable clinical improvement after discontinuation of heparin and initiation of argatroban. There are several potential options for anticoagulation in patients with HIT-induced thrombosis, including direct thrombin inhibitor (DTI), fondaparinaux, danaparoid, and direct oral anticoagulants (DOACs) [16]. There is no preferred agent for AC, but argatroban (DTI) is preferred by many experts in the acute setting due to its shorter duration of effect [17].

4. Conclusion

HIT is a rare but life-threatening prothrombotic state leading to thrombosis in several distinct locations. CVST is a rare manifestation of HIT requiring prompt discontinuation of heparin and initiation of nonheparin AC to prevent catastrophic consequences. The diagnosis and workup of HIT should be promptly pursued in patients with CVST, thrombocytopenia, and recent exposure to heparin products. In cases where heparin was started for the treatment of CVST and new occurrence of thrombocytopenia, HIT should be strongly suspected. Discontinuation of heparin and initiation of nonheparin AC are the key management steps. Currently, no agent is superior to other, but large prospective studies are needed to better identify the agent of choice.

References

[1] G. Saposnik, F. Barinagarrementeria, R. D. Brown et al., "Diagnosis and management of cerebral venous thrombosis: a statement for healthcare professionals from the American Heart Association/American Stroke Association," *Stroke*, vol. 42, no. 4, pp. 1158–1192, 2011.

[2] K. M. Einhaupl, A. Villringer, S. Mehraein et al., "Heparin treatment in sinus venous thrombosis," *The Lancet*, vol. 338, no. 8767, pp. 597–600, 1991.

[3] S. K. Lee, R. Willinsky, and K. Terbrugge, "Dural sinus thrombosis complicated with heparin induced thrombocytopenia and thrombosis (HITT)," *Interventional Neuroradiology: Journal of Peritherapeutic Neuroradiology, Surgical Procedures and Related Neurosciences*, vol. 8, no. 1, pp. 77–80, 2002.

[4] S. F. T. M. de Bruijn and J. Stam, "Clinical features and prognostic factors of cerebral venous sinus thrombosis in a prospective series of 59 patients," *Journal of Neurology, Neurosurgery & Psychiatry*, vol. 70, no. 1, pp. 105–108, 2001.

[5] B. Dhakal, L. B. Kreuziger, L. Rein et al., "Disease burden, complication rates, and health-care costs of heparin-induced thrombocytopenia in the USA: a population-based study," *The Lancet Haematology*, vol. 1, pp. e220–31, 2018.

[6] T. E. Warkentin, J. A. I. Sheppard, C. S. Sigouin, T. Kohlmann, P. Eichler, and A. Greinacher, "Gender imbalance and risk factor interactions in heparin-induced thrombocytopenia," *Blood*, vol. 108, no. 9, pp. 2937–2941, 2006.

[7] N. Martel, J. Lee, and P. S. Wells, "Risk for heparin-induced thrombocytopenia with unfractionated and low-molecular-weight heparin thromboprophylaxis: a meta-analysis," *Blood*, vol. 106, no. 8, pp. 2710–2715, 2005.

[8] G. M. Arepally and D. B. Cines, "Pathogenesis of heparin-induced thrombocytopenia," *Translational Research*, vol. 225, pp. 131–140, 2020.

[9] M. M. J. Bauman, R. M. Naylor, and E. F. Wijdicks, "HIT in the head: a systematic review of cerebral venous sinus thrombosis in classical and autoimmune heparin-induced thrombocytopenia," *Journal of Thrombosis and Thrombolysis*, vol. 52, no. 3, pp. 952–961, 2021.

[10] A. Cuker, G. M. Arepally, B. H. Chong et al., "American Society of Hematology 2018 guidelines for management of venous thromboembolism: heparin-induced thrombocytopenia," *Blood Advances*, vol. 2, no. 22, pp. 3360–3392, 2018.

[11] A. M. Pishko, S. Fardin, D. S. Lefler et al., "Prospective comparison of the HEP score and 4Ts score for the diagnosis of heparin-induced thrombocytopenia," *Blood Advances*, vol. 2, no. 22, pp. 3155–3162, 2018.

[12] E. J. Favaloro, G. McCaughan, and L. Pasalic, "Clinical and

laboratory diagnosis of heparin induced thrombocytopenia: an update," *Pathology*, vol. 49, no. 4, pp. 346–355, 2017.

[13] M. Nagler, L. M. Bachmann, H. Ten Cate, and A. ten Cate-Hoek, "Diagnostic value of immunoassays for heparin-induced thrombocytopenia: a systematic review and meta-analysis," *Blood*, vol. 127, no. 5, pp. 546–557, 2016.

[14] T. E. Warkentin, D. M. Arnold, I. Nazi, and J. G. Kelton, "The platelet serotonin-release assay," *American Journal of Hematology*, vol. 90, no. 6, pp. 564–572, 2015.

[15] E. Gleichgerrcht, M. Y. Lim, and T. N. Turan, "Cerebral venous sinus thrombosis due to low-molecular-weight heparin-induced thrombocytopenia," *The Neurologist*, vol. 22, no. 6, pp. 241–244, 2017.

[16] G. M. Arepally, "Heparin-induced thrombocytopenia," *Blood*, vol. 129, no. 21, pp. 2864–2872, 2017.

[17] B. Tardy-Poncet, P. Nguyen, J. C. Thiranos et al., "Argatroban in the management of heparin-induced thrombocytopenia: a multicenter clinical trial," *Critical Care*, vol. 11, 2015.

Acute Portal Vein Thrombosis during COVID-19 Convalescent Phase

Shoja Rahimian, Tushar Pawar, Ian Garrahy, and Andrew Rettew

Department of Hematology & Oncology, Reading Hospital, West Reading, PA, USA

Correspondence should be addressed to Shoja Rahimian; shorahimian@gmail.com

Academic Editor: Gergely Feher

Acute portal vein thrombosis represents a less common type of venous thromboembolism, even among the prothrombotic complications of coronavirus disease 2019 (COVID-19). Such complications are primarily reported during the active phase of infection. The case here describes acute portal vein thrombosis following resolution of COVID-19 in a 44-year-old male who presented with abdominal pain. Abdominal imaging identified portal and other splanchnic vein thromboses. Studies for hypercoagulable conditions were negative. Polymerase chain reaction was negative for severe acute respiratory syndrome coronavirus-2; however, IgG serology was positive. The case highlights the importance of considering thrombotic complications, particularly splanchnic vein thromboses, in patients with recent COVID-19.

1. Background

Coronavirus disease 2019 (COVID-19) caused by severe acute respiratory syndrome corovirus-2 (SARS-CoV-2) has been associated with hypercoagulability, with recent literature identifying arterial and venous thromboembolism as potential complications [1]. There have also been several case studies that describe portal vein thrombosis (PVT) complicating COVID-19, most of which occurred at the time of acute respiratory illness [2–11]. We present a case of acute portal vein thrombosis in the convalescent phase as identified by the presence of SARS-CoV-2 IgG antibodies.

2. Case Presentation

A 44-year-old Hispanic male with no significant past medical history presented to the emergency department with severe intermittent abdominal pain of four-week duration with acute worsening prior over 3-4 days. He had experienced fever, nausea, anosmia, and dry cough four weeks prior at which time he self-quarantined for 14 days, given that concern for COVID-19. SARS-CoV-2 testing was not performed at that time. His symptoms resolved within one week of isolation. On arrival, he was afebrile (38.2°C), tachycardic (115 beats per minute), and with normal blood pressure (124/74 mmHg). Oxygen saturation was 94% on room air. He endorsed worsening generalized abdominal pain, but denied nausea, vomiting, or diarrhea. Comprehensive metabolic panel was significant for elevated AST of 44 (range: 13–39 IU/L) and ALT of 172 (range: 7–52 IU/L). CBC was unremarkable. Acute hepatitis panel and serum lipase were negative, while AFP tumor marker was undetectable. Other pertinent labs included elevated CRP, 8.60 (range: <1 mg/dL); ESR, 18 (range: 0–15 mm/hr); ferritin, 385 (range: 24–336 ng/ml); and D-dimer 14,540 (normal <500 ug/L). Given his recent symptoms, a nasal swab SARS-CoV-2 RNA polymerase chain reaction (PCR) was ordered which was negative.

A computed tomographic (CT) scan of abdomen with contrast (Figure 1) demonstrated dilation with heterogeneous density involving the portal and splenic veins associated with surrounding inflammation concerning for portal vein thrombosis. Subsequent magnetic resonance imaging of the abdomen/pelvis (Figure 2) revealed findings consistent with extensive thrombosis of the portal vein extending from the superior mesenteric and splenic veins

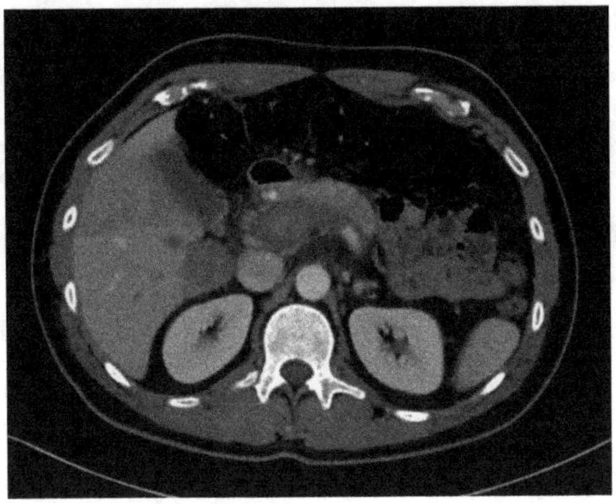

FIGURE 1: CT scan of abdomen/pelvis showing portal vein thrombosis.

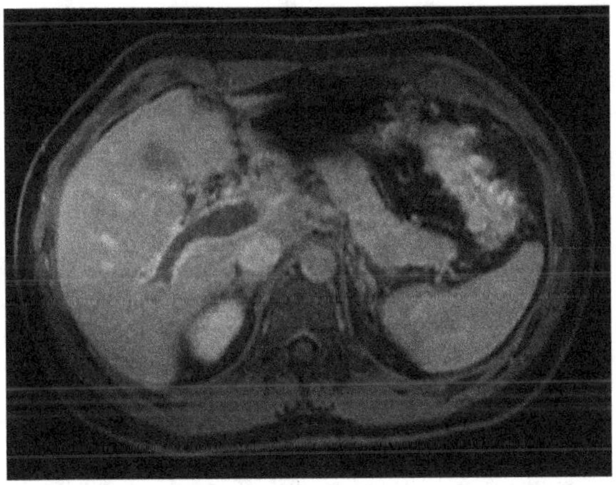

FIGURE 2: MRI of abdomen and pelvis with portal vein thrombosis.

through to the intrahepatic branches most pronounced within the right hepatic lobe. Given his extensive PVT, absence of personal or family history of thrombosis, and no evidence for underlying malignancy, further workup for hypercoagulable state was commenced. Myeloproliferative neoplasm panel was negative for JAK2 V617F, JAK2 exon 12–14, CALR, and MPL mutations. High sensitivity flow cytometry for paroxysmal nocturnal hemoglobinuria was also negative. Other pertinent negatives included factor V Leiden mutation, prothrombin gene mutation, anti-cardiolipin antibodies, beta-2 glycoprotein antibodies, and lupus anticoagulant.

Given the negative workup and considering his prior illness suspicious for COVID-19, a SARS-CoV-2 IgG antibody test was ordered which returned positive, signifying prior disease in this patient who had not been vaccinated. He was initially started on enoxaparin 1 mg/kg twice daily and then transitioned to rivaroxaban at discharge. He completed 6 months of oral anticoagulation with complete resolution of thrombosis on posttreatment CT abdomen with no plan for further anticoagulation given the provoked nature of the thrombosis in the setting of COVID-19.

3. Discussion

The clinical presentation of COVID-19 infection is variable, ranging from a flu-like syndrome with mild respiratory symptoms to viral pneumonia with acute respiratory failure, multiorgan dysfunction, and death. Studies and clinical experience identify that patients with COVID-19 infection have an acquired hypercoagulable state with predisposition to thrombotic events [12].

Case reports have documented a tendency of SARS-CoV-2 to induce a hypercoagulable state, including the formation of in situ pulmonary embolism. Several cases of PVT associated with COVID-19 have been reported in the literature to date. The prevalence of PVT in the general population is rare at around 1% as evidenced in a Swedish study where 23,796 consecutive autopsies demonstrated presence of PVT in 254 patients. 28% of these cases were associated with liver cirrhosis, 44% primary and secondary hepato-biliary malignancies, 10% abdominal infections, 3% in myeloproliferative neoplasms, and 14% idiopathic [13]. PVT with COVID-19 represents a less common association, but one that requires further review and acknowledgement. Our case represents the ninth such reported COVID-19-associated PVT [2–9].

An in-depth review of the other eight case reports showed that most PVT occurred while the patients were hospitalized. Similar to the case described by Franco-Moreno et al., our case is unique in which the portal vein thrombosis occurred after resolution of his respiratory symptoms several weeks prior. PCR testing was negative, and the diagnosis of COVID-19-associated portal vein thrombosis was made using antibody testing in an individual who had not been previously vaccinated.

The highly inflammatory potential of SARS-CoV-2 is thought to be related to its prothrombotic pathogenicity. It has been shown that the virus binds to the transmembrane angiotensin-converting enzyme 2 (ACE2) protein to enter type II pneumocytes, macrophages, and other cell types. In humans, an abundant expression of ACE2 receptors on endothelial cells enhances their vulnerability to SARS-CoV-2 binding, membrane fusion, and viral entry causing vascular injury [14–16]. SARS-CoV-2 infection of the host can affect the ACE/ACE2 ratio, leading to downregulation of ACE2 [17]. An increase in the ACE/ACE2 ratio is profibrotic and proinflammatory. Most viral infections lead to host cell death leading to the local intense inflammatory response that may become systemic because of the potent proinflammatory cytokines, such as interleukin-1β and interleukin-18 [18]. The ACE2-facilitated inflammatory response can lead to development of hepatic portal venous gas in COVID-19 which is a possible finding in the patients with abdominal pain [19].

Platelets represent the interplay between hemostasis and the immune system. The potent local and systemic cytokine production leads to platelet activation and interaction with neutrophils. Leukocyte activation, specifically neutrophils, through various vascular and platelet pathways, may promote neutrophil extracellular trap (NET) formation. NETs are large, extracellular, weblike structures composed of cytosolic and granule proteins assembled on a scaffold of decondensed chromatin [20]. NETs are an ideal foundation for binding activated platelets, erythrocytes, and leukocytes, and activating factor XI, and generating thrombin for fibrin production. Panigada et al. assessed several coagulation parameters in patients with COVID-19 [21]. Using whole blood thromboelastography, the authors identified hypercoagulability features, such as a decrease in time to fibrin formation, a decrease in time to clot formation, and increase in clot strength. Using thromboelastographic analysis, other authors found low lysis at 30 minutes, which is suggestive of fibrinolysis shutdown. The excess of fibrin deposition and fibrinolysis shutdown leads to intravascular thrombosis and, finally, to clinical thromboembolic complications.

4. Conclusion

Acute thrombotic complication associated with COVID-19 has been reported in the literature with most cases occurring within the COVID-19 hospitalization and consists mainly of deep vein thrombosis and pulmonary embolism. This case gives an insight into rare thrombotic complication of PVT occurring in relatively mild COVID-19, and a few weeks after resolution of his infection-associated symptoms. This case highlights the importance of considering thrombotic complications in patients with ongoing or recent COVID-19 and thus a low threshold for imaging studies and treatment as indicated.

Consent

Patient privacy: Identifiable information and dates have been removed from this report to protect patient privacy. As such no written consent has been obtained from the patient as there is no patient identifiable data included in this case report.

References

[1] D. Bari, S. Paul, W. Reese, K. Danny, and S. K. Douglas, "Hypercoagulability in COVID-19: identification of arterial and venous thromboembolism in the abdomen, pelvis, and lower extremities," *American Journal of Roentgenology*, vol. 216, 2021.

[2] A. Ofosu, D. Ramai, A. Novikov, and V. Sushma, "Portal vein thrombosis in a patient with COVID-19," *American Journal of Gastroenterology*, vol. 115, no. 9, pp. 1545-1546, 2020.

[3] V. La Mura, A. Artoni, I. Martinelli et al., "Acute portal vein thrombosis in SARS-CoV-2 infection: a case report," *American Journal of Gastroenterology*, vol. 115, no. 7, pp. 1140–1142, 2020.

[4] K. W. Abeysekera, H. Karteszi, A. Clark, and F. H. Gordon, "Spontaneous portomesenteric thrombosis in a non-cirrhotic patient with SARS-CoV-2 infection," *BMJ Case Reports*, vol. 13, no. 12, Article ID e238906, 2020.

[5] A. Franco-Moreno, E. Piniella-Ruiz, J. Montoya-Adarraga et al., "Portal vein thrombosis in a patient with COVID-19," *Thrombosis Research*, vol. 194, pp. 150–152, 2020.

[6] R. Borazjani, S. R. Seraj, M. J. Fallahi, and Z. Rahmanian, "Acute portal vein thrombosis secondary to COVID-19: a case report," *BMC Gastroenterology*, vol. 20, no. 1, p. 386, 2020.

[7] S.-W. Low, K. L. Swanson, J. D. McCain, A. Sen, A. Kawashima, and S. F. Pasha, "Gastric ischemia and portal vein thrombosis in a COVID-19-infected patient," *Endoscopy*, vol. 52, no. 12, pp. E465–E466, 2020.

[8] B. Singh, P. Kaur, and M. Maroules, "Splanchnic vein thrombosis in COVID-19: a review of literature," *Digestive and Liver Disease*, vol. 52, no. 12, pp. 1407–1409, 2020.

[9] S. H. Jafari, R. Naseri, N. Khalili, S. Haseli, and M. Bahmani, "Portal vein thrombosis associated with COVID-19: points to consider," *BJR case reports*, vol. 6, no. 3, Article ID 20200089, 2020.

[10] W. Hassan and H. K.-A. Ramadan, "COVID-19 as a novel etiology of portal vein thrombosis: change in the current management concepts," *Infectious Diseases*, vol. 53, no. 2, pp. 148–150, 2021.

[11] P. Keshavarz, F. Rafiee, H. Kavandi, S. Goudarzi, F. Heidari, and A. Gholamrezanezhad, "Ischemic gastrointestinal complications of COVID-19: a systematic review on imaging presentation," *Clinical Imaging*, vol. 73, pp. 86–95, 2021.

[12] J. M. Connors and J. H. Levy, "COVID-19 and its implications for thrombosis and anticoagulation," *Blood*, vol. 135, no. 23, pp. 2033–2040, 2020.

[13] M. Ögren, D. Bergqvist, M. Björck, S. Acosta, H. Eriksson, and N. H. Sternby, "Portal vein thrombosis: prevalence, patient characteristics and lifetime risk: a population study based on 23 796 consecutive autopsies," *World Journal of Gastroenterology*, vol. 12, no. 13, pp. 2115–2119, 2006.

[14] N. Tang, H. Bai, X. Chen, J. Gong, D. Li, and Z. Sun, "Anticoagulant treatment is associated with decreased mortality in severe coronavirus disease 2019 patients with coagulopathy," *Journal of Thrombosis and Haemostasis*, vol. 18, no. 5, pp. 1094–1099, 2020.

[15] T. Iba, M. Levi, and J. H. Levy, "Sepsis-induced coagulopathy and disseminated intravascular coagulation," *Seminars in Thrombosis and Hemostasis*, vol. 46, no. 1, pp. 89–95, 2020.

[16] P. Zhou, X. L. Yang, X. G. Wang et al., "A Pneumonia outbreak associated with a new coronavirus of probable bat origin," *Nature*, vol. 579, pp. 270–273, 2020.

[17] H. Kai and M. Kai, "Interactions of coronaviruses with ACE2, angiotensin II, and RAS inhibitors-lessons from available evidence and insights into COVID-19," *Hypertension Research*, vol. 43, no. 7, pp. 648–654, 2020.

[18] Z. Varga, A. J. Flammer, P. Steiger et al., "Endothelial cell infection and endotheliitis in COVID-19," *The Lancet*, vol. 395, no. 10234, pp. 1417-1418, 2020.

[19] N. Mumoli, S. Cerutti, and A. Mazzone, "Man with fever, cough, and weakness," *Journal of the American College of Emergency Physicians Open*, vol. 1, no. 6, pp. 1755-1756, 2020.

[20] V. Brinkmann, U. Reichard, C. Goosmann et al., "Neutrophil extracellular traps kill bacteria," *Science*, vol. 303, no. 5663, pp. 1532–1535, 2004.

[21] M. Panigada, N. Bottino, P. Tagliabue et al., "Hypercoagulability of COVID-19 patients in intensive care unit: a report of thromboelastography findings and other parameters of hemostasis," *Journal of Thrombosis and Haemostasis*, vol. 18, no. 7, pp. 1738–1742, 2020.

26

Aggressive Central Nervous System Relapse after Autologous Stem Cell Transplant in Multiple Myeloma: Case Reports and Literature Review

Rui Bergantim,[1,2,3,4] Juliana Bastos,[1,4] Maria José Soares,[1,5] Bruno Carvalho,[4,6] Pedro Soares,[7] Cristina Marques,[8] Jennifer Costa,[9] José Eduardo Guimarães,[1,2,3,4] and Fernanda Trigo[1]

[1]*Hematology Department, Centro Hospitalar São João, Porto, Portugal*
[2]*i3S—Instituto de Investigação e Inovação em Saúde, Universidade do Porto, Porto, Portugal*
[3]*Cancer Drug Resistance Group, IPATIMUP—Institute of Molecular Pathology and Immunology of the University of Porto, Porto, Portugal*
[4]*Hematology & Oncology Unit, Department of Medicine, Faculty of Medicine of University of Porto, Porto, Portugal*
[5]*Cytogenetics Laboratory, Hematology Department, Centro Hospitalar São João, Porto, Portugal*
[6]*Neurosurgery Department, Centro Hospitalar São João, Porto, Portugal*
[7]*Radiotherapy Department, Centro Hospitalar São João, Porto, Portugal*
[8]*Flow Cytometry Laboratory, Clinical Pathology Department, Centro Hospitalar São João, Porto, Portugal*
[9]*Pathologic Anatomy Department, Centro Hospitalar São João, Porto, Portugal*

Correspondence should be addressed to Rui Bergantim; rui.bergantim@gmail.com

Academic Editor: Vincent Ribrag

Extramedullary disease is an aggressive presentation at diagnosis and relapse for multiple myeloma (MM) patients. Central nervous system (CNS) is a very rare manifestation of the extramedullary disease, accounting for less than 1% of MM on diagnosis and relapse. Neurological symptoms are unspecific and usually attributed to other causes. We present two patients with CNS-MM at relapse after autologous stem cell transplant highlighting the importance of clinical suspicion and interdisciplinarity at diagnostic workup as well as the need for intensive therapeutic options on such rare and aggressive cases. The presence of neurological abnormalities in anamnesis and physical examination on a patient with MM should always prompt to suspect of a CNS involvement, and active investigation must be undertaken. MRI is the standard radiological method to detect CNS-MM, with histopathological corroboration by stereotactic biopsy and CSF evaluation alongside. Treatment of CNS-MM should include two essential approaches—be able to cross the BBB and treat the systemic disease. There is no standard therapy for this extramedullary relapse, and a tailored and multiple therapy should be promptly started—intrathecal therapy, radiotherapy, and systemic therapy, including an immunomodulator.

1. Introduction

Despite novel agents and increased better outcomes over the last years, multiple myeloma (MM) is still an incurable disease marked by a relapse-remission pattern [1]. Mainly characterized as a medullary monoclonal proliferation, some cases present as extramedullary disease. At diagnosis, the extramedullary disease is found in 6 to 8% of patients [2, 3], while another 10 to 30% may develop extramedullary lesions later in their disease course [4, 5]. Central nervous system (CNS) is a very rare manifestation of the extramedullary disease, accounting for less than 1% of MM on diagnosis and relapse [6, 7]. CNS involvement is defined by the presence of monoclonal malignant plasma cells in the cerebrospinal fluid or by magnetic resonance imaging revealing the bone-derived contiguous intraparenchymal mass, isolated intraparenchymal tumors, and leptomeningeal involvement [7–9]. Neurological symptoms are unspecific and usually attributed to other causes [8]. CNS-MM confers a dismal prognosis, with median survival of less than six months, being a final event in the majority of these patients [9, 10]. Approach and therapeutic options are not established for these patients, and many data rely on case reports and small series [9, 11, 12]. We present two patients with CNS-MM at relapse after autologous stem cell transplant, highlighting the importance of clinical suspicion and interdisciplinarity at diagnostic workup as well as the need for intensive therapeutic options on such rare and aggressive cases.

2. Case 1

A 49-year-old man with no relevant past clinical history was diagnosed with MM IgG/lambda, Durie–Salmon stage IIIA, and International Staging System (ISS) stage III in August 2011. He presented with anemia and extensive lytic bone lesions. His bone marrow assessment showed 33% of abnormal plasma cells, CD38+ve, CD19−ve, CD56+ve, CD45−ve, and lambda+ve and no alterations on fluorescence in situ hybridization (FISH) of selected plasma cells. He was treated with bortezomib and dexamethasone (VD) for four cycles, achieving a very good partial response (VGPR), followed by stem cell mobilization with an intermediate dose of cyclophosphamide (4 g/m^2) collecting enough cells for two grafts, and he underwent his first autologous stem cell transplant (ASCT), after high-dose melphalan (200 mg/m^2) in January 2012. He maintained a VGPR at day 100 assessment.

In August 2014, he presented with severe back pain leading to a progression evaluation. He had new lytic bone lesions on the skull and lumbar vertebrae, hypercalcemia, anemia, and acute renal failure. A new bone marrow assessment was performed with 40% of abnormal plasma cells and no FISH abnormalities identified. He was treated with bortezomib, thalidomide, and dexamethasone (VTD) for four cycles reaching only a partial response (PR), followed by high-dose melphalan and was submitted to a second ASCT in January 2015. At day 100, he had a VGPR and was kept on observation.

Nine months after the second ASCT, he was admitted to the emergency room in a comatose status (Glasgow Coma Scale 9). His blood workup was normal without anemia, hypercalcemia, or acute renal failure. Brain computed tomography showed two large extra-axial lesions (a right one with 3.5 cm in the coronal plane and a left one with 1.4 cm in the coronal plane), spontaneously hyperdense and with strong contrast enhancement, a posterior extension of the lesion with dura mater infiltration, and diffuse involvement of the calvaria. Due to rapid neurological deterioration, the patient was operated by neurosurgery with resection of the right frontoparietal lesion with invaded dura and bone flap. The anatomopathological exam showed an extensive collection of plasma cells with high mitotic activity, multiple apoptotic bodies, and extension to the adjacent bone. FISH analysis of the excised cerebral mass showed del17p13.2 (72%) and del1q21 (30%). His bone marrow had no plasma cells, no FISH abnormalities, and no serum or urine monoclonal component, besides the serum immunofixation Ig/lambda and abnormal free light chain ratio (Figure 1). After recovery from surgery, he started DPACE (dexamethasone, 40 mg/day; cisplatin, 10 mg/m^2/day; doxorubicin, 10 mg/m^2/day; cyclophosphamide, 400 mg/m^2/day; and etoposide, 40 mg/m^2/day from days 1 to 4) completing 2 cycles, simultaneous cranial radiotherapy (RT) 40 Gy (2.5 Gy per day for 16 sessions and a photon energy of 6 Mv), and started lenalidomide plus dexamethasone until progression. He completed 14 cycles. Although he had never achieved a complete remission, there was full recovery of functional and cognitive status with a performance status ECOG of zero by the time he was on the second cycle of lenalidomide. He progressed in May 2017 with a new lumbar extramedullary disease and was put on daratumumab, bortezomib, and dexamethasone (DVD) and simultaneous lumbar RT (3 Gy per day for ten sessions and photon energy 6 Mv). He completed 10 cycles of DVD, progressing again with extensive bone disease and rapid deterioration of his performance and was referred to palliative care.

3. Case 2

A 66-year-old man with no relevant past clinical history was diagnosed with MM IgA/lambda, Durie–Salmon stage IIIA, and ISS stage III in December 2014. He presented with anemia, hypercalcemia, and extensive lytic bone lesions on skull, thoracic, and lumbar vertebrae and long bones. His bone marrow showed 40% of plasma cells, CD38+ve, CD138+ve, CD19−ve, CD56−ve, and CD45+ve, with del13q (87%). He was treated with bortezomib, thalidomide, and dexamethasone for four cycles, achieving a complete remission (CR). He was proposed for ASCT with stem cell collection after steady mobilization with G-CSF and underwent high-dose melphalan (200 mg/m^2) followed by ASCT in May 2015. On day 100 evaluation, he remained in CR.

In November 2015, he went to the daycare hospital with refractory nausea, holocranial headaches, confusion, diplopia, and loss of muscle strength in the upper right limb with three days duration. His blood workup was normal without anemia, hypercalcemia, or acute renal failure. A cerebral scan was performed showing spontaneous hypodense areas with intense cortical contrast enhancement in the bilateral insula, anterior temporal predominance of the left sulci, engorgement of the left choroid plexus, right cerebellar tentorium, right prepontine cistern and pituitary gland, supratentorial ventricular dilatation with transependymal edema, extensive leptomeningeal infiltration, and focal low density on the sphenoid body. A lumbar puncture was performed with the cerebrospinal fluid (CSF) analysis showing 39 cells, of which 88.7% were monoclonal plasma cells CD38+ve, CD19−ve, CD56−ve, and CD45-het, with lambda restriction and all with del1q21 on FISH. His bone marrow had no plasma cells, no FISH abnormalities, and no serum or urine monoclonal component, besides the

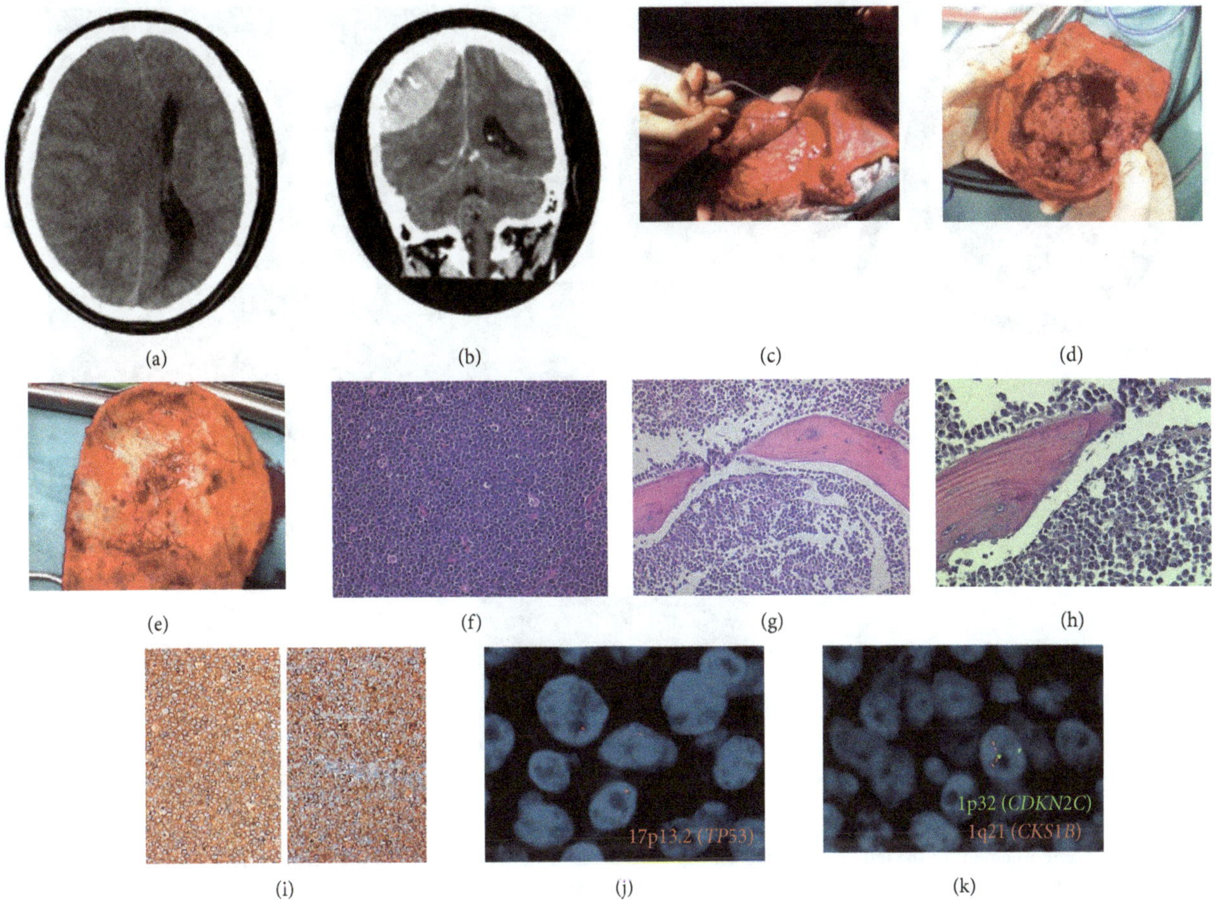

Figure 1: (a, b) Two massive extra-axial tissue lesions (right: 3.5 cm in the coronal plane; left: 1.4 cm in the coronal plane), spontaneously hyperdense and with strong contrast enhancement; posterior extension of the lesion with dura infiltration; diffuse involvement calvaria; (c–e) surgical removal of the frontoparietal bone flap with adherent soft tissue lesion and dura mater; (f–i) plasma cells with high mitotic activity and apoptotic bodies. (HE, 200x); invasion of the bone. (HE, 400x); (j, k) 1p32/1q21 and 17p13.2 (TP53) copy number changes evaluated by FISH: (j) (17p13.2, red), (k) (1p32, green and 1q21, red), (j) del17p13.2 (30%), and (k) 1q21 gain (72%).

reappearance of serum immunofixation IgA/lambda and abnormal free light chain ratio (Figure 2). He received intrathecal therapy with methotrexate, cytarabine, and dexamethasone until plasma cell clearance that was achieved after 10 IT administrations followed by neuroaxial RT 16.5 Gy (1.5 Gy per day for 11 sessions with photon energy 6 MvM; this was suspended due to severe pancytopenia). Poor performance status at that point did not allow him to start systemic cytotoxic therapy, and he was treated with lenalidomide plus dexamethasone until progression. He completed ten cycles, with biochemical and imagiological criteria of CR and improved performance status, recovering his autonomy in most of all daily tasks. He progressed on September 2016 with new lumbar and cutaneous extramedullary disease and started daratumumab and dexamethasone, without response at the second cycle and deterioration of performance status being referred to palliative care.

4. Discussion

Both cases represented great challenges in clinical practice. No guidelines and recommendations are evident in how to approach or treat CNS-MM. In the past years, many reports suggest that extramedullary disease, including CNS-MM, increased with the use of novel agents and autologous stem cell transplant [4, 13]. So far, no plausible or physiopathological explanation supports this inference. Novel agents and ASCT are nowadays standard in clinical practice and better outcomes achieved with first-line therapies with longer disease-free survival and overall survival probably allow for appearance of new patterns of relapse and clinical manifestations [10, 14].

Clinical manifestations are usually unspecific and heterogeneous, like headaches and cognitive dysfunction, resembling other common neurological diseases or chemotherapy-related side effects making the differential diagnosis hard in clinical practice [7, 8]. The presence of neurological abnormalities in anamnesis or physical examination on a patient with MM should always prompt to suspect CNS involvement, and active investigation must be undertaken.

Contrast-enhanced MRI is the standard radiological method to detect CNS-MM, but sensitivity is lower for hematological malignancies (20–37%) than for solid tumors (85%) [15]. Moreover, patterns are diverse and difficult to

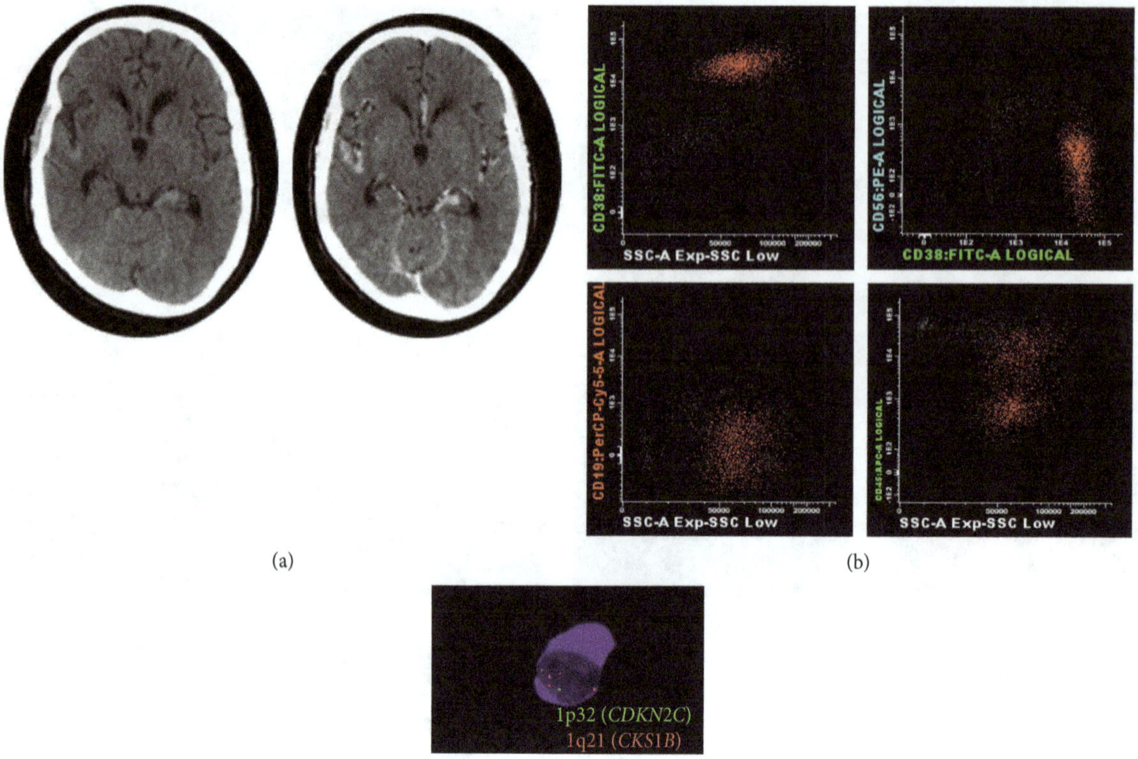

(a) (b) (c)

FIGURE 2: (a) Spontaneous hypodense areas with intense cortical contrast enhancement in bilateral insulae, anterotemporal predominance of the left grooves, engorgement of the left choroid plexus, right cerebellar tent, the right side of the prepontine cistern and pituitary gland, supratentorial ventricular dilatation with transependymal edema, focal area of lower density in the body of sphenoid, and extensive leptomeningeal infiltration. (b) 35 cells (87% neoplastic plasma cells). (c) 1p32/1q21 copy number changes evaluated by FISH: 1p32, green; 1q21, red and 1q21 gain (100%).

interpret with most series accounting 10% of false negatives [6, 15–17]. Consequently, it is recommended to perform histopathological corroboration and CSF evaluation alongside, whenever possible. Stereotactic biopsy is not always possible due to location of infiltration, patient limitations, or the urgency of treatment initiation. Nonetheless, it should always be considered. The isolated presence of MM cells is not enough to assume CNS involvement, as in other hematologic diseases [16]. However, when it happens in a patient with MM that confers a high suspicion of effective CNS-MM. CSF protein is often increased while glucose is low on CNS-MM [7]. The recent use of abnormal free light chain detection on CSF is an attractive complementary diagnostic tool as it appears to be more reliable than cytology and could be used in patients with other equivocal test results and allowing therapy monitoring additionally [18–20]. The opposite is also possible, and patients have been described with intraparenchymal and dura lesions but with no plasma cells on CSF [17, 21]. Our two patients illustrate these disparities of findings. One had a massive involvement of CSF with a meningeal enhancement on MRI, but with no intracerebral mass to biopsy, while the other had an evident intraparenchymal infiltration with extension to dura mater and adjacent bone, evident on radiological studies, which was surgically approached. On clinical practice, all data available should be integrated to assure a reliable and safe diagnosis of CNS-MM.

There is no independent prognostic factor for the development of MM-CNS. Some reports show that the high-risk patients share some classic features related to adverse prognosis such as lambda and IgD subtype, high-burden disease, stage III by Salmon–Durie, high lactate dehydrogenase (LDH), and high beta2-microglobulin [7, 14, 22–24]. Extramedullary disease, rather than CNS, is often associated with the development of CNS-MM. Plasma cell leukemia (PCL) is a rare extramedullary MM characterized by >20% or 2000/mL monoclonal plasma cells in peripheral blood. Some series assume this as a significant factor for CNS involvement [7, 9]. More recently, the use of circulating plasma cells on peripheral blood also showed a higher burden disease and risk for adverse relapse [25]. Unfavorable chromosomal abnormalities are related to various extramedullary sites, indicating they may drive different clonal architecture between the bone marrow and extramedullary disease, mainly a possible role of p53 mutations/del17p13 [16, 26–28]. CD56 is an adhesion molecule involved in plasma cell migration from the bone marrow, and its downregulation could promote MM cells to escape their natural environment and establish a plasma cell metastasis at distance [16]. Chang et al. reported that the expression of CD56 was detected in 80% of patients with non-CNS-MM ($n = 84$) and was absent in 62.5% of the bone marrow and 88% of CSF with CNS-MM ($n = 8$) [29]. Nonetheless, other reports failed to demonstrate this [6]. Despite these risk factors, many cases of CNS-MM are characterized by a low degree of bone marrow infiltration [16], as in our 2 cases. The role of a CNS assessment in high-risk patients and concurrently prophylactic intrathecal chemotherapy is debatable, but it should be considered individually in the future patients.

There are some hypotheses that emerge as an explanation of CNS involvement by MM. The first hypothesis relates to the hematogenous spread in which plasma cells and earlier cells with a specific phenotype can induce metastasis to distant places as extramedullary disease including the CNS [14, 16]. In some series, the negativity of CD56 is appointed as a hallmark to CNS-MM, as its function is essential on the cell-cell adhesion as exposed previously [29, 30]. Bladé and colleagues in a report demonstrated that decreased expression of adhesion molecules on myelomatous cells over time would promote egress from the BM environment [4]. The presence of circulating plasma cells, and in an extreme phase as plasma cell leukemia, is also appointed to support this hypothesis. A report showed that 40% of PCL patients had some CNS involvement [9]. None of our patients had negativity to CD56 or circulating plasma cells. Autopsy studies in MM patients revealed that circulating plasma cells can infiltrate the arachnoid veins diffusely leading to the destruction of the arachnoid trabeculae and continuously spread to CSF [8, 16]. A second hypothesis, mainly in patients with parenchymal infiltration, is related to the extension of tissue infiltration of adjacent skull lytic lesions or plasmacytomas, varying from 39% to 65% in some cohorts [9, 14]. A third hypothesis relies on the continuous growth of plasma cell nesting in CNS, as the sanctuary site compared to lymphoblastic leukemia, during treatment, as most of the MM drugs used do not cross the brain-blood barrier (BBB) [7, 10]. Finally, the clonal heterogeneity of MM could play a role on this rare relapse, in which there is emergence of a clone population resistant to the treatment used on previous lines [14, 16, 31, 32]. Our patients showed high-risk features of the parenchymal tumor and CSF that were not present at diagnosis, hypothesizing that probably the relapse arose from a different clone rather than the one present at diagnosis.

Regarding the treatment of CNS-MM, significant data are sparse, and there is no standard of care advised for these cases [6, 9, 18]. Treatment of CNS-MM should include two essential approaches—be able to cross the BBB and treat the systemic disease.

Immunomodulators can cross the BBB. Thalidomide can be detected on CSF after an oral administration of 100 mg/day, peaking a concentration of 30% to 60% as compared to the plasma [33–35]. However, its neurological side effects, low efficacy on del17p patients, and the long time to an actual drug effect make its use less appealing. Lenalidomide and pomalidomide also showed to penetrate the BBB in animal studies [36–38]. Recent data showed that lenalidomide and pomalidomide have a moderate effect displaying a 30 to 40% penetration but enough to be effective in clearance of neoplastic cells from CSF in both lymphomas and myeloma [39–41]. This effect can also be seen with other disease markers and patients with POEMS exhibited a reduction of CSF VEGF when treated with lenalidomide as well as patients with astrocytoma, endorsing the use of IMIDs as antiangiogenic agents with the ability to cross the BBB [42].

Bortezomib has a limited penetration through the BBB in animal models, with few reports showing its inefficacy in CNS-MM patients [43], and there are no data on ixazomib. Marizomib is the only proteasome inhibitor known to be able to cross the BBB, even though it has so far not proved to be of use on MM. Radiolabeled marizomib showed 30% CNS biodistribution compared to blood levels on animal models. In a case report, two patients were treated with marizomib with reduction of CSF plasmacytosis as well as symptoms and had radiological improvement. Nonetheless, its activity in systemic myeloma is yet to be determined [44]. No precise data are supporting the use of daratumumab on CNS-MM, and the case report on marizomib also showed that the clearance of CD38 cells from CSF suggested that daratumumab may also cross the BBB and recently a case report showed a successful outcome with the monoclonal antibody [44, 45].

Intrathecal chemotherapy (ITC) is mostly used in several hematological malignancies with CNS involvement with diverging results [9]. The intrathecal agents are normally used in combination with systemic therapy that theoretically penetrates the BBB, and its use in monotherapy may be ineffective. Several reports show that patients that received ITC have a longer survival of 7.2 to 20 months versus 1.4 to 5 months for the patients who did not receive ITC [18, 19]. In Case 2, with myelomatous meningitis, no systemic therapy was administrated due to the patient's bad performance status. As a bridge to start chemotherapy, intrathecal administration of recognized agents is quickly done and usually fast on malignant cells clearance. Some series showed that ITC and IMIDs containing regimens had higher median survival comparing to IMID's monotherapy or other drugs (17.1 months versus 4.6 months) [9].

Brain and neuraxial radiation, as there is a well-known pattern of plasma cell radiosensitivity, seems an essential coadjuvant therapy in CNS-MM [9]. Nonetheless, it carries significant toxicity and its application may be limited to older patients and with a bad performance status. In the literature review, radiation was the only treatment option which showed to be associated with prolonged survival, presenting a median survival of 3 months versus 0.81 months (without radiation) [18]. Nonetheless, in other reports, RT improved survival was evident only when combined with new agents as a coadjuvant treatment [24].

Standard chemotherapy used on MM as alkylating agents penetrates the BBB very poorly, with only 10% of melphalan levels found at LCR of treated patients [7]. The intensive chemotherapy combinations such as PACE are useful as salvage regimens in refractory/relapsed MM and PCL and appear to be a robust approach to systemic treatment to prevent further hematogenous spread to CNS and elimination of residual clones [46]. As a sole treatment for CNS disease, it is insufficient. The combination with immunomodulators and proteasome inhibitors such as VTD (bortezomib, thalidomide, and dexamethasone)-PACE and

VRD (bortezomib, lenalidomide, and dexamethasone)-PACE are attractive choices for this aggressive manifestation of MM [26, 35].

Our patients were treated according to presentation and performance status. In Case 1, the exuberance of presentation demanded a life-saving approach with the surgical approach, systemic therapy, radiotherapy, and immunomodulators. In Case 2, due to the absence of intraparenchymal tumor, the patient was treated with intrathecal chemotherapy, radiotherapy, and immunomodulators. We believe that the aggressive management of these patients followed by a continuous therapy with an agent that cross the BBB improved their survival comparing to published data.

Prognosis of CNS-MM is dismal across all series and case reports, with a post-CNS-MM survival of 3 to 6 months and does not appear to be different in patients treated with novel agents compared to those treated with conventional drugs [6, 7, 14, 18, 24]. In our cases, both patients had a surprising progression-free survival (PFS) of 14 and ten months, respectively, on Case 1 and 2. As prognostic factors are at relapse to post-CNS-MM survival, extramedullary disease and LDH continue to be strong predictors showing a tendency for more aggressive disease, demanding a closer follow-up [14]. The normal LDH and absence of other disease manifestations, including bone marrow infiltration, may influence the long PFS in our two patients.

These cases illustrate unusual patterns of CNS-MM involvement that could envisage two different hypotheses for CNS relapses such as the direct contiguous spread from the eroded lytic lesions of the skull (more probable in Case 1) and hematogenous spread of plasma cells (more probable in Case 2). Although rare, CNS involvement by MM should be considered in MM patients with neurological deficits/symptoms. There is no standard therapy for this extramedullary relapse, and a tailored aggressive therapy should be promptly started—ICT, RT, and systemic therapy, including an IMID. Even in the era of novel therapies, the prognosis of CNS involvement remains dismal, highlighting the need for adequate CNS penetration in MM novel drug development to improve these patients' outcomes.

Consent

Verbal and written consent was obtained from the patients for using this case for publication purposes. All data used in this case report were anonymized.

Authors' Contributions

RB was the patient's primary hematologist and performed data collection and wrote the manuscript. MJS, JC, CM, PS, and BC were involved in diagnostic tests and treatment plan and revised the data and the drafted paper. JEG and FT revised and supervised the drafted paper.

References

[1] S. K. Kumar, V. Rajkumar, R. A. Kyle et al., "Multiple myeloma," *Nature Reviews Disease Primers*, vol. 3, no. 1, pp. 1–20, 2017.

[2] B. Wirk, J. R. Wingard, and J. S. Moreb, "Extramedullary disease in plasma cell myeloma: the iceberg phenomenon," *Bone Marrow Transplantation*, vol. 48, no. 1, pp. 10–18, 2013.

[3] M. Varettoni, A. Corso, G. Pica, S. Mangiacavalli, C. Pascutto, and M. Lazzarino, "Incidence, presenting features and outcome of extramedullary disease in multiple myeloma: a longitudinal study on 1,003 consecutive patients," *Annals of Oncology*, vol. 21, no. 2, pp. 325–330, 2010.

[4] J. Bladé, C. Fernández de Larrea, L. Rosiñol, M. T. Cibeira, R. Jiménez, and R. Powles, "Soft-tissue plasmacytomas in multiple myeloma: incidence, mechanisms of extramedullary spread, and treatment approach," *Journal of Clinical Oncology*, vol. 29, no. 28, pp. 3805–3812, 2011.

[5] C. Varga, P. Xie, J. Laubach et al., "Development of extramedullary myeloma in the era of novel agents: No evidence of increased risk with lenalidomide-bortezomib combinations," *British Journal of Haematology*, vol. 169, no. 6, pp. 843–850, 2015.

[6] A. Jurczyszyn, A. Gozzetti, A. Cerase et al., "Central Nervous System Involvement by Multiple Myeloma: a Multi-Institutional Retrospective Study of 172 Patients," *Clinical Lymphoma Myeloma and Leukemia*, vol. 15, pp. e128–e129, 2015.

[7] L. Nieuwenhuizen and D. H. Biesma, "Central nervous system myelomatosis: review of the literature," *European Journal of Haematology*, vol. 80, no. 1, pp. 1–9, 2008.

[8] A.-o. Abdallah, S. Atrash, Z. Shahid et al., "Patterns of central nervous system involvement in relapsed and refractory multiple myeloma," *Clinical Lymphoma Myeloma and Leukemia*, vol. 14, no. 3, pp. 211–214, 2014.

[9] C. I. Chen, E. Masih-Khan, H. Jiang et al., "Central nervous system involvement with multiple myeloma: long term survival can be achieved with radiation, intrathecal chemotherapy, and immunomodulatory agents," *British Journal of Haematology*, vol. 162, no. 4, pp. 483–488, 2013.

[10] S. A. Gangatharan, D. A. Carney, H. M. Prince et al., "Emergence of central nervous system myeloma in the era of novel agents," *Hematological Oncology*, vol. 30, no. 4, pp. 170–174, 2012.

[11] C. Touzeau and P. Moreau, "How i treat extramedullary myeloma," *Blood*, vol. 127, no. 8, pp. 971–976, 2017.

[12] G. Varga, G. Mikala, L. Gopcsa et al., "Multiple myeloma of the central nervous System: 13 cases and review of the literature," *Journal of Oncology*, vol. 2018, Article ID 3970169, 7 pages, 2018.

[13] R. Ali, F. Ozkalemkas, A. Ozkan et al., "Bortezomib and extramedullary disease in multiple," *British Leukemia Research*, vol. 31, no. 8, pp. 1153–1155, 2007.

[14] E. Katodritou, E. Terpos, E. Kastritis et al., "Lack of survival improvement with novel anti-myeloma agents for patients with multiple myeloma and central nervous system involvement: the Greek myeloma study group experience," *Annals of Hematology*, vol. 94, no. 12, pp. 2033–2042, 2015.

[15] S. Ginkel, T. J. Snijders, N. W. C. J. Donk, C. J. M. Klijn, and M. L. D. Broekman, "Progressive neurological deficits in multiple myeloma: meningeal myelomatosis without MRI abnormalities," *Journal of Neurology*, vol. 259, no. 6, pp. 1231–1233, 2012.

[16] A. Marini, G. Carulli, T. Lari et al., "Myelomatous meningitis evaluated by multiparameter flow cytometry : report of a case and review of the literature," *Journal of Clinical and Experimental Hematopathology*, vol. 54, no. 2, pp. 129–136, 2014.

[17] A. Cerase, A. Tarantino, A. Gozzetti et al., "Intracranial involvement in plasmacytomas and multiple myeloma: a pictorial essay," *Neuroradiology*, vol. 50, no. 8, pp. 665–674, 2008.

[18] N. Majd, X. Wei, A. Demopoulos, A. Hormigo, A. Chari et al., "Characterization of central nervous system multiple myeloma in the era of novel therapies," *Leukemia & Lymphoma*, vol. 57, no. 7, pp. 1709-1713, 2016.

[19] D. Lee, A. Kalff, M. Low et al., "Central nervous system multiple myeloma—potential roles for intrathecal therapy and measurement of cerebrospinal fluid light chains," *British Journal of Haematology*, vol. 162, no. 3, pp. 371–375, 2013.

[20] M. Ise, C. Sakai, and K. Kumagai, "Meningeal myelomatosis developed after treatment with novel agents," *International Journal of Hematology*, vol. 98, no. 3, pp. 271-272, 2013.

[21] C. E. Méndez, B. J. Hwang, S. Destian, A. Mazumder, S. Jagannath, D. H. Vesole et al., "Intracranial multifocal dural involvement in multiple myeloma: case report and review of the literature," *Clinical Lymphoma Myeloma and Leukemia*, vol. 10, no. 3, pp. 220–223, 2010.

[22] R. Velasco, J. Petit, R. Llatjós, A. Juan, and J. Bruna, "Can leptomeningeal myelomatosis be predicted in patients with IgD multiple myeloma?" *Journal of Clinical Neuroscience*, vol. 17, no. 8, pp. 1071-1072, 2010.

[23] N. Ochiai, C. Shimazaki, A. Okano et al., "Meningeal relapse after double peripheral blood stem cell transplantation in IgD myeloma," *Leukemia & Lymphoma*, vol. 43, no. 3, pp. 641–643, 2002.

[24] A. Gozzetti, A. Cerase, F. Lotti et al., "Extramedullary intracranial localization of multiple myeloma and treatment with novel agents: a retrospective survey of 50 patients," *Cancer*, vol. 118, no. 6, pp. 1574–1584, 2012.

[25] R. Chakraborty, E. Muchtar, S. K. Kumar et al., "Serial measurements of circulating plasma cells before and after induction therapy have an independent prognostic impact in patients with multiple myeloma undergoing upfront autologous transplantation," *Haematologica*, vol. 102, no. 8, pp. 1439–1145, 2017.

[26] J. Lee, D. Smith, N. Rabin, J. Tobias, and K. Yong, "17P deleted multiple myeloma presenting with intracranial disease: durable remission after tailored management," *Hematological Oncology*, vol. 34, no. 3, pp. 165–170, 2016.

[27] A. B. T. Fassas, S. Ward, F. Muwalla et al., "Myeloma of the central nervous system: strong association with unfavorable chromosomal abnormalities and other high-risk disease features," *Leukemia & Lymphoma*, vol. 45, no. 2, pp. 291–300, 2004.

[28] H. Chang, S. Sloan, D. Li, and A. K. Stewart, "Multiple myeloma involving central nervous system: high frequency of chromosome 17p13.1 (p53) deletions," *British Journal of Haematology*, vol. 127, no. 3, pp. 280–284, 2004.

[29] H. Chang, E. S. Bartlett, B. Patterson, C. I. Chen, and Q. L. Yi, "The absence of CD56 on malignant plasma cells in the cerebrospinal fluid is the hallmark of multiple myeloma involving central nervous system," *British Journal of Haematology*, vol. 129, no. 4, pp. 539–541, 2005.

[30] I. M. S. Dahl, T. Rasmussen, A. Husebekk, and G. Kauric, "Differential expression of CD56 and CD44 in the evolution of extramedullary myeloma," *British Journal of Haematology*, vol. 116, no. 2, pp. 273–277, 2002.

[31] J. J. Keats, M. Chesi, J. B. Egan et al., "Clonal competition with alternating dominance in multiple myeloma," *Blood*, vol. 120, no. 5, pp. 1067–1076, 2012.

[32] Y. A. Wang, X. Yu, P. M. Silverman, R. L. Harris, and H. Edward, "The structure of F-pili," *Journal of Molecular Biology*, vol. 385, no. 1, pp. 22–29, 2010.

[33] Y. Hattori, M. Yabe, S. Okamoto, K. Morita, Y. Tanigawara, and Y. Ikeda, "Thalidomide for the treatment of leptomeningeal multiple myeloma," *European Journal of Hematology*, vol. 76, no. 4, pp. 358-359, 2006.

[34] P. Vicari, C. Ribas, and M. Sampaio, "Can thalidomide be effective to treat plasma cell leptomeningeal infiltration?" *European Journal of Haematology*, vol. 70, no. 3, pp. 198-199, 2003.

[35] H. Nahi, E. Svedmyr, R. Lerner et al., "Bendamustine in combination with high-dose radiotherapy and thalidomide is effective in treatment of multiple myeloma with central nervous system involvement," *European Journal of Haematology*, vol. 92, no. 5, pp. 454-455, 2014.

[36] C. E. Devoe, J. Y. Li, and A. M. Demopoulos, "The successful treatment of a recurrent intracranial, dural-based plasmacytoma with lenalidomide," *Journal of Neuro-Oncology*, vol. 119, no. 1, pp. 217–220, 2014.

[37] J. A. Muscal, Y. Sun, J. G. Nuchtern et al., "Plasma and cerebrospinal fluid pharmacokinetics of thalidomide and lenalidomide in nonhuman primates," *Cancer Chemotherapy and Pharmacology*, vol. 69, no. 4, pp. 943–947, 2012.

[38] A. Mussetti, S. Dalto, and V. Montefusco, "Effective treatment of pomalidomide in central nervous system myelomatosis," *Leukemia & Lymphoma*, vol. 54, no. 4, pp. 864–866, 2013.

[39] M. C. Cox, G. Mannino, L. Lionetto, V. Naso, M. Simmaco, and M. A. A. Spiriti, "Lenalidomide for aggressive B-cell lymphoma involving the central nervous system?" *American Journal of Hematology*, vol. 86, no. 11, p. 957, 2011.

[40] S. Anwer, F. Collings, K. Trace, Y. Sun, and A. Sternberg, "Cerebrospinal fluid penetrance of lenalidomide in meningeal myeloma," *British Journal of Haematology*, vol. 162, no. 2, pp. 281-282, 2013.

[41] Z. Li, Y. Qiu, D. Personett et al., "Pomalidomide shows significant therapeutic activity against CNS lymphoma with a major impact on the tumor microenvironment in murine models," *PLoS One*, vol. 8, no. 8, Article ID e71754, 2013.

[42] C. Briani, R. Manara, F. Lessi, V. Citton, R. Zambello, and F. Adami, "Pachymeningeal involvement in POEMS syndrome: dramatic cerebral MRI improvement after lenalidomide therapy," *American Journal of Hematology*, vol. 87, no. 5, pp. 539–541, 2012.

[43] G. Mele, S. Pinna, E. Alloro, M. C. Brocca, M. R. Coppi, and G. Quarta, "Inefficacy of bortezomib therapy for CNS involvement of refractory multiple myeloma," *Leukemia Research*, vol. 31, no. 5, pp. 721–723, 2007.

[44] A. Z. Badros, Z. Singh, B. Dhakal et al., "Marizomib for CNS-multiple myeloma," *Blood*, vol. 128, no. 22, p. 2118, 2016.

[45] E. Elhassadi, M. Murphy, D. Hacking, and M. Farrell, "Durable treatment response of relapsing CNS plasmacytoma using intrathecal chemotherapy, radiotherapy, and Daratumumab," *Clinical Case Reports*, vol. 6, no. 4, pp. 723–728, 2018.

[46] A. Lakshamn, P. P. Singh, S. V. Rajkumar et al., "Efficacy of VDT PACE-like regimens in treatment of relapsed/refractory multiple myeloma," *American Journal of Hematology*, vol. 93, no. 2, pp. 179–186, 2018.

It is very important to confirm the author(s) last and first names in order to be displayed correctly on our website as well as in the indexing databases:

Author 1
Given Names: Rui
Last Name: Bergantim

Author 2
Given Names: Juliana
Last Name: Bastos

Author 3
Given Names: Maria José
Last Name: Soares

Author 4
Given Names: Bruno
Last Name: Carvalho

Author 5
Given Names: Pedro
Last Name: Soares

Author 6
Given Names: Cristina
Last Name: Marques

Author 7
Given Names: Jennifer
Last Name: Costa

Author 8
Given Names: José Eduardo
Last Name: Guimarães

Author 9
Given Names: Fernanda
Last Name: Trigo

It is also very important for each author to provide an ORCID (Open Researcher and Contributor ID). ORCID aims to solve the name ambiguity problem in scholarly communications by creating a registry of persistent unique identifiers for individual researchers.

To register an ORCID, please go to the Account Update page (http://mts.hindawi.com/update/) in our Manuscript Tracking System and after you have logged in click on the ORCID link at the top of the page. This link will take you to the ORCID website where you will be able to create an account for yourself. Once you have done so, your new ORCID will be saved in our Manuscript Tracking System automatically.

27

Pancytopenia with Development of Persistent Neutropenia Secondary to COVID-19

Kathie Wu[1] **Yvonne Dansoa**[1,2] **and Priyanka Pathak**[1,2]

[1]*Geisinger Medical Center, 100 N Academy Ave, Danville 17822, PA, USA*
[2]*Department of Hematology/Oncology, 100 N Academy Ave, Danville17822, PA, USA*

Correspondence should be addressed to Kathie Wu; kwu1@geisinger.edu

Academic Editor: Pier Paolo Piccaluga

Viral infections have long been linked to hematologic dysfunction. With the rapid spread of COVID-19, various hematologic manifestations have emerged. While there have been several reports of immune thrombocytopenic purpura from SARS-CoV-2, concurrent lymphopenia and anemia have sparse. We describe a case of COVID-induced pancytopenia that presented months after initial COVID infection that initially responded to IVIG and steroids, but now with persistent neutropenia.

1. Introduction

Pancytopenia describes a condition in which there are simultaneous decreases in all three cell lines and can be attributed to a number of causes including nutritional deficiency, medications, malignancy, autoimmune disease, and infection. Viruses especially have long been associated with hematologic dysfunction, and the emersion of COVID-19 proved no exception [1]. There have been reports of isolated cell lines being impacted by COVID [2, 3], but we present a unique case of late onset pancytopenia in an immunocompetent patient, complicated by the development of unresolved neutropenia secondary to COVID.

2. Case Presentation

A 64-year-old female, with the medical history significant for only a remote history of breast cancer that was treated with lumpectomy in 2010, presented initially to the primary care office with concerns of petechiae of her oral mucosa. A few months prior, she got routine testing for COVID through work and found she was positive for COVID but was asymptomatic at that time. Routine blood work was obtained which revealed significant leukopenia and thrombocytopenia with WBC of 1.82 and platelets less than 3. Patient was given 2 units of platelet transfusion and admitted to the hospital.

On hospital day one, labs showed still worsening leukopenia with white count dropping further to 1.58. Despite the 2 units of platelet transfusion prior, platelet levels were still undetectable. Patient had no signs of active bleeding, but hemoglobin levels were still noted to drop by almost a gram from 11.8 to 10.9. Given high suspicion for an immune-mediated etiology of the pancytopenia, patient was started on dexamethasone 40 mg for 4 days and 2 doses of IVIG therapy. By hospital day four, patient continued to show rebound in her white count and platelet levels and her hemoglobin levels were starting to plateau off (Figures 1–3). Various tests were sent to determine underlying etiology of the pancytopenia. Laboratory tests including viral hepatitis, HIV, parvovirus, and rheumatological markers were unremarkable. Blood work was not consistent with a consumptive coagulopathy or thrombotic microangiopathy, and peripheral smear showed no blasts or schistocytes. A direct Coombs test, however, was positive with warm agglutinin, but the patient had nonelevated total or direct bilirubin levels at any point during her hospitalization that would have been suggestive of hemolytic anemia.

On one week follow-up, the patient had repeat blood work that showed sharp decline in both her white cell and

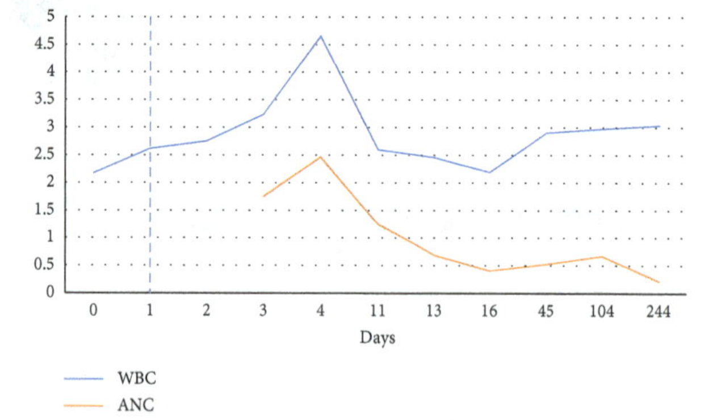

FIGURE 1: Trend in white blood cell count (WBC) in units of 10^9 L. Dashed line represents administration of IVIG and steroid therapy.

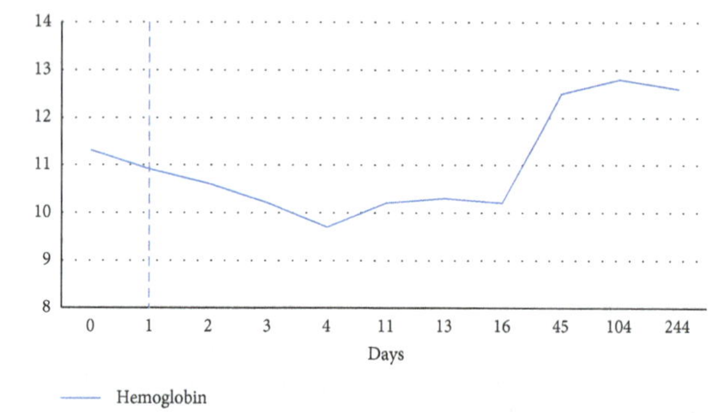

FIGURE 2: Trend in hemoglobin in units of g/dL. Dashed line represents administration of IVIG and steroid therapy.

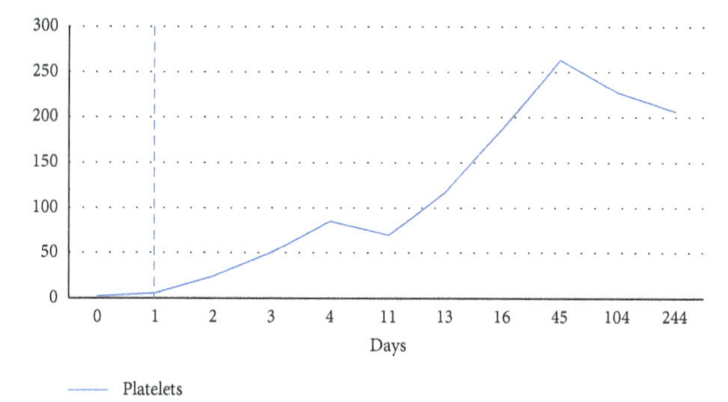

FIGURE 3: Trend in platelets in units of 10^4 μL. Dashed line represents administration of IVIG and steroid therapy.

platelet levels (Figure 1 and Figure 3). A bone marrow biopsy was pursued which revealed no concerning abnormalities. A few months later, blood work showed resolution of the anemia and thrombocytopenia, but patient was noted to have persistent leukopenia with ANC as low as 210 (Figure 3). As patient was otherwise asymptomatic, no further steroids or IVIG therapy was administered, but patient remains under close surveillance.

3. Discussion

Pancytopenia can result in the setting of nutrition deficiency, medications, or autoimmune processes, but with the improvement of the white count, hemoglobin, and platelets with IVIG and steroids, the positive Coombs, and considering a largely otherwise negative work up, the etiology of this patient's pancytopenia was thought to be immune mediated from her recent COVID infection. The effects of viral infections on hematopoiesis are well known, but the exact etiology by which viruses impact hematopoiesis are still under investigation. Various mechanisms including direct suppression of hematopoiesis by the virus, production of proinflammatory cytokines in response to viral infections, and invasion of the infection into the bone marrow have been hypothesized [4, 5]. Interestingly, there have been case reports published which have demonstrated infiltration of COVID-19 into the bone marrow that has tested positive via viral PCR [6].

COVID-19 causes a profound inflammatory response, and our patient initially responded well to steroid therapy to suppress inflammation which likely explains the initial improvement in her cell lines. As she only received four days of steroids which was a relatively short course, there may have been smoldering inflammation that was not adequately sequestered, allowing proinflammatory cytokines to damage the bone marrow. The initial bone marrow biopsy was unrevealing, but it may have been obtained early enough that the development of fibrosis was not yet detected. As our patient showed no infectious symptoms, there was no role for the use of granulocyte colony stimulating factor (G-CSF).

4. Conclusion

There have been emerging reports of a few cases of immune-mediated thrombocytopenia due to COVID-19, but literature has still been sparse, and most effects were seen in patients acutely hospitalized with COVID-19 infection, unlike our patient who presented months after initial resolution of the virus [7]. Again, there are many postulated mechanisms for etiology of disease, but what has been consistent across literature has been the response of COVID-19-induced pancytopenia to short courses of corticosteroids and intravenous immunoglobulin. Though there appears to be appropriate response to treatment, the progression of disease can be unpredictable as seen in our patient who initially improved with the same therapy then rebounded. The duration of the inflammatory effects of COVID-19 is unknown, but our patient's persistent neutropenia suggests that patients who have hematologic involvement during COVID-19 may benefit from longer courses of steroids. Though the bone marrow biopsy did not formally show bone marrow fibrosis, a longer course of steroids may help to reduce the activity of proinflammatory cytokines for longer periods of time and diminish possible long-term damage to the bone marrow. This case indicates that we may see lingering effects of COVID-19 well beyond the pulmonary manifestations of the disease and active surveillance must be maintained.

Consent

Patient consent was obtained for this study.

References

[1] A. Gupta, M. V. Madhavan, K. Sehgal et al., "Extrapulmonary manifestations of COVID-19," *Nature Medicine*, vol. 26, no. 7, pp. 1017–1032, 2020.
[2] S. Letícia de Oliveira Toledo, L. Sousa Nogueira, M. das Graças Carvalho, D. Romana Alves Rios, and M. de Barros Pinheiro, "COVID-19: review and hematologic impact," *Clinica Chimica Acta*, vol. 510, pp. 170–176, 2020.
[3] G. Lazarian, A. Quinquenel, M. Bellal et al., "Autoimmune haemolytic anaemia associated with COVID-19 infection," *British Journal of Haematology*, vol. 190, no. 1, pp. 29–31, 2020.
[4] M. F. Pascutti, M. N. Erkelens, and M. A. Nolte, "Impact of viral infections on hematopoiesis: from beneficial to detrimental effects on bone marrow output," *Frontiers in Immunology*, vol. 7, p. 364, 2016.
[5] Y. Zhao, J. He, J. Wang et al., "Development of pancytopenia in a patient with COVID-19," *Journal of Medical Virology*, vol. 93, no. 3, pp. 1219-1220, 2021.
[6] J. M. Hernandez, R. Quarles, S. Lakshmi et al., "Pancytopenia and profound neutropenia as a sequela of severe SARS-CoV-2 infection (COVID-19) with concern for bone marrow involvement," *Open Forum Infectious Diseases*, vol. 8, no. 2, Article ID ofab017, 2021.
[7] S. Bhattacharjee and M. Banerjee, "Immune thrombocytopenia secondary to COVID-19: a systematic review," *SN Comprehensive Clinical Medicine*, vol. 2, pp. 2048–2058, 2020.

28

Double-Hit Primary Plasma Cell Leukemia with *IGH/MYC* and *IGH/CCND1* Translocations

Masato Yasumi,[1] Takaya Endo,[1] Hiroshi Sata,[2] and Takahiro Karasuno[1]

[1]*Department of Hematology, Rinku General Medical Center, Izumisano, Japan*
[2]*Division of Hematology, Department of Internal Medicine, Daini Osaka Police Hospital, Osaka, Japan*

Correspondence should be addressed to Masato Yasumi; m-yasumi@rgmc.izumisano.osaka.jp

Academic Editor: Sergio Storti

Primary plasma cell leukemia (pPCL) is an aggressive variant of multiple myeloma (MM). Immunoglobulin heavy chain (*IgH*) translocations are found in a majority of pPCL cases, supporting a central relation to pathogenesis of pPCL. However, two independent *IgH* translocations are barely detected at the onset of pPCL, and their significance is yet to be elucidated. Here, we report a case of an aggressive pPCL with simultaneous *IGH/MYC* and *IGH/CCND1* translocations. A 73-year-old man was referred to our hospital with back pain and diagnosed as having pPCL with more than 50% circulating plasma cells. Cytogenetic analysis revealed 47, Y, t (X; 8;14) (q24; q24; q32), t (11; 14) (q13; q32), and +18. *IGH/MYC* and *IGH/CCND1* translocations were confirmed by fluorescence in situ hybridization analysis. Bortezomib and dexamethasone treatment achieved rapid elimination of peripheral malignant plasma cells, and the patient maintained a partial response for 18 months. After biological relapse, he received salvage therapy with ixazomib, lenalidomide, and dexamethasone, followed by pomalidomide and dexamethasone, and exhibited stable disease for an additional 14 months. Although *IGH/MYC* translocation in association with dysregulation of antiapoptotic pathway leads to worse prognosis in lymphomas, the novel agent-based regimen showed good efficacy, suggesting that *IGH/MYC* plays a different role in the pathogenesis of MM. *IGH/CCND1* and *IGH/MYC* translocations may have contributed to abrupt onset of pPCL in this case.

1. Introduction

Plasma cell leukemia (PCL) is a rare and aggressive form of multiple myeloma (MM), and the incidence of PCL was reported to be less than 1% of MM cases [1]. PCL is classified into two clinical types: primary PCL (pPCL) and secondary PCL [2]. In the former type, presentation is de novo and the prognosis is poor, with median overall survival (OS) of 4 months due to being refractory to various chemotherapies [1].

Recurrent immunoglobulin heavy chain (*IgH*) gene translocations involving *CCND1*, *FGFR3* and *MMEST*, *CCND3*, *MAF*, and *MAFB* are important oncogenic pathways observed in about 40% of MM and in 87% of pPCL cases [3]. Among them, *CCND1* is the most prevalent partner of *IgH* translocation, detected in 20–71% of pPCL cases [4]. Because most of these primary *IgH* translocations are speculated to be mediated by errors in *IgH* class switch recombination during B cell maturation, they are considered to be an early oncogenic event [3]. On the other hand, *IgH* translocations that target *MYC* are thought to be a very late and progressive event in the course of MM and rarely identified at the onset of MM, especially in pPCL [5].

Here, we report a case of an aggressive pPCL with simultaneous *IGH/MYC* and *IGH/CCND1* translocations.

2. Case Report

A 73-year-old man was referred to our hospital with a history of back pain for one month. Laboratory findings were as follows: a white blood cell count of 8.9 × 109/L with 55.0% of atypical plasma cells, hemoglobin level of 8.1 g/dL, platelet count of 55 × 109/L, lactate dehydrogenase level of 326 IU/L, creatinine level of 1.03 mg/dL, and blood urea nitrogen of 30.6 mg/dL. IgG was elevated at 4847 mg/dL with low levels of IgA and IgM (31 mg/dL and 9 mg/dL, respectively), and free light chain (FLC) analysis demonstrated a slight increase in free λ chain: κ FLC of 3.1 mg/dL, λ FLC of 50.8 mg/dL, and κ/λ ratio of 0.06.

Immunoelectrophoresis of serum identified IgG-λ monoclonal protein. Bone marrow examination revealed an infiltration of atypical plasma cells, comprising 55% of overall cellularity. Cytogenetic analysis revealed 47, Y, t (X; 8; 14) (q24; q24; q32), t (11; 14) (q13; q32), and +18 in 2 of the 20 cells studied. On immunohistochemistry, atypical plasma cells were strongly positive for cyclin D1 and partially weakly positive for MYC (Figure 1). We confirmed *IGH/MYC* and *IGH/CCND1* translocations by fluorescence in situ hybridization (FISH) analysis at the first relapse (Figure 2). Thus, he was diagnosed as having IgG-λ type primary plasma cell leukemia with *IGH/MYC* and *IGH/CCND1* translocations.

Initially, the patient was treated by Bd therapy (1.3 mg/m2 of bortezomib administered subcutaneously on days 1, 8, and 15 every 28 days, with 20 mg dexamethasone administered orally on days 1–2, 8–9, and 15–16). Malignant plasma cells rapidly disappeared from peripheral blood after one cycle of Bd therapy. He achieved a partial response after three cycles of Bd therapy. His IgG level was stable at around 1200 mg/dL for 18 months; however, it increased to 3083 mg/dL after 15 cycles of Bd therapy. As second-line therapy, IRd therapy (4 mg of ixazomib given orally on days 1, 8, and 15 every 28 days in addition to reduced doses of lenalidomide (10 mg daily on days 1–21) and 20 mg of dexamethasone weekly) was administered. IRd therapy was effective, and his IgG level decreased to 1380 mg/dL after five cycles. He achieved a partial response again. Unfortunately, he fractured the right femoral neck after 12 cycles of IRd therapy. He also developed severe pneumonia; therefore, we discontinued IRd therapy. Thereafter, bone marrow examination was performed, which revealed increased atypical plasma cells, and additional aberrations, including der (11)t (11; 14) and der (14)t (8; 14), were found on cytogenetic analysis (Figure 2(b) and Table 1). Due to his poor performance status and cytopenia, reduced-dose Pd therapy (1 mg of pomalidomide administered daily on days 1–14 every 28 days with 8 mg of dexamethasone weekly) was started. His IgG level had been stable at around 2000 mg/dL for 5 months. However, he developed recurrent infections and became bedridden, and then, he received palliative care and died 36 months after diagnosis.

3. Discussion

We report a case of pPCL harboring *IGH/MYC* and *IGH/CCND1* translocations at onset that showed a good response to novel agent-based treatment.

There are two main types of primary cytogenetic abnormalities in MM: hyperdiploidy and primary *IgH* translocations. In pPCL, *IgH* translocations were observed in 87%, and *CCND1* was the most common translocation partner observed in 20–71% [4], supporting a central role of *IGH/CCND1* translocation in the pathogenesis of pPCL. Recently, as high *BCL2/BCL-*X_L and *MCL-1* expression ratios were reported in t (11; 14) MM, *IGH/CCND1* translocation may contribute to plasma cell survival by altering the antiapoptotic pathway [7].

MYC is dysregulated or overexpressed in most human cancers and contributes to cell activation, cell proliferation, and apoptosis [8]. In MM, upregulation of *MYC* is involved in the progression from MGUS to MM [9] and also associated with leukemic and extramedullary presentation [10]. *MYC* is dysregulated by genetic rearrangements, such as translocations and amplifications, and is also modulated by deregulation of upstream pathways such as IRF4, DIS3/LIN28B/let-7, or MAPK [11].

Ig translocation with *MYC* is speculated to be a late and progressive event [12] and has been reported in 2.4% of newly diagnosed MM cases and rarely reported at the onset of pPCL [5]. To our knowledge, double translocations of *IgH* with *MYC* and *CCND1* were reported in only six cases of newly diagnosed MM, and this is the second case in pPCL [5, 13–16]. Nakayama et al. reported a 76-year-old patient with double-hit nonsecretory pPCL who had advanced disease [16], and Ji et al. described a 51-year-old patient with double-hit IgD myeloma who exhibited an aggressive clinical course and became refractory to conventional chemotherapy 18 months after the diagnosis [13]. However, there was no description of the detailed clinical course in other previously reported myeloma cases. Therefore, this is the first report of a clinical response to novel agent-based treatment.

Double-hit lymphoma with rearrangements of *MYC* and *BCL2* is recognized as a distinct entity under the WHO 2016 and known to have very poor prognosis [17]. Concomitant dysregulation of antiapoptotic molecule *BCL2* may counteract the proapoptotic function of *MYC*, resulting in rapid cell growth and resistance to therapy [18]. However, the prognosis of a double-hit case with rearrangements of *MYC* and *CCND1* in pPCL is not known, especially when treated with novel agent-based regimens. Despite leukemic presentation, frailty, as well as *MYC* and *CCND1* rearrangements, doublet and triplet regimens of novel agents had good efficacy in the patient and responded to treatment for more than 30 months after diagnosis. Recently, it was reported that *IGH/MYC* translocations in MM have extragenic *IGH* breakpoints, which are distinct from other B cell malignancies that usually have breakpoints in *IGH* switch regions [6]. These genetic alterations and cell differentiation states may contribute to affect the relatively good treatment response in *IGH/MYC*-possessing MM.

Interestingly, a previous study observed that cyclin *D* genes (cyclin D1, D2, and D3) were ectopically expressed in almost all MM cases from an early stage, implying a unifying and initial oncogenic event in MM [19]. In this case, juxtaposition of *CCND1* and *MYC* to the *IgH* gene enhancer may lead to simultaneous activation of initiating and progressive oncogenic pathways, resulting in abrupt onset of aggressive pPCL.

We also observed the accumulation of *IGH/MYC and IGH/CCND1* translocations over time during treatment, which suggested that *MYC* and *CCND1* signaling play a role in disease progression. There were discrepancies between

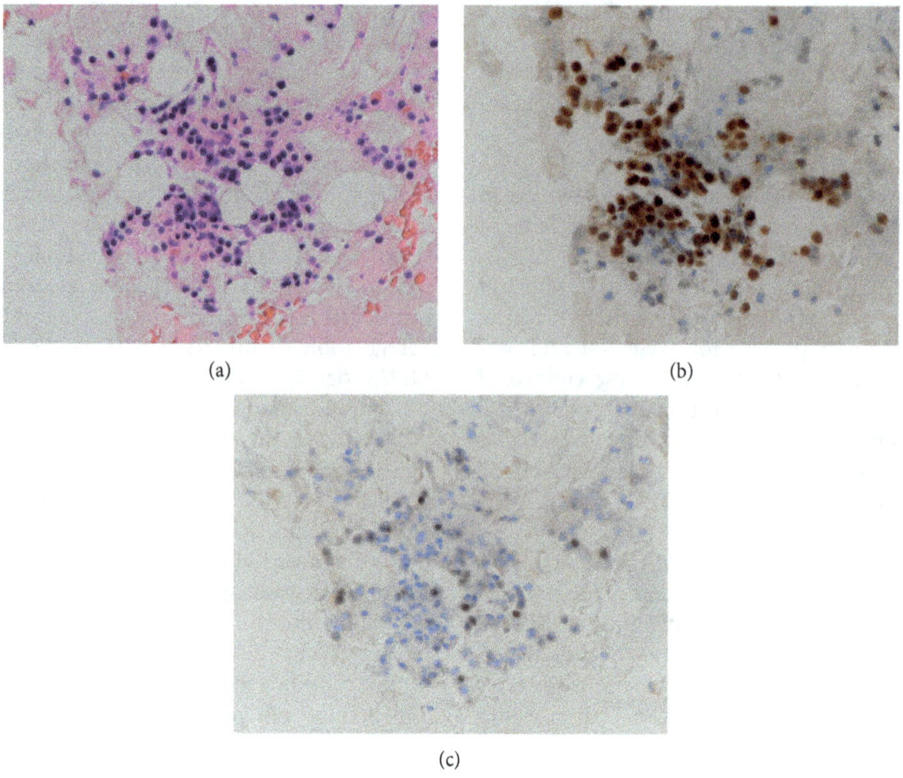

Figure 1: Pathological and immunohistochemical findings of bone marrow clot samples. (a) Hematoxylin and eosin staining showing infiltration of small-sized atypical plasma cells with eccentric nuclei. (b) Plasma cells were strongly positive for cyclin D1. (c) Plasma cells exhibited partial and weak MYC expression. Magnification: 400x.

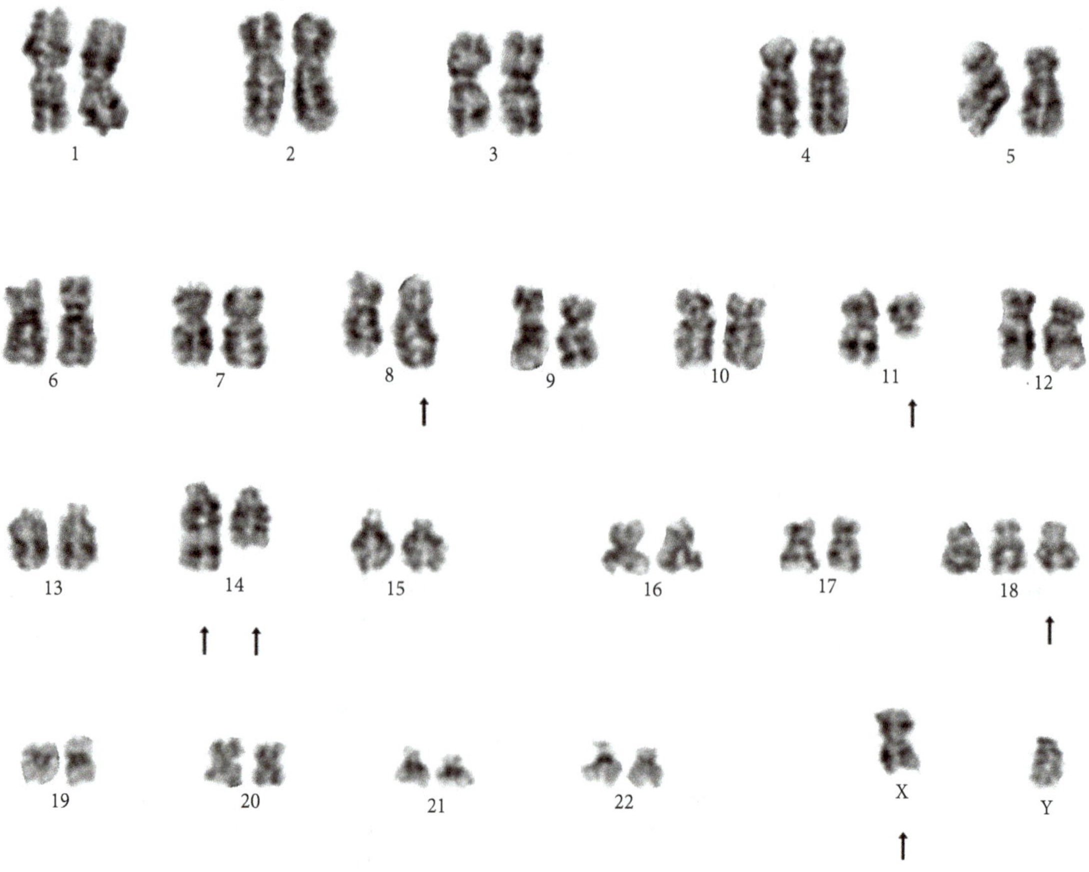

(a)
Figure 2: Continued.

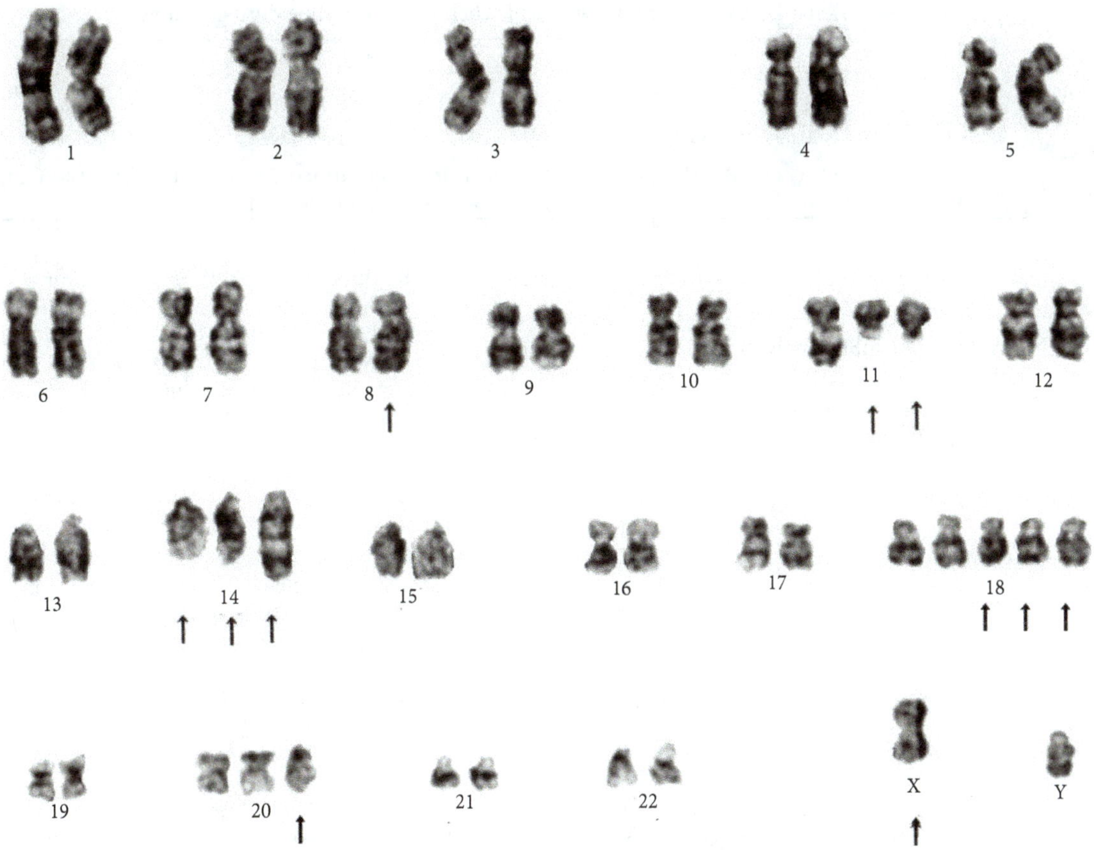

(b)

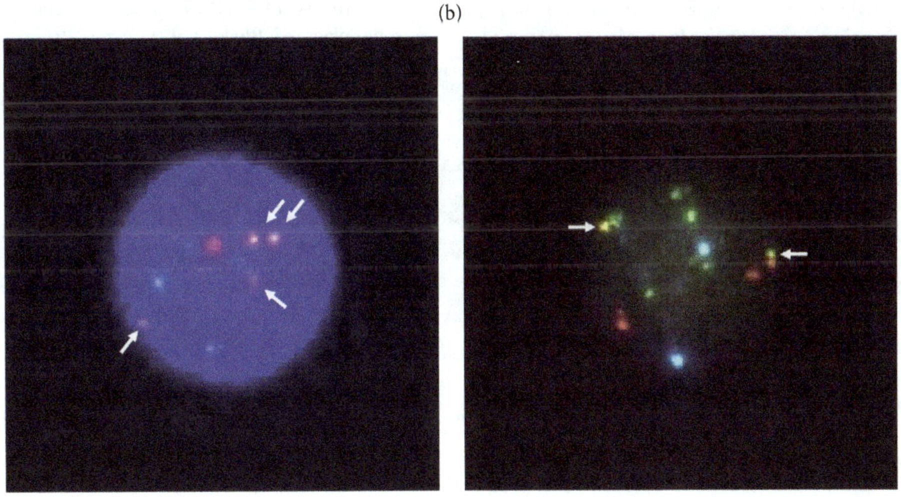

(c) (d)

FIGURE 2: Karyotype of metaphase chromosomes and interphase fluorescence in situ hybridization (FISH) analysis obtained from the bone marrow. (a) The following complex karyotypes were observed at diagnosis: 47, Y, t (X; 8; 14) (q24; q24; q32), t (11; 14) (q13; q32), and +18. The arrows indicate the abnormal chromosomes. (b) Additional karyotype aberrations, including der (11)t (11; 14) and der (14)t (8; 14), were observed after IRd therapy. (c) FISH analysis was performed using a vysis LSI IGH/CCND1 dual color, dual fusion translocation probe. The orange signal represents CCND1, and the green signal represents IGH. Four fusion signals were observed. (d) FISH analysis was performed using a vysis LSI IGH/MYC/CEP 8 tri-color dual fusion probe. The orange signal represents MYC, the green signal represents IGH, and the aqua signal represents alpha satellite sequences on 8q11.1. Two fusion signals were visible.

Table 1: Development of cytogenetic aberrations over time during treatment.

Period	Karyotype Result
At onset	47, Y, t (X; 8; 14) (q24; q24; q32), t (11; 14) (q13; q32), +18 [2]/46, XY [6]
At first relapse (after Bd therapy)	51, Y, t (X; 8; 14) (q24; q24; q32), −5, t (11; 14) (q13; q32), +12,−17, +18 + 20, +4mar [1]/46, XY[5]
After IRd therapy	52, Y, t (X; 8; 14) (q24; q24; q32), +der (11)t (11; 14) (q13; q32), t (11; 14), +der (14)t (8; 14) (q24; q32),+18, +18, +18, +20 [4]/46, XY [3]

cytogenetic analysis and FISH analysis in the time period and number of additional translocations. These may reflect the high sensitivity of FISH analysis in detecting chromosomal translocations [20].

Here, we described a case of double-hit primary plasma cell leukemia with *IGH/MYC* and *IGH/CCND1* successfully treated with novel agent-based regimens.

It is important to evaluate the *MYC* and *CCND1* signaling in the pathogenesis of pPCL for further understanding and identifying new therapeutic targets of pPCL.

References

[1] W. I. Gonsalves, S. V. Rajkumar, R. S. Go et al., "Trends in survival of patients with primary plasma cell leukemia: a population-based analysis," *Blood*, vol. 124, no. 6, pp. 907–912, 2014.

[2] International Myeloma Working Group, "Criteria for the classification of monoclonal gammopathies, multiple myeloma and related disorders: a report of the international myeloma working group," *British Journal Haematology*, vol. 121, pp. 749–757, 2003.

[3] M. Chesi and P. L. Bergsagel, "Molecular pathogenesis of multiple myeloma: basic and clinical updates," *International Journal of Hematology*, vol. 97, no. 3, pp. 313–323, 2013.

[4] C. F. De Larrea, R. A. Kyle, B. G. M. Durie et al., "Plasma cell leukemia: consensus statement on diagnostic requirements, response criteria, and treatment recommendations by the international myeloma working group (IMWG)," *Leukemia*, vol. 27, pp. 780–791, 2013.

[5] H. Avet-Loiseau, F. Gerson, F. Magrangeas, S. Minvielle, J. L. Harousseau, and R. Bataille, "Rearrangements of the c-myc oncogene are present in 15% of primary human multiple myeloma tumors," *Blood*, vol. 98, no. 10, pp. 3082–3086, 2001.

[6] B. G. Barwick, P. Neri, N. J. Bahlis et al., "Multiple myeloma immunoglobulin lambda translocations portend poor prognosis," *Nature Communications*, vol. 10, no. 1, p. 1911, 2019.

[7] S. Kumar, J. L. Kaufman, C. Gasparetto, J. Mikhael et al., "Efficacy of venetoclax as targeted therapy for relapsed/refractory t (11; 14) multiple myeloma," *Blood*, vol. 130, no. 22, pp. 2401–2409, 2017.

[8] C. V. Dang, "Myc on the path to cancer," *Cell*, vol. 149, no. 1, pp. 22–35, 2012.

[9] W.-J. Chng, G. F. Huang, T. H. Chung et al., "Clinical and biological implications of MYC activation: a common difference between MGUS and newly diagnosed multiple myeloma," *Leukemia*, vol. 25, no. 6, pp. 1026–1035, 2011.

[10] I. C. Glitza, G. Lu, R. Shah et al., "Chromosome 8q24.1/c-MYCabnormality: a marker for high-risk myeloma," *Leukemia & Lymphoma*, vol. 56, no. 3, pp. 602–607, 2014.

[11] K. K. Jovanovic, C. Roche-Lestienne, I. M. Ghobrial, T. Facon, B. Quesnel, and S. Manier, "Targeting MYC in multiple myeloma," *Leukemia*, vol. 32, pp. 1295–1306, 2018.

[12] A. Dib, A. Gabrea, O. K. Glebov, P. L. Bergsagel, and W. M. Kuehl, "Characterization of MYC translocations in multiple myeloma cell lines," *JNCI Monographs*, vol. 2008, no. 39, pp. 25–31, 2008.

[13] M. Ji, S. Jang, J.-H. Lee, and E.-J. Seo, "Double-hit myeloma with IGH/MYC and IGH/CCND1 translocations," *Annals of Hematology*, vol. 92, no. 8, pp. 1129–1131, 2013.

[14] N. V. Smadja, C. Bastard, C. Brigaudeau, D. Leroux, and C. Fruchart, "Hypodiploidy is a major prognostic factor in multiple myeloma," *Blood*, vol. 98, no. 7, pp. 2229–2238, 2001.

[15] J. L. Lai, L. Michaux, N. Dastugue et al., "Cytogenetics in multiple myeloma: a multicentric study of 24 patients with t (11; 14) (q13; q32) or its variant," *Cancer Genet Cytogenet* vol. 104, pp. 133–138, 1998.

[16] S. Nakayama, T. Oda, S. Minabe et al., "Primary nonsecretory plasma cell leukemia with multiple chromosomal abnormalities: a case report," *Archives of Iranian Medicine*, vol. 21, no. 1, pp. 41–43, 2018.

[17] S. H. Swerdlow, E. Campo, S. A. Pileri et al., "The 2016 revision of the world health organization classification of lymphoid neoplasms," *Blood*, vol. 127, no. 20, pp. 2375–2390, 2016.

[18] G. Ott, "Impact of MYC on malignant behavior," *Hematology* vol. 2014, no. 1, pp. 100–106, 2014.

[19] P. L. Bergsagel, W. M. Kuehl, F. Zhan, J. Sawyer, B. Barlogie, and J. Shaughnessy, "Cyclin D dysregulation: an early and unifying pathogenic event in multiple myeloma," *Blood* vol. 106, no. 1, pp. 296–303, 2005.

[20] K. Nishida, A. Tamura, N. Nakazawa et al., "The Ig heavy chain gene is frequently involved in chromosomal translocations in multiple myeloma and plasma cell leukemia as detected by in situ hybridization," *Blood*, vol. 90, no. 2, pp. 526–534, 1997.

29

De Novo Acute Myeloid Leukemia with Combined *CBFB-MYH11* and *BCR-ABL1* Gene Rearrangements: A Case Report and Review of Literature

Venkata Rakesh Sethapati, Ra'ed Jabr, Leyla Shune, Wissam El Atrouni, Patrick R. Gonzales, Wei Cui, and Shivani Golem

University of Kansas Medical Center, Kansas City, KS, USA

Correspondence should be addressed to Shivani Golem; sgolem@kumc.edu

Academic Editor: Sudhir Tauro

Acute myeloid leukemia (AML) with inv(16)(p13.1q22) resulting in *CBFB-MYH11* fusion is associated with a favorable prognosis. The presence of a KIT mutation modifies it to an intermediate prognosis. Additionally, inv(16) can cooperate with other genetic aberrations to further increase cell proliferation. Coexistence of inv(16) and t(9;22) is extremely rare (20 cases). We present a case of a 55-year-old male with elevated white blood cell count. Bone marrow evaluation and flow cytometry analysis were compatible with AML with monocytic features. Cytogenetic studies revealed two-related clones, a minor clone with inv(16) and a major clone with concurrent inv(16) and t(9;22) rearrangements. Fluorescent in situ hybridization studies confirmed these rearrangements. Molecular analysis detected a p190 *BCR-ABL1* transcript protein. *KIT* mutations were negative. The patient was initially treated with standard induction regimen; 7 daily doses of cytarabine from day 1–day 7, 3 daily doses of daunorubicin from day 1–day 3, and 1 dose of Mylotarg (gemtuzumab ozogamicin) on day 1. The detection of t(9;22) led to the addition of daily doses of dasatinib (tyrosine kinase inhibitor) from day 7 onwards. The patient achieved complete remission on day 45. During his treatment course, he acquired disseminated *Fusarium* infection. Day 180 bone marrow evaluation revealed florid relapse with 64% blasts. Cytogenetic study showed clonal evolution of the inv(16) clone with no evidence of the t(9;22) subclone. Eventually, bone marrow transplantation was contraindicated, and the patient was transferred to palliative care. Literature review revealed that AML with co-occurrence of *CBFB-MYH11* and *BCR-ABL1* gene rearrangements was involved by only a small number of cases with de novo and therapy-related AML. Most cases were in myeloid blast crisis of chronic myeloid leukemia (CML). Treatment and prognosis among the de novo AML cases varied and majority of them achieved clinical remission. In contrast, these cytogenetic abnormalities in the blast phase of CML had a poor prognosis. As the prognosis and management of AML is dependent upon the underlying genetic characteristics of the neoplasm, it is imperative to include clinical outcome with such rare combinations of genetic alterations.

1. Introduction

Acute myeloid leukemia (AML) is one of the most commonly encountered types of leukemias in adults. AML is characterized by clonal expansion of undifferentiated myeloid blasts and consequentially results in impaired hematopoiesis and bone marrow failure. It is a heterogenous disease clinically, morphologically, and genetically. Cytogenetic aberrations and gene mutations play critical roles in the pathogenesis of AML. There are many driver mutations, and the disease can evolve to accumulate more competing clones.

Core binding factor (CBF) leukemias include t(8;21)/*RUNX1-RUNX1T1* and inv(16)/t(16;16)/*CBFB-MYH11* and are classified as AML with recurrent genetic abnormalities under the World Health Organization (WHO) classification [1, 2]. Inv(16) is found in 5–8% of younger patients with AML and accounts for around 7–10% of all patients with de novo AML [1, 3]. This abnormality results in the fusion of myosin heavy chain 11 gene (*MYH11*) at 16p13 and the core binding factor beta subunit gene (*CBFB*) at 16q12. This gene fusion results in chimeric proteins that suppress transactivation mediated by CBF and lead to impaired hematopoietic differentiation [3]. A bone marrow biopsy typically shows an acute myelomonocytic leukemia, accompanied with atypical eosinophils classified as the FAB subtype $M4_{Eo}$ [3]. Chromosome abnormalities involving CBF rearrangements are associated with a favorable prognosis, except when a *KIT* mutation is present [1].

In addition, genetic alterations can also activate signal transduction pathways and confer a proliferation advantage on hematopoietic cells. *BCR-ABL1* is one such example. *BCR-ABL1* translocation, also known as the Philadelphia (Ph) chromosome, results from a reciprocal translocation between chromosomes 9 and 22: t(9;22)(q34; q11.2). This translocation is necessary in defining chronic myeloid leukemia (CML) and is also responsible for a subset of B cell acute lymphoblastic leukemia (B-ALL) and less commonly in de novo AML [4]. The most common form of *BCR-ABL1* fusion (b2a2 or b3a2) in CML and blast phase of CML results in a 210 kDa product (Major breakpoint), whereas in B-ALL, the main fusion form (e1a2) results in a 190 kDa product (minor breakpoint) [5].

We report a case with combined occurrence of inv(16) and *BCR-ABL1* rearrangements, presenting as de novo AML. Our case also utilized the 190 kDa *BCR-ABL1* fusion protein. With only 20 cases of AML described in literature with similar coexisting inv(16) and *BCR-ABL1* rearrangements, there is a greater need to report such cases.

2. Case Presentation

A 55-year-old male presented with worsening fatigue. Upon evaluation, he had leukocytosis (white blood cell count—103×10^9/L), thrombocytopenia (platelets—25×10^9/L), and anemia (hemoglobin—7.6 g/dL). Review of the peripheral blood smear revealed 57% circulating blasts, and flow cytometry was compatible with AML with monocytic features. Myeloblasts comprised 15% of cells and showed expression of CD13, CD33, CD117, CD34, HLA-DR, partial CD123, minimal CD64, CD38, and partial cMPO; the blasts were negative for CD56, CD15, CD11b/C, CD14, TdT, and B and T cell markers. There were around 8% immature monocytic cells present which expressed dim CD45, CD13, CD117, CD33, CD15, partial CD11b, and partial CD64 and were negative for CD34. There were also 14% mature monocytic cells.

A comprehensive bone marrow evaluation was diagnostic for acute myeloid leukemia involving a hypercellular bone marrow (100%) with decreased erythropoiesis, decreased megakaryopoiesis, increased eosinophils, 19% monocytes, and 24% blasts and promonocytes. Morphologically, the blasts appeared large, with irregular and convoluted nuclear contours, dispersed chromatin, and small amounts of basophilic cytoplasm. They were admixed with an increased number of promonocytes that had delicately folded nuclei, dispersed chromatin, inconspicuous nucleoli, and finely granulated cytoplasm. Importantly, there were increased eosinophils that had increased and coarse basophilic granules (Figure 1). Flow cytometry evaluation of the bone marrow biopsy yielded a hemodiluted specimen with myeloblasts expressing CD34, CD13, CD33, CD117, and HLA-DR comprising 1.1% of total cells.

Conventional cytogenetics at diagnosis demonstrated two-related clones. Two metaphases had pericentric inversions of chromosome 16 (Figure 2(a)). The second related clone was observed in majority of the metaphases, and each had a Philadelphia chromosome with the classic (9;22) translocation along with an inversion 16 abnormality (Figure 2(b)). Fluorescence in situ hybridization (FISH) assays were positive for *CBFB* rearrangement and *BCR/ABL1* translocation in 94.0~95.0% of the interphase nuclei (Figures 3(a) and 3(b)). A FISH assay for rearrangement of *RUNX1T1/RUNX1* was normal (Figure 3(c)).

A qualitative reverse transcriptase polymerase chain reaction (RT-PCR) was positive for an e1a2 *BCR-ABL1* fusion transcript coding for the 190 kDa *BCR-ABL1* fusion protein. A hematologic neoplasm next generation sequencing (NGS) 141 gene panel that was obtained based on the first bone marrow reported only two mutations of unknown significance in *TET2* (p.L1322R) and *P2RY2* (p.V77A). There were no pathogenic variants detected for *FLT3* exon 14 (internal tandem duplication), *FLT3* exon 20 (tyrosine kinase domain), *NPM1* exon 11, *CEBPA*, and *KIT* exon 17 p.D816V at a minimum allelic fraction of 1.0%.

The patient was initially treated with a 7 + 3 cytarabine-based induction regimen: seven daily doses of cytarabine (100 mg/m^2) from day 1 to day 7, three daily doses of daunorubicin (90 mg/m^2) from day 1 to day 3, and a single dose of Mylotarg (gemtuzumab ozogamicin, 4.5 mg/m^2) on day 1. The detection of p190 *BCR-ABL1* transcript at day 5 led to the addition of daily doses of 100 mg of dasatinib (tyrosine kinase inhibitor, TKI) from day 7 onwards. Intrathecal cytarabine therapy was omitted due to a low number of platelets. The patient was pancytopenic and needed multiple red blood cells and platelets transfusions. On day 14, peripheral blood showed severe pancytopenia and bone marrow showed a hypocellular (<5%) bone marrow with decreased trilineage hematopoiesis and 1% blasts. Although flow cytometry evaluation revealed a negative immunophenotypic study, FISH studies were positive for t(9;22) and inv(16) in 25.1–27.1% of the interphase cells. Conventional cytogenetics did not yield enough metaphases for a complete study. Dasatinib was stopped on day 21 due to persistent leukopenia. G-colony stimulating factor was given once on day 21 and on day 23. Notably on day 20, the patient's clinical course was complicated by a skin ulceration in his toes that later resulted in disseminated *Fusarium* infection (Figure 4). Unable to obtain a bone marrow biopsy to evaluate for hematopoietic recovery, dasatinib was restarted on day 34. On day 45, peripheral blood was significant for absolute lymphopenia and monocytosis. Day 45 bone marrow biopsy showed a hypercellular marrow (80%), increased trilineage hematopoiesis, and less than 1% blasts. Flow cytometry on the same specimen was reported as a negative immunophenotypic study. The conventional cytogenetic study showed normal karyotype,

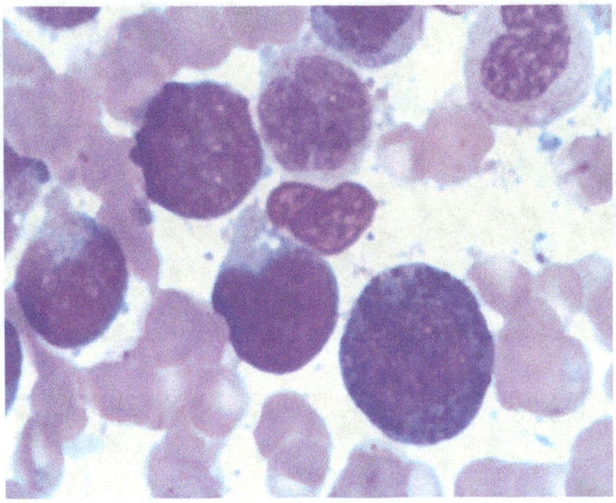

FIGURE 1: Bone marrow morphology: increased blasts, promonocytes, and atypical eosinophils with large basophilic granules.

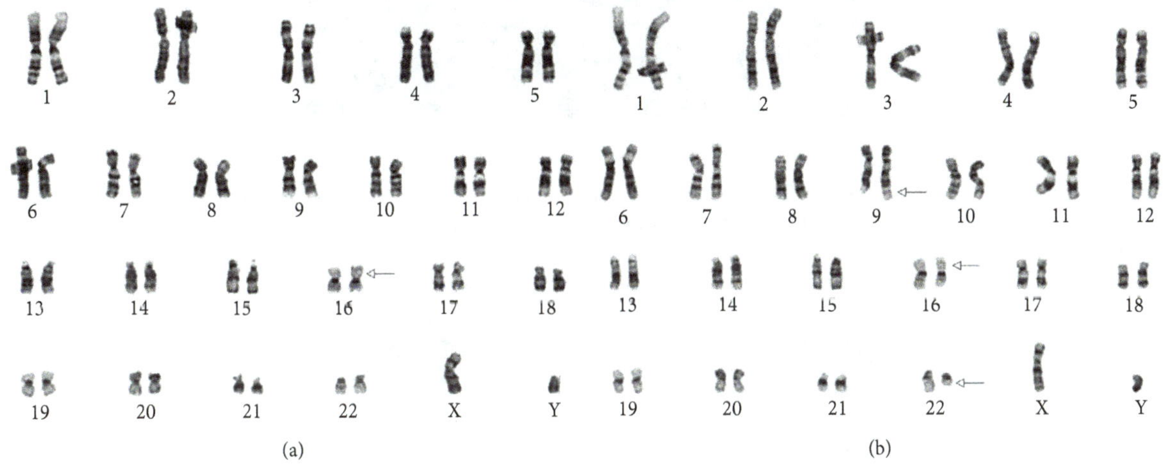

FIGURE 2: Representative G-banded karyogram showing (a) the inv(16)(p13.1q22) as a sole abnormality and (b) co-occurrence of inv(16)(p13.1q22) and t(9;22)(q34; q11.2). The arrows indicate the rearranged chromosomes.

and RT-PCR analysis for p190 *BCR/ABL1* transcript was undetectable. His clinical status was in complete remission (CR), and the patient was eventually discharged on day 60.

Patient was kept on a continued daily dose of 100 mg of dasatinib. However, the patient had gradually increasing Fungitell values and eventually developed fulminant *Fusarium* infection. He was admitted for bilateral pneumonia on day 120 and was treated with amphotericin (5 mg/kg). He was later enrolled on a clinical trial for an alternative oral-based antifungal medication therapy. His fungal infection was reported to have improved with decreased pulmonary infiltrates and a healed foot wound. The patient returned on day 180 for bone marrow transplant evaluation. His peripheral blood smear was remarkable for pancytopenia and 9% circulating blasts. His bone marrow showed persistent AML with 64% blasts and blast equivalents involving a mildly hypercellular bone marrow (50–60%) with decreased trilineage hematopoiesis. The corresponding flow cytometry on the bone marrow specimen revealed 30% of aberrant myeloid blasts that were positive for CD45 (dim), CD34, CD117, HLA-DR, CD13, CD33, and CD38. Chromosome study showed complete resolution of the t(9;22) subclone (negative by FISH and RT-PCR); however, the inv(16) clone resurfaced with other additional abnormalities significant for clonal evolution (Figure 5). Fungitell values were again high, and CT scan showed findings consistent with pneumonia and pansinusitis. Bronchial lavage cultures and blood cultures were negative for microorganism growth. Bone marrow hematopoietic stem cell transplantation (HSCT) was eventually contraindicated. The patient preferred hospice care and died two months after.

3. Discussion

An inv(16) abnormality is found in 5–8% of younger patients with AML, while the Ph chromosome is a rare event in AML with a reported incidence ranging from 0.5% to 3% [1, 6]. *BCR-ABL1* AML is now included as a new provisional entity in the 2017 revised WHO classification of hematopoietic malignancies [1, 7]. This entity excludes cases with evidence

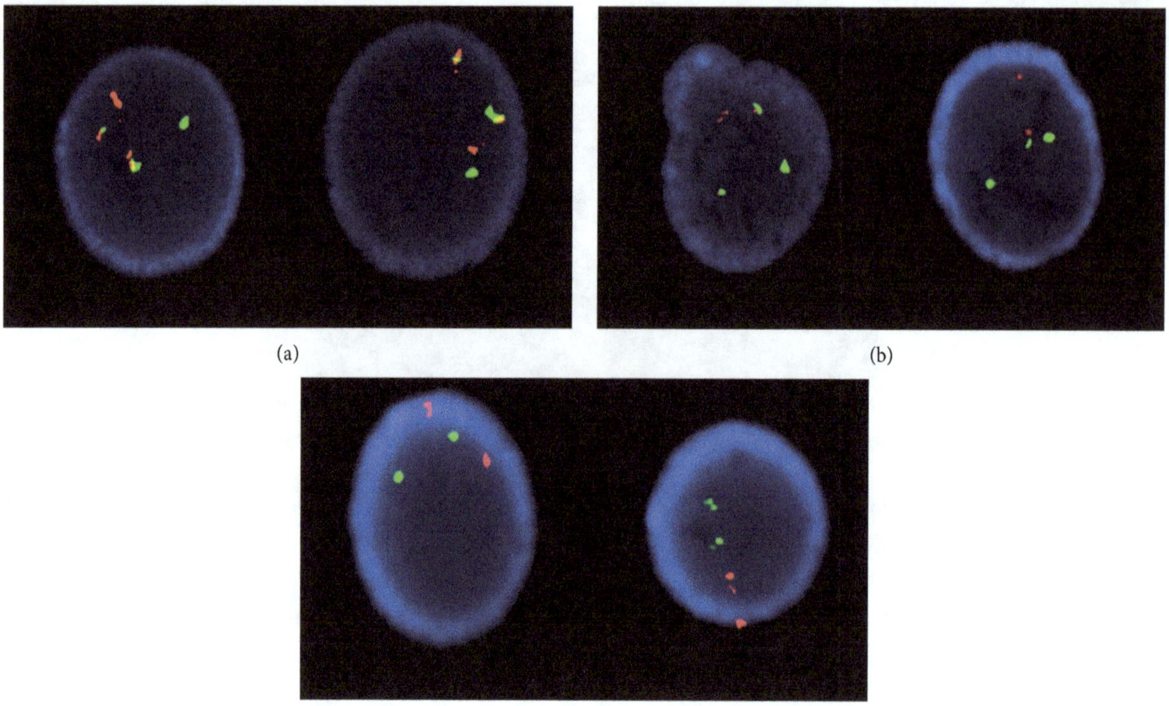

(a) (b) (c)

Figure 3: Fluorescence in situ hybridization (FISH) studies on interphase cells showing (a) *CBFB* and *MYH11* rearrangement, dual fusion probe (Cytocell); (b) *BCR/ABL1* translocation, dual fusion probe (Cytocell); and (c) normal FISH signal pattern for *RUNX1T1/RUNX1* rearrangement, dual fusion probe (Abbott molecular).

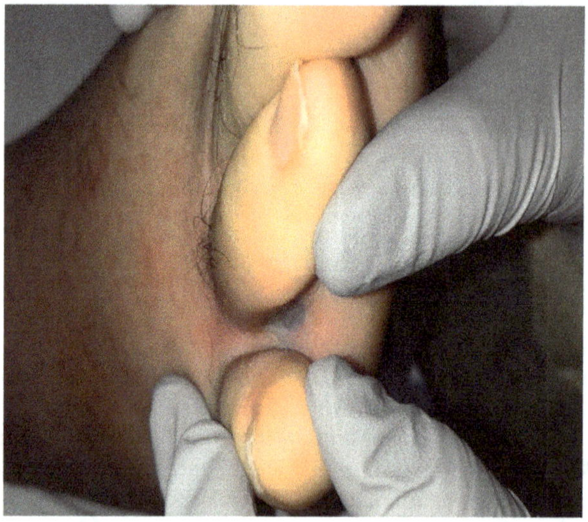

Figure 4: Fusarium infection presenting as a skin ulceration in his toes.

of the history of CML. Literature review describes a limited number of cases with AML with *BCR-ABL1* translocation that tend to incorporate additional distinct genetic aberrations including inv(16), t(8;21)/*RUNX1-RUNX1T1*, t(15;17)/*PML-RARA*, inv(3), 5q deletion, and *NPM1* mutation [8, 9]. Our case report similarly illustrates a patient with de novo AML with combined *BCR-ABL1* (p190 form) and inv(16) abnormalities.

The Ph chromosome was observed as a subclone in our patient suggestive for "real AML" as Bacher et al. described in his case series [8]. In case #2, their patient had Ph chromosome-positive subclones as a secondary genetic alternation along with inv(16) at initial diagnosis. The patient was treated with hydroxycarbamide and daunorubicin/cytarabine followed by a TKI, imatinib. The patient went into remission but relapsed three months later. At relapse, cytogenetics showed 22 metaphases carrying an inv(16), two of which had an additional t(9;22). The first relapse was treated by intensified chemotherapy using fludarabine, cytarabine, G-CSF, and idarubicin, and again complete

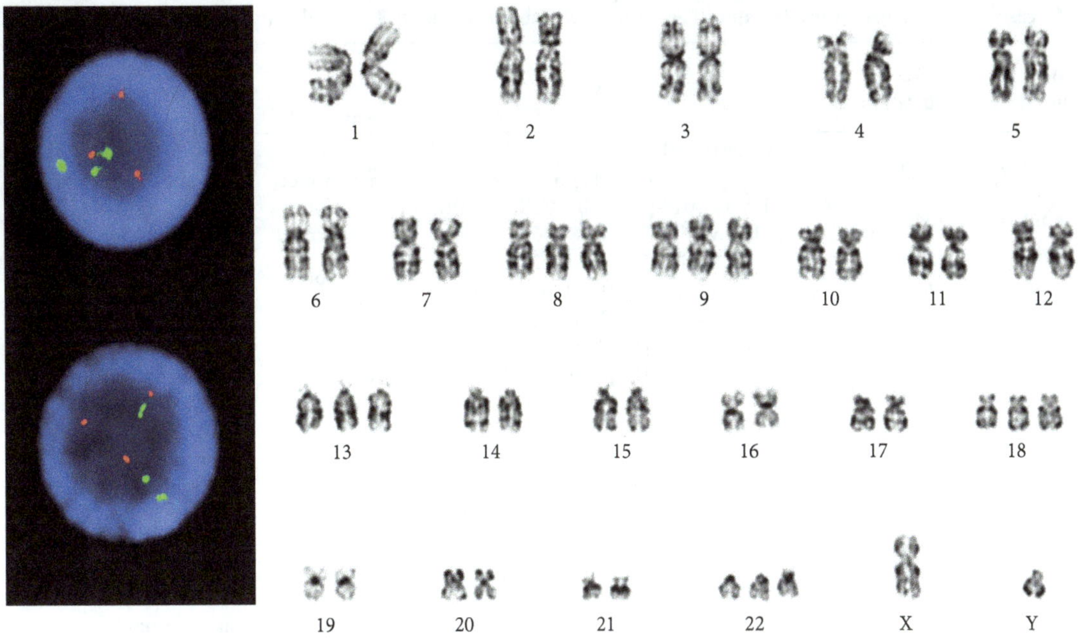

(a) (b)

FIGURE 5: (a) Fluorescence in situ hybridization (FISH) studies on interphase cells showing *BCR* and *ABL1* FISH probe signals, dual fusion probe (Cytocell) and (b) representative *G*-banded karyogram showing relapsed clone of the inv(16)(p13.1q22) primary clone.

remission was achieved. A second relapse occurred ten months from initial diagnosis where 10 of 18 metaphases showed inv(16), while the other eight had evidence of both inv(16) and t(9;22). Their patient's clinical status after the second relapse is unknown. In contrast, our case at relapse showed complete resolution of the t(9;22) subclone (negative FISH and RT-PCR for *BCR-ABL1*), but the inv(16) clone resurfaced with other additional abnormalities significant for clonal evolution. This finding substantiates the efficacy of a TKI inhibitor in cases of Ph-positive AML.

Similar de novo and therapy-related AML cases with concurrent inv(16) and *BCR-ABL1* rearrangements are compared in Table 1 [10–14]. Bustamante and team described a rapid response to single agent treatment with imatinib and demonstrated a negative finding of *BCR-ABL1* fusion by FISH or RT-PCR after 3 weeks of therapy. Salem et al. included one patient with de novo AML and one with initial AML with *CBFB* rearrangement but subsequently acquired a *BCR-ABL1* translocation [4]. The former received induction therapy with FLAG-IDA (fludarabine, cytarabine, idarubicin, and G-CSF) regimen and dasatinib with clinical remission in 21 months, and the latter received an induction with 7 + 3 regimen and dasatinib but relapsed after 8 months and died 2 years after initial diagnosis [4]. Miura et al. and Secker-Walker et al. reported stable remissions up to 70 months were achieved after allogenic stem cell transplantation.

We also know that the Ph chromosome can pair up with other abnormalities in AML. Han JY and team presented an AML case with a known prognostically adverse aberration inv(3) and monosomy 7 with Ph chromosome as a secondary abnormality at diagnosis [15]. The patient was treated with induction chemotherapy, but the patient's course was complicated by neutropenic fever and acute renal failure. Repeated bone marrow examinations showed the presence of persistent leukemia, and the patient subsequently went into hospice care. Mozziconacci et al. described two cases, one in which *BCR-ABL1* translocation was in combination with inv(3) where the patient did not respond to initial treatment and died [9]. The other case was a more favorable rearrangement involving acute promyelocytic leukemia where a total of 100 mitoses were analyzed and two metaphases with t(15;17) and t(9;22) were found. The patient was treated with all-trans retinoic acid and chemotherapy and achieved complete remission on day 30. At 3 months, a very low level of MBCR (b2a2) transcript was detected. RT-PCR was still positive at 4 months but negative at 9, 14, 17, and 30 months. 4 years after diagnosis, the patient was still in remission. These findings suggest prognosis of AML with Ph-positive subclones can be associated with the corresponding cytogenetic abnormality.

Interestingly, cases with CML in the blast phase that acquire an inv(16) aberration have a poor prognosis. Salem et al. studied ten patients with combined inv(16) and *BCR-ABL1* cytogenetic abnormalities and seven of which were CML cases [4]. In the seven patients, six died with a median overall survival time of 14 months despite intensive chemotherapy and targeted therapy with TKI [4]. Analyzing these cases and cases from Table 1, we can conclude that the p210 form was found in CML cases that transformed into the blast phase, and the p190 form was found in 'true AML' with the exception of the case by Ninomiya et al. [16]. The p190 isoform is also more commonly associated with leukemogenesis leading to *BCR-ABL1*-positive acute lymphoblastic

Table 1: AML cases with concurrent inv(16) and BCR-ABL genetic abnormalities in this study and selected cases from literature review.

Sex/age	AML subtype	FAB classification	Karyotype	Other mutation assay(s)	Clinical course	PMID
M/40	De novo	M4eo	46,XY,inv(16)(p13q22)[17]/46,XY,idem,t(9;22)(q34:q11)[3]	Not performed	Chemotherapy and HSCT; stable remission	8250017
F/9	De novo	M4eo	46,XX,inv(16)(p13q22)[21]/46,XX,t(9;22)(q34;q11),inv(16)(p13q22)[8]/46,XX [10]	Not performed	Chemotherapy and HSCT; died soon after HSCT	1728947
M/13	De novo	M4	46,XY,inv(16)(p13.1q22)[2]/ 46,idem,del(7)(q22q32)[16]/46,idem,t(9;22;19)(q34;q11.2;p13.1)[2]	Not performed	Cytarabine, daunomycin, etoposide + gemtuzumab	20513535
F/40	De novo	M1	46,XX,inv(16)(p13q22)[4]/46,XX,t(9;22)(q34;q11),inv(16)(p13q22)[18]	Not performed	One cycle of conventional induction therapy	11368385
M/63	De novo	M4eo	At diagnosis: 46,XY,inv(16)(p13q22)[20]/ 46,XY,t(9;22)(q34;q11),inv(16)(p13q22)[2] At last relapse: 46,XY,inv(16)(p13q22)[10]/ 46,XY,+8,t(9;22)(q34;q11),inv(16)(p13q22)[8]	Not performed	Hydroxycarbamide, daunorubicin/ cytarabine and imatinib with relapse in 3 months. Fludarabine, cytarabine, G-CSF and Idarubicine with complete remission but relapsed 10 months later	21275954
F/49	Therapy-related	M4eo	46,XX,inv(16)(p13.1q22)[5]/46,XX,t(9;22)(q34;q11.2)[7]/46,XX[8]	Not performed	Imatinib; remission in 3 weeks	22370710
M	De novo	M4eo	46,XY,inv(16)(p13.1q22)[3]/46,idem,t(9;22)(q34;q11.2)[17]	None (NGS, multiple genes)	Fludarabine, cytarabine, G-CSF and Idarubicine + dasatinib; stable remission	28253536
M/55	De novo	M4eo	At Diagnosis: 46,XY,inv(16)(p13.1q22)[2]/ 46,sl,t(9;22)(q34;q11.2)[20]/46,XX[1].nuc ish(MYH11,CBFB)x3(MYH11 con CBFBx2) [190/200]/(ABL1,BCR)x3(ABL1 con BCRx2) [188/200] 13-day follow-up: 46,XY[2].nuc ish(ABL1,BCR) x3(ABL1 con BCRx2)[88/350]/(MYH11,CBFB) x3(MYH11 con CBFBx2)[95/350] 45-day follow-up: 46,XY[20] 188-day follow-up: 51,XY,+8,+9,+13,inv(16)(p13.1q22),+18,+22 [19]/46,XY[1].nuc ish(MYH11,CBFB) x3(MYH11 con CBFBx2)[155/200]/ (ABL1x2~3,BCRx2~3)[372/500]	None (NGS, multiple genes)	Gemtuzumab ozogamicin induction + Dasatinib; a first relapse diagnosed 6 months from initial diagnosis. Hospice.	Current case

leukemia than AML [17, 18]. However, the immunophenotypic study from our case is against a lymphoblastic or mixed phenotypic leukemia.

Due to the rarity of this disease, the prognosis is difficult to determine. *CBFB* rearrangement in AML with no additional mutation is known to have a favorable prognosis. A study with 201 de novo AML patients indicated that the 5-year survival probability was 43% for *CBFB-MYH11* rearrangements [19]. Ph-positive AML appears to be an aggressive disease with poor response to traditional AML therapy or TKI alone [1, 4]. Additionally, only limited cases in literature included multigene mutation analysis in these rare co-occurring inv(16) and *BCR-ABL1* abnormalities. Our case and the study by Salem et al. did not detect any pathogenic variants. This indicates that these co-occurring abnormalities act independently of other commonly seen mutations in myeloid neoplasms. Our patient had initially shown a favorable response to treatment and achieved CR by day 45 postdiagnosis. He later developed disseminated *Fusarium* infection, which compromised his leukemic treatment. Incidence of *Fusarium* spp. infection in patients with acute leukemia is 0.06% and the survival rate is 4% [20]. Despite enrolling in an investigational antifungal clinical trial, his fungal infection persisted and was not a suitable candidate for HSCT. Overall, we feel that the combination of inv(16) and *BCR-ABL1* genetic abnormalities confers an intermediate prognosis.

De novo AML patients with combined inv(16) and t(9;22) cytogenetic abnormalities seem to benefit from intensive chemotherapy and targeted TKIs. Decisions about HSCT in intermediate-risk AML were less clear-cut in the past, and nowadays, most patients are considered for HSCT in their first CR [21]. Patient fitness, availability of a sibling donor or an alternative donor, a clinical trial option, and the transplant center experience must be considered when making a decision about HSCT. It is important to note that a longer duration of *BCR-ABL1* fusion transcript surveillance can be used to establish a standard of care for such Ph-positive AML patients with additional rearrangements [7].

4. Conclusion

Molecularly defined genetic abnormalities in AML have a significant impact on a patient's management and prognosis. AML presenting with both inv(16) and t(9;22) abnormalities confers an intermediate prognosis. The pathognomic effect of the occurrence of these abnormalities acts independent of other common molecular mutations seen in myeloid neoplasms. These cases are rare and need to be documented and studied further to formulate better management strategies. Such cases may benefit from intensive chemotherapy and TKIs as a bridge to stem cell transplantation. Comorbidities and infectious diseases arising from an immunocompromised state must be taken into consideration when planning treatment regimens to prevent doing more harm than benefit to the patient.

References

[1] S. H. Swerdlow, E. Campo, N. L. Harris et al., Eds., *WHO Classification of Tumors of Hematopoietic and Lymphoid Tissues*, International Agency for Research on Cancer, Lyon, France, 4th edition, 2017.

[2] M. L. Wang, N. G. Bailey, and N. Bailey, "Acute myeloid leukemia genetics: risk stratification and implications for therapy," *Archives of Pathology & Laboratory Medicine*, vol. 139, no. 10, pp. 1215–1223, 2015, PMID 26414465.

[3] S. Schnittger, U. Bacher, C. Haferlach, W. Kern, and T. Haferlach, "Rare CBFB-MYH11 fusion transcripts in AML with inv(16)/t(16;16) are associated with therapy-related AML M4eo, atypical cytomorphology, atypical immunophenotype, atypical additional chromosomal rearrangements and low white blood cell count: a study on 162 patients," *Leukemia*, vol. 21, no. 4, pp. 725–731, 2007, PMID—17287858.

[4] A. Salem, S. Loghavi, G. Tang et al., "Myeloid neoplasms with concurrent BCR-ABL1 and CBFB rearrangements: a series of 10 cases of a clinically aggressive neoplasm," *American Journal of Hematology*, vol. 92, no. 6, pp. 520–528, 2017.

[5] E. Jabbour and H. Kantarjian, "Chronic myeloid leukemia: 2016 update on diagnosis, therapy, and monitoring," *American Journal of Hematology*, vol. 91, no. 2, pp. 252–265, 2016, PMID—26799612.

[6] S. Konoplev, C. C. Yin, S. M. Kornblau et al., "Molecular characterization OFDE novo Philadelphia chromosome-positive acute myeloid leukemia," *Leukemia & Lymphoma*, vol. 54, no. 1, pp. 138–144, 2013.

[7] N. R. Neuendorff, T. Burmeister, B. Dörken, and J. Westermann, "BCR-ABL-positive acute myeloid leukemia: a new entity? Analysis of clinical and molecular features," *Annals of Hematology*, vol. 95, no. 8, pp. 1211–1221, 2016.

[8] U. Bacher, T. Haferlach, T. Alpermann et al., "Subclones with the t(9;22)/BCR-ABL1 rearrangement occur in AML and seem to cooperate with distinct genetic alterations," *British Journal of Haematology*, vol. 152, no. 6, pp. 713–720, 2011, PMID— 21275954.

[9] M.-J. Mozziconacci, D. Sainty, J. Gabert et al., "The Philadelphia chromosome as a secondary abnormality in two cases of acute myeloid leukemia," *British Journal of Haematology*, vol. 102, no. 3, pp. 873–875, 1998, PMID—9722319.

[10] D. Bustamante, K. R. Chan, D. R. Czuchlewski, and A. A. Al Saadi, "Patterns of *BCR* breakpoints in patients with coexisting inv(16)(p13.1q22) and t(9;22)(q34;q11.2)," *International Journal of Hematology*, vol. 95, no. 3, pp. 324–326, 2012, PMID—22370710.

[11] I. Miura, H. Takatsu, A. Yamaguchi et al., "Standard Ph chromosome, t(9;22)(q34;q11), as an additional change in a patient with acute myelomonocytic leukemia (M4Eo) associated with inv(16)(p13q22)," *American Journal of Hematology*, vol. 45, no. 1, pp. 94–96, 1994, PMID—8250017.

[12] L. M. Secker-Walker, G. J. Morgan, T. Min et al., "Inversion of chromosome 16 with the Philadelphia chromosome in acute myelomonocytic leukemia with eosinophilia. Report of two cases," *Cancer Genetics and Cytogenetics*, vol. 58, no. 29, 34 pages, 1992, PMID—1728947.

[13] M. Svaldi, A. Lanthaler, R. Venturi, P. Coser, and M. Mitterer, "Simultaneous occurrence of BCR-ABL and inv16 in a case of M1 acute myeloid leukemia," *Leukemia*, vol. 15, no. 4, p. 695, 2001, PMID—11368385.

[14] C. A. Tirado, F. Valdez, L. Klesse et al., "Acute myeloid leukemia with inv(16) with CBFB-MYH11, 3′CBFB deletion, variant t(9;22) with BCR-ABL1, and del(7)(q22q32) in a pediatric patient: case report and literature review," *Cancer Genetics and Cytogenetics*, vol. 200, no. 1, pp. 54–59, 2010, PMID: 20513535.

[15] J.-Y. Han and K. S. Theil, "The Philadelphia chromosome as a secondary abnormality in inv(3)(q21q26) acute myeloid leukemia at diagnosis: confirmation of p190 BCR-ABL mRNA by real-time quantitative polymerase chain reaction," *Cancer Genetics and Cytogenetics*, vol. 165, no. 1, pp. 70–74, 2006, PMID: 16490599.

[16] S. Ninomiya, N. Kanemura, H. Tsurumi et al., "Coexistence of inversion 16 and the Philadelphia chromosome comprising P190 BCR/ABL in chronic myeloid leukemia blast crisis," *International Journal of Hematology*, vol. 93, no. 6, pp. 806–810, 2011, PMID—21523337.

[17] X. Thomas and M. Heiblig, "The development of agents targeting the BCR-ABL tyrosine kinase as Philadelphia chromosome-positive acute lymphoblastic leukemia treatment," *Expert Opinion on Drug Discovery*, vol. 11, no. 11, pp. 1061–1070, 2016, PMID: 27548716.

[18] R. Vinhas, A. Lourenço, S. Santos et al., "A novel *BCR-ABL1* mutation in a patient with Philadelphia chromosome-positive B-cell acute lymphoblastic leukemia," *OncoTargets and Therapy*, vol. 11, pp. 8589–8598, 2018, PMID: 30584318; PMCID: PMC 6280987.

[19] C. Sinha, L. C. Cunningham, and P. P. Liu, "Core binding factor acute myeloid leukemia: new prognostic categories and therapeutic opportunities," *Seminars in Hematology*, vol. 52, no. 3, pp. 215–222, 2015, Epub 2015 Apr 7. PMID: 26111469; PMCID: PMC 4484884.

[20] Y.-S. Liu, N.-C. Wang, R.-H. Ye, and W.-Y. Kao, "Disseminated Fusarium infection in a patient with acute lymphoblastic leukemia: a case report and review of the literature," *Oncology Letters*, vol. 7, no. 2, pp. 334–336, 2014.

[21] A. A. Kassim and B. N. Savani, "Hematopoietic stem cell transplantation for acute myeloid leukemia: a review," *Hematology/Oncology and Stem Cell Therapy*, vol. 10, no. 4, pp. 245–251, 2017 Dec, Epub 2017 Jun 20. PMID: 28666104.

30

Management of Allogeneic Stem Cell Transplantation for High-Risk AML following SARS-CoV-2 Associated Pancytopenia with Marked Bone Marrow Biopsy Alterations

Maria Kaparou, Zbigniew Rudzki, Hannah Giles, Vidhya Murthy, Swathy Srinath, Rebecca Lloyd, Maria Zahid Ahmed, Beena Salhan, Saleena Chauhan, Bhuvan Kishore, Richard Lovell, Claire Horgan, Shankara Paneesha, Evgenia Xenou, Anand Lokare, Joanne Ewing, Hansini Dassanayake, Emmanouil Nikolousis, and Alexandros Kanellopoulos

University Hospitals Birmingham NHS Foundation Trust, London, UK

Correspondence should be addressed to Alexandros Kanellopoulos; akanell@hotmail.com

Academic Editor: Håkon Reikvam

The present study describes a patient aged 70 with very high-risk AML who successfully received a nonmyeloablative matched unrelated donor allograft shortly following SARS-CoV-2 infection, which manifested with mild cough, interstitial abnormalities on chest CT, and pancytopenia with profound bone marrow biopsy histological alterations. In parallel, our study provides bone marrow biopsy data in a series of contemporary patients with serious haematological diseases who had a bone marrow biopsy performed within two weeks of PCR confirmation of SARS-CoV-2 infection. This study is notable because there are no published data describing the bone marrow biopsy changes observed in patients with haematological malignancies and SARS-CoV-2 infection. Finally, it is suggested that nonmyeloablative hematopoietic stem cell transplantation for very high-risk haematological malignancies can be successfully performed following recovery from SARS-CoV-2 infection.

1. Case Report

Corona virus disease 2019 (COVID-19), which is caused by the severe acute respiratory syndrome corona virus 2 (SARS-CoV-2), has infected millions of people all over the world and over one million deaths reported [1].

Individuals infected by SARS-CoV-2 experience a broad spectrum of symptoms, ranging from mild respiratory symptoms to severe respiratory and multiorgan failure [2]. Pathological findings precipitated by the SARS-CoV-2 virus are under intense study, but there is a paucity of data with regards to bone marrow involvement [3]. Herein, we describe the case of a 70-year-old female patient with acute myeloid leukaemia (AML) who had clinically mild COVID-19 infection pretransplant, which resulted in new onset cytopenias and novel bone marrow morphological changes in the absence of disease relapse.

The patient was diagnosed with AML with myelodysplastic changes based on myelodysplastic syndrome-(MDS-) related cytogenetic features but with no morphological evidence of dysplasia in December 2019. She had no significant comorbidities. The immunophenotype of the neoplastic cells at diagnosis was CD34+/CD117+/CD13+/HLA-DR+/nTdt+/CD33-/MPO weak. The karyotype and next generation sequencing panel showed an abnormal karyotype with trisomy13/add(17p) and clinically significant variants in ASXL1, RUNX1, IDH2, and BCOR, respectively.

The patient was treated with two cycles of CPX-351 (liposomal cytarabine/daunorubicin), which were completed in February 2020 and resulted in complete remission. Bone marrow biopsy after cycle two of induction chemotherapy showed prominent postchemotherapy damage and dysplastic megakaryocytes but no excess of blasts, consistent with a dysplastic remission. Karyotype was normal, consistent with cytogenetic remission. The complete blood count (CBC) at that time was Hb 85 g/L, WBC 4.34×10^9/L, neutrophils 1.24×10^9/L, and platelets 85×10^9/L.

Based on the very high-risk genetic profile and taking into account patient fitness and preference, a fully matched volunteer unrelated donor (MUD) hematopoietic stem cell transplant, conditioned with fludarabine/cyclophosphamide/total body irradiation 2 Gy with post-transplant cyclophosphamide/tacrolimus/mycophenolate mofetil for primary graft versus host disease prophylaxis, was deployed for consolidation due to the high-relapse risk and the low rates of chronic graft-versus-host disease observed with this T-replete nonmyeloablative conditioning regimen [4].

The patient had a screening nasopharyngeal swab for SARS-CoV-2 before the planned admission date for the transplant, which was reported as positive. The transplant was therefore postponed. Apart from mild fatigue and mild dry cough, the patient did not report significant symptoms. CRP was only mildly elevated, peak level recorded 39 mg/L. Over the next two weeks, the patient became more pancytopenic and required transfusion support with packed red cells and platelets (CBC at the end of April: Hb 67 g/L, WBC 2.30×10^9/L, neutrophils 0.81×10^9/L, and platelets 7×10^9/L). Repeat bone marrow biopsy showed no evidence of relapse, but accentuated myelodysplasia-related findings including striking erythroid hyperplasia, megaloblastic features (folate 2.4 μg/L and vitamin B12 371 ng/L), extreme "stress-type" arrangement of erythroid cells, myeloid suppression, reduced numbers of megakaryocytes with megakaryocytic atypia, and increased histiocytes (confirmed on CD163 and CD68/PGM1 immunostaining) in conjunction with other features of stromal damage, consistent with very pronounced toxic-type injury (Figure 1). The aspirate showed abundant foamy macrophages with markedly reduced megakaryocytes, some haemophagocytosis, and mild erythroid dysplasia. Liver function tests confirmed elevated bilirubin and ferritin at 31 μmol/L and 1854 ng/mL, respectively, with normal enzymes. The patient was afebrile and did not have any organomegaly. The karyotype was normal. Serology was negative for HIV, hepatitis B/C/E, and oarvovirus, whereas the patient was negative for EBV and CMV by PCR. PT was only mildly prolonged at 15 seconds and APTT was never prolonged; D-dimer and fibrinogen were not measured. High resolution CT scan of the chest demonstrated bilateral air space opacities, with ground glass changes and interlobular septal thickening in the right lower lobe. The patient underwent bronchoalveolar lavage which did not isolate any other viral, fungal, or bacterial pathogen. In all, there were neither respiratory sequelae (other than the mild cough), nor any need to treat with remdesivir or steroids, as repeat SARS-CoV-2 nasopharyngeal swabs were negative and there was improvement in the findings in the follow-up high resolution CT scan of the chest. The patient therefore proceeded with the planned nonmyeloablative MUD allogeneic stem cell transplant. The peritransplant period was complicated by a single episode of culture negative febrile neutropenia and delayed engraftment (neutrophils-platelets engrafted on days +25 and +45, respectively). The patient remains well, disease-free (100% chimerism), without infective concerns, or active GvHD as of the time of writing this report, on day +180 out from transplant.

2. Discussion

This case describes an individual who was incidentally diagnosed with SARS-COV-2 infection before a planned bone marrow transplant for high-risk AML with MDS-related changes. At the time of SARS-CoV-2 infection, the patient was in complete remission with near normal counts, but the virus triggered new onset transfusion-dependent cytopenias. The transplant was therefore deferred by four weeks. Bone marrow biopsy two weeks after SARS-COV-2 infection diagnosis revealed marked changes (i.e., exacerbated dysplasia in hematopoietic cells, abundant histiocytes, and toxic stromal changes). To date, there are no data from patient series with regards to SARS-CoV-2-induced bone marrow biopsy changes although there have been scant data about bone marrow haemophagocytosis in bone marrow aspirates in patients with severe SARS-CoV-2 infection [5].

The haematological manifestations in patients with symptomatic SARS-CoV-2 infection have been widely reported and include leukopenia with lymphopenia and mild thrombocytopenia. However, the exact mechanisms causing these cytopenias are unclear and might involve both peripheral destruction/consumption and medullary dysfunction [6].

Cytopenias may be caused by a reduction in CD34+ cells, which may occur due to a variety of mechanisms. The SARS-CoV-2 virus can bind to the ACE2 receptor on the surface of hematopoietic cells and be internalized into CD34+ cells, resulting in viral replication and apoptosis. This process may be facilitated by CD13 and CD66a (EACAMIa) receptors, which are present on the surface of human bone marrow CD34+ cells. It has been also proposed that autoantibodies targeting CD34+ bone marrow cells may be produced in some individuals with SARS-CoV-2 infection [7, 8]. SARS-CoV-2 may also affect bone marrow stromal cells, leading to an altered bone marrow microenvironment.

Patients with severe SARS-CoV-2 infection experience an excessive inflammatory response characterized by high levels of cytokines, profound lymphopenia, and substantial mononuclear cell infiltration in the lungs, heart, spleen lymph nodes, and kidneys [9]. Destruction of bone marrow progenitor cells by the cytokine storm could overwhelm the rate of blood cell production, resulting in cytopenias [10]. Macrophages are key players as they can be evaded directly by the virus and activated by inflammatory signals, such as type I interferon, with recruitment to inflamed tissues via chemokine receptor CCR-2 [11, 12]. This explains the accumulation of histiocytes and stromal abnormalities observed in this patient's bone marrow biopsy after infection with the SARS-CoV-2 virus. Similar changes also were observed in two other patients in our centre who were diagnosed with COVID-19 as discussed in Table 1 (patient number six who died of COVID-19 after BEAM-autologous stem cell for nodular lymphocyte predominant Hodgkin lymphoma and case two with newly

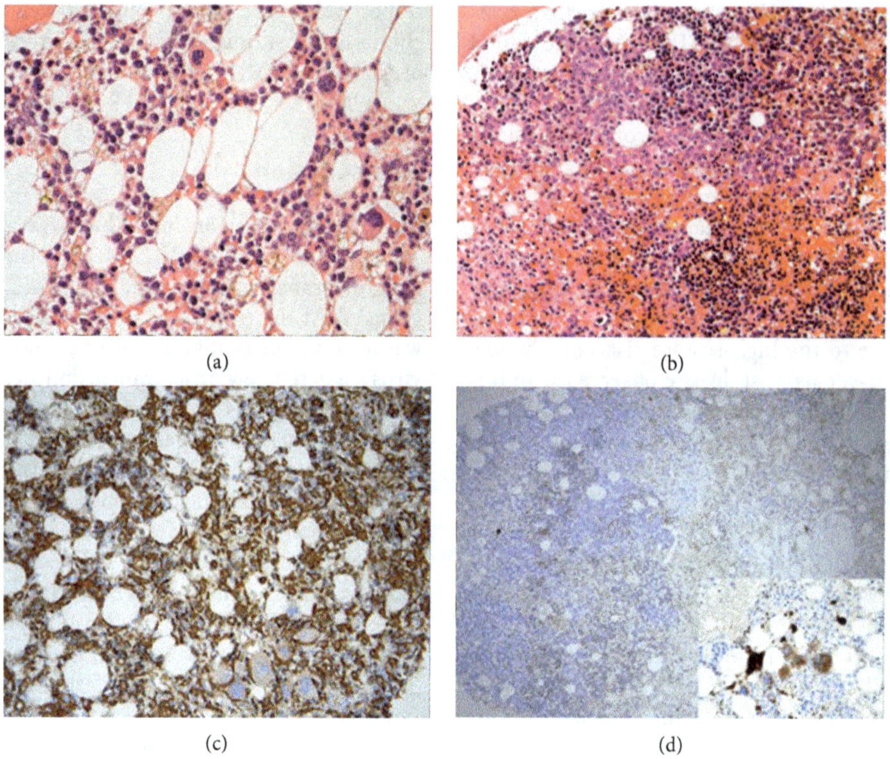

FIGURE 1: Bone marrow biopsy findings before and after COVID-19 diagnosis. (a) Before SARS-CoV-2 detection, all three main hematopoietic lineages were visible. There was no significant dysplasia. Erythroid cells were relatively scant and scattered. There was subtle stromal damage. (b) Following SARS-CoV-2 infection, prominent erythroid hyperplasia and signs of stromal damage were observed. Large clusters of erythroid cells were locally synchronised at the same maturational stage ("stress erythropoiesis"). Proerythroblasts showed megaloblastoid features. Erythroid cells approached the trabecular bone. (c) An excess of stromal histiocytes on CD163 immunostaining after SARS-CoV-2 infection. (d) On CD61 immunostaining, profound megakaryocytic deficit and atypia were illustrated after SARS-CoV-2 infection.

TABLE 1: Characteristics of haematology patients with SARS-CoV-2 infection who had simultaneous bone marrow biopsy.

Patient	Age	Gender	Diagnosis	Stage of disease	Date of bone marrow biopsy compared to most recent COVID PCR positivity	Bone marrow findings	Full blood count	Coagulation results	Outcome
Case described	70	Female	AML	In CR1, after 2 cycles of induction chemotherapy (CPX-351)	After 8 days	Suppressed myelopoiesis. No excess of blasts. Hyperplastic erythropoiesis with stress-type arrangement. Young forms appear megaloblastic. Reduced megakaryocytes with atypia. Many foamy histiocytes	Hb 86 g/L, WCC 2.36×10^9/L, neutrophils 1.10×10^9/L, lymphocytes 0.74×10^9/L, monocytes 0.43×10^9/L, platelets 15×10^9/L	PT NA, APTT NA, fibrinogen NA, D-dimer NA	Now COVID-19 negative and has engrafted post-allogeneic stem cell transplant

Table 1: Continued.

Patient	Age	Gender	Diagnosis	Stage of disease	Date of bone marrow biopsy compared to most recent COVID PCR positivity	Bone marrow findings	Full blood count	Coagulation results	Outcome
2	68	Female	Multiple myeloma	Diagnosis	N/A	Severely reduced megakaryocytes, erythropoiesis, and myelopoiesis. >90% blastoid plasma cells	Hb 76 g/L, WCC 7.88×10^9/L, neutrophils 2.44×10^9/L, lymphocytes 3.58×10^9/L, monocytes 1.79×10^9/L, platelets 129×10^9/L	PT 16.2 seconds, APTT 28.8 seconds, fibrinogen NA, D-dimer NA	Now COVID-19 negative. Ongoing induction chemotherapy
2	68	Female	Multiple myeloma	Midthird cycle of chemotherapy	After 3 days	Globally reduced megakaryocytes with nonspecific atypia. Normal myelopoiesis with scattered hyperplastic areas. Normal erythropoiesis with scattered hyperplastic areas. Postnecrotic scarring with numerous histiocytes and a few clusters of histiocytes. Scattered residual blastoid plasma cells	Hb 89 g/L, WCC 4.2 × 109/L, neutrophils 2.99 × 109/L, lymphocytes 0.71 × 109/L, monocytes 0.47 × 109/L, platelets 13 × 109/L	PT 12.65 seconds, APTT 28.35 seconds, fibrinogen 4.00 g/L, D-dimer 2034 ng/ml	Now COVID-19 negative. Ongoing induction chemotherapy
3	47	Male	Aplastic anaemia	Diagnosis	After 1 day	Myelopoiesis almost completely absent. Erythropoiesis almost completely absent. Megakaryocytes completely absent. Scattered increase in mast cells, which are very granulated. Less than 5% bone marrow cellularity	Hb 56 g/L, WCC 3.98×10^9/L, neutrophils 0.5×10^9/L, lymphocytes 3.36×10^9/L, monocytes 0.11×10^9/L, platelets 23×10^9/L	PT 12.7 seconds, APTT 27.8 seconds, fibrinogen NA, D-dimer NA	Now COVID-19 negative. Awaiting allogeneic stem cell transplant for very severe aplastic anaemia
4	88	Male	MDS with multilineage dysplasia	Diagnosis	After 2 days	Suppressed left shifted myelopoiesis. 1–2% blasts. Dysplastic, hyperplastic erythropoiesis. Increased megakaryocytes with numerous dysplastic micromegakaryocytes. Moderate excess of mast cells that are degranulated	Hb 78 g/L, WCC 3.7×10^9/L, neutrophils 0.48×10^9/L, lymphocytes 2.90×10^9/L, monocytes 0.32×10^9/L, platelets 32×10^9/L	PT 14.6 seconds, APTT NA, fibrinogen NA, D-dimer NA	Now COVID-19 negative. Ongoing support with G-CSF and erythropoietin

Table 1: Continued.

Patient	Age	Gender	Diagnosis	Stage of disease	Date of bone marrow biopsy compared to most recent COVID PCR positivity	Bone marrow findings	Full blood count	Coagulation results	Outcome
5	79	Male	Primary myelofibrosis	Suspected disease progression	After 7 days	Suppressed myelopoiesis. 8% blasts. Dysplastic erythropoiesis. Increased megakaryocytes which look dysplastic, including micromegakaryocytes. Diffuse stromal fibrosis, Bauermeister 3+	Hb 70 g/L, WCC 3.21×10^9/L, neutrophils 1.76×10^9/L, lymphocytes 0.91×10^9/L, monocytes 0.52×10^9/L, platelets 56×10^9/L	PT 15.0 seconds, APTT 29.9 seconds, fibrinogen 4.17 g/L, D-dimer 1519 ng/ml	COVID-19 negative on discharge. Died of progressive disease
6	41	Male	Nodular lymphocyte predominant Hodgkin lymphoma	3 months after BEAM autograft	Before 4 days	Normal myelopoiesis. Normal erythropoiesis. Reduced megakaryocytes but no dysplastic features. Extensive stromal oedema and expansion of loose pathological extracellular matrix. No pathological lymphoid infiltrate	Hb 123 g/L, WCC 3.36×10^9/L, neutrophils 2.80×10^9/L, lymphocytes 0.43×10^9/L, monocytes 0.13×10^9/L, platelets 17×10^9/L	PT 15.8 seconds, APTT 26.8 seconds, fibrinogen 5.31 g/L, D-dimer 11380 ng/ml	Died of COVID-19
7	65	Female	AML with MDS-related changes	6 weeks after allogeneic stem cell transplant	Before 13 days	Chaotic myelopoiesis. Normal erythropoiesis. Increased megakaryocytes, which are mostly small and dysplastic. 30–40% blasts. Widespread stromal oedema	Hb 85 g/L, WCC 1.45×10^9/L, neutrophils 0.61×10^9/L, lymphocytes 0.5×10^9/L, monocytes 0.28×10^9/L, platelets 33×10^9/L	PT NA, APTT NA, fibrinogen NA, D-dimer NA	Died of disease relapse

diagnosed blastoid plasma cell myeloma who also developed severe thrombocytopenia amidst velcade/thalidomide/dexamethasone induction treatment). The remaining patients described in Table 1 had newly diagnosed haematological disorders and the causative role of the SARS-CoV-2 infection in their abnormal bone marrow histology is felt less likely.

The patient described in this report had been diagnosed with high-risk AML with MDS-related changes The bone marrow microenvironment in MDS is characterized by higher levels of inflammatory cytokines and upregulation of cell surface receptors for proinflammatory molecules [13], such as TGF-beta, IL-1-beta and, danger-associated molecular pattern (DAMP) proteins. Therefore, the "dysplastic" hematopoietic progenitor cells and their bone marrow niche inflicted severe dysfunction during an otherwise mild COVID-19.

The immunocompromised nature of patients with haematological malignancies, including patients undergoing allogeneic stem cell transplantation, could have a negative impact on clearance of the SARS-CoV-2 virus. On the other hand, it might play an important role in later phases of the disease, by regulating inflammatory processes [14].

There is a dilemma regarding the appropriate management of transplant candidates who have been infected with the SARS-CoV-2 virus as there is insufficient evidence to support whether stem cell transplantation should be postponed or not. The European Society for Blood and Marrow Transplantation (EBMT) recommendations advise that deferral of the transplant procedure should be considered in patients who are PCR positive for SARS-CoV-2 infection [15]. However, they acknowledge that this decision should be individualised, taking into account the risk of progression of the underlying disease. They advise that patients with high risk disease who have tested positive for SARS-CoV-2 should have their transplant procedure deferred for a minimum of 14 days and that they should be asymptomatic and have had two negative PCR tests for the SARS-CoV-2 virus that have been taken at least 24 hours apart [15]. In keeping with this guidance, the transplant procedure was deferred by four weeks in the case described in this report. We proceeded once PCR negativity for SARS-CoV-2 infection was confirmed and the CT changes were resolving [15].

3. Conclusion

To the best of our knowledge, this is the first report focusing on bone marrow architectural changes in the context of SARS-CoV-2 infection, in addition to the feasibility of proceeding to a nonmyeloablative allogeneic stem cell transplant with post-transplant cyclophosphamide for an elderly individual with high-risk AML less than one month following SARS-CoV-2 infection. Our report describes how the virus might precipitate marked bone marrow pathology in patients predisposed to inflammatory bone marrow states (e.g., postchemotherapy or in myelodysplasia). In view of the very limited number of patients and the heterogeneity of haematological diagnoses of the patients described in this report, further multicentre clinical studies are warranted to best evaluate the bone marrow changes induced by SARS-CoV-2 infection and to inform the optimal peritransplant management of patients with recent SARS-CoV-2 infection.

Abbreviations

AML: Acute myeloid leukaemia
CR: Complete remission
CPX-351: Liposomal daunorubicin/cytarabine
Hb: Haemoglobin
WCC: White cell count
PT: Prothrombin time
PTT: Partial thromboplastin time
COVID-19: Corona virus disease 2019
MDS: Myelodysplasia
BEAM: Carmustine/etoposide/cytarabine/melphalan.

Consent

No written consent has been obtained from the patients as there is no patient identifiable data included in this case report.

Authors' Contributions

AK, MN, HG, and MK conceived and designed the study. MK, AK, HG, ZR, and MN wrote the manuscript. All authors were involved in data collection and patient management and provided crucial intellectual input.

References

[1] Q. Li, X. Guan, P. Wu et al., "Early transmission dynamics in wuhan, China, of novel coronavirus-infected pneumonia," *New England Journal of Medicine*, vol. 382, no. 13, pp. 1199–1207, 2020.

[2] N. Chen, M. Zhou, X. Dong et al., "Epidemiological and clinical characteristics of 99 cases of 2019 novel coronavirus pneumonia in Wuhan, China: a descriptive study," *The Lancet*, vol. 395, no. 10223, pp. 507–513, 2020.

[3] T. Menter, J. D. Haslbauer, R. Nienhold et al., "Post-mortem examination of COVID19 patients reveals diffuse alveolar damage with severe capillary congestion and variegated findings of lungs and other organs suggesting vascular dysfunction," *Histopathology*, vol. 3, 2020.

[4] Y. L. Kasamon, R. F. Ambinder, E. J. Fuchs et al., "Prospective study of nonmyeloablative, HLA-mismatched unrelated BMT with high-dose posttransplantation cyclophosphamide," *Blood Advances*, vol. 1, no. 4, pp. 288–292, 2017.

[5] A. Debliquis, I. Harzallah, J. Y. Mootien et al., "Haemophagocytosis in bone marrow aspirates in patients with COVID-19," *British Journal of Haematology*, vol. 190, no. 2, pp. e70–e3, 2020.

[6] A. Amgalan and M. Othman, "Exploring possible mechanisms for COVID-19 induced thrombocytopenia: unanswered questions," *Journal of Thrombosis and Haemostasis*, vol. 18, no. 6, pp. 1514–1516, 2020.

[7] Y. Zhang, X. Zeng, Y. Jiao et al., "Mechanisms involved in the development of thrombocytopenia in patients with COVID-19," *Thrombosis Research*, vol. 193, pp. 110–115, 2020.

[8] W. Chen, Z. Li, B. Yang et al., "Delayed-phase thrombocytopenia in patients of coronavirus disease 2019 (COVID-19)," *British Journal of Haematology*, vol. 190, pp. 174–184, 2020.

[9] M. Merad and J. C. Martin, "Pathological inflammation in patients with COVID-19: a key role for monocytes and macrophages," *Nature Reviews Immunology*, vol. 20, no. 6, pp. 355–362, 2020.

[10] P. Xu, Q. Zhou, and J. Xu, "Mechanism of thrombocytopenia in COVID-19 patients," *Annals of Hematology*, vol. 99, no. 6, pp. 1205–1208, 2020.

[11] I. Hamming, W. Timens, M. Bulthuis, A. Lely, G. Navis, and H. van Goor, "Tissue distribution of ACE2 protein, the functional receptor for SARS coronavirus. A first step in understanding SARS pathogenesis," *The Journal of Pathology*, vol. 203, no. 2, pp. 631–637, 2004.

[12] B. M. Henry, M. H. S. De Oliveira, S. Benoit, M. Plebani, and G. Lippi, "Hematologic, biochemical and immune biomarker abnormalities associated with severe illness and mortality in coronavirus disease 2019 (COVID-19): a meta-analysis," *Clinical Chemistry and Laboratory Medicine (CCLM)*, vol. 58, no. 7, pp. 1021–1028, 2020.

[13] A. J. Li and L. M. Calvi, "The microenvironment in myelodysplastic syndromes: niche-mediated disease initiation and progression," *Experimental Hematology*, vol. 55, pp. 3–18, 2017.

[14] A. Niu, A. McDougal, B. Ning et al., "COVID-19 in allogeneic stem cell transplant: high false-negative probability and role of CRISPR and convalescent plasma," *Bone Marrow Transplant*, vol. 34, 2020.

[15] P. Ljungman, M. Mikulska, M. Mikulska et al., "The challenge of COVID-19 and hematopoietic cell transplantation; EBMT recommendations for management of hematopoietic cell transplant recipients, their donors, and patients undergoing CAR T-cell therapy," *Bone Marrow Transplantation*, vol. 55, no. 11, pp. 2071–2076, 2020.

31

Nonimmunoglobulin Crystal-Storing Histiocytosis (CSH): Case Report and Literature Review

Manuel Beltran,[1] Sharad Khurana,[2] Yennifer Gil,[3] Jason T. Lewis,[4] Rohit Kumar,[5] and James M. Foran[6]

[1]*Division of General Internal Medicine, Mayo Clinic, Jacksonville, FL, USA*
[2]*Division of Hematology & Oncology, University of Arizona Cancer Center, Tucson, AZ, USA*
[3]*Department of Anesthesia and Preoperative Medicine, Mayo Clinic, Jacksonville, FL, USA*
[4]*Department of Pathology, Mayo Clinic, Jacksonville, FL, USA*
[5]*Division of Medical Oncology and Hematology, University of Louisville, Louisville, KY, USA*
[6]*Department of Hematology & Oncology, Mayo Clinic, Jacksonville, FL, USA*

Correspondence should be addressed to James M. Foran; foran.james@mayo.edu

Academic Editor: Masayuki Nagasawa

Crystal-storing histiocytosis (CSH) is an uncommon condition in which histiocytes accumulate a crystalline matter within their cytoplasm. Generally, those crystals are composed of either monoclonal or polyclonal immunoglobulin chains, which have a strong association with an underlying lymphoproliferative or plasma cell disorder (LP-PCD). Rarely, CSH has been reported as local or generalized manifestation of a variety of benign disorders. These cases are associated with crystals composed of nonimmunoglobulin substances. We are reporting an exceptional case of a local colonic CSH with Charcot–Leyden crystals. This patient underwent a screening colonoscopy that detected some polyps. The biopsy reported tubular adenomas, with a markedly dense, transmural inflammatory infiltrates, which were predominantly composed of eosinophils and crystal-storing histiocytes containing Charcot–Leyden crystals. The patient had a negative workup for LP-PCD and autoimmune conditions, including a normal skeletal survey and bone marrow aspirate/biopsy. The only positive laboratory workup was an elevated absolute eosinophil count and a positive IgG anti-*Strongyloides* antibody. Giving those findings, this parasitic infection is the most likely etiology of the CSH in our patient. Although there was an initial negative evaluation for LP-PCD, close monitoring of patients with either immunoglobulin or nonimmunoglobulin CSH is recommended.

1. Introduction

Crystal-storing histiocytosis (CSH) is a unique entity presenting as sheets of histiocytes with accumulation of crystalline matter within the cytoplasm. It can present as either a localized or generalized disease and has a variable outcome depending on the underlying CSH etiology [1]. Most often, the crystals are composed of monoclonal or polyclonal immunoglobulin light or heavy chains and have a strong association with an underlying lymphoproliferative or plasma cell disorder (LP-PCD) [1–3]. Rarely, the crystals are composed of nonimmunoglobulin substances such as clofazimine, cystine, silica, or Charcot–Leyden crystals and are often seen in association with a variety of benign disorders [1]. Literature on nonimmunoglobulin CSH is scarce. We discuss here a case of presentation with a colonic-only nonimmunoglobulin CSH with Charcot–Leyden crystals, along with a review of literature on this rare disease.

2. Case Description

A 55-year-old man with a history of hypertension, hyperlipidemia, gout, recurrent *H. pylori* gastritis, gastroesophageal reflux with reflux esophagitis and esophageal stricture underwent a screening colonoscopy which showed polyps along with white nodular submucosa in the proximal ascending colon. Biopsy confirmed tubular adenomas, with a markedly dense, transmural inflammatory infiltrates predominantly composed of eosinophils and crystal-storing histiocytes containing Charcot–Leyden crystals (Figures 1 and 2). Besides the recurrent dyspeptic symptoms and dysphagia, he denied any other gastrointestinal symptoms such as cramping, diarrhea, or constipation. Review of system was negative for any fatigue, recurrent infections, bony pain, or easy bleeding/bruising. Laboratory workup showed an elevated absolute eosinophil count of 500 cells/μl and a positive IgG anti-*Strongyloides* antibody. Serum evaluation for a monoclonal protein, serum free light chains, lactate dehydrogenase (LDH), and beta-2 microglobulin was normal. Tryptase levels and *CHIC2*, *PDGFRA*, and *FIP1L1* gene regions were normal as well. A negative autoimmune workup was noted. Skeletal survey showed no lytic or blastic bony lesions, and CT scan of the chest, abdomen, and pelvis showed no lymphadenopathy or hepatosplenomegaly. Bone marrow aspirate/biopsy did not show any evidence of an underlying plasma cell disorder or any mast cell disorder. The patient was treated with ivermectin for *Strongyloides stercoralis* infection and continued to follow-up with gastroenterology for his antibiotic and pantoprazole-treated *H. pylori* gastritis and esophagitis. He continued to follow closely with hematology for monitoring of development of any LP-PCD in future.

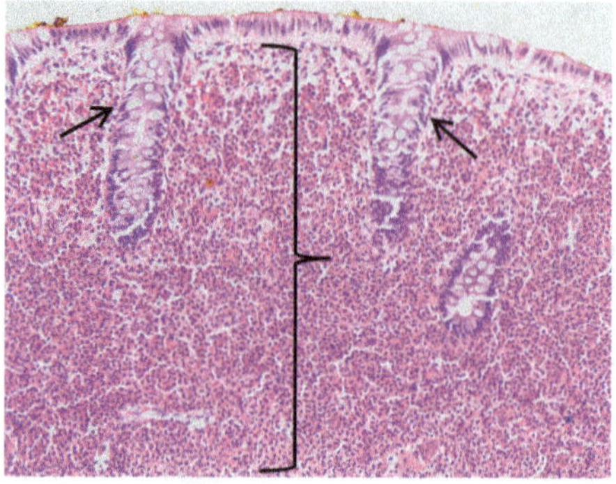

Figure 1: Medium power H&E of the colonic mucosa demonstrating a diffuse expansion of the lamina propria by eosinophils (denoted by black bracket). There is displacement of the colonic crypts (black arrows). No other inflammatory cell types are seen.

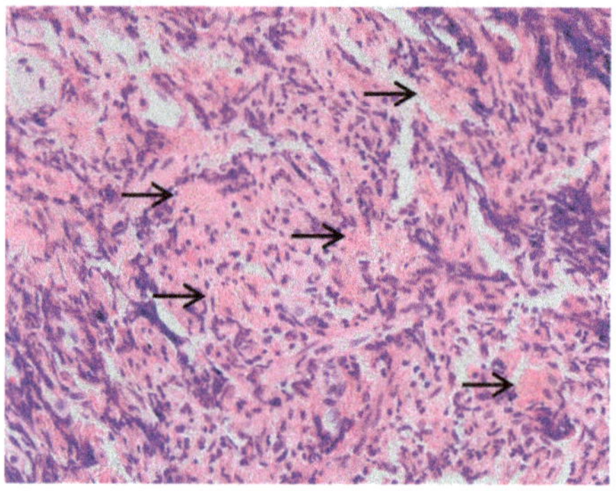

Figure 2: High power H&E showing aggregates of histiocytes within the muscularis mucosa and superficial submucosa. The cytoplasm of the histiocytes contains eosinophilic Charcot–Leyden crystals which are present in the form of fine, granular, and needle-shaped deposits within the macrophage cytoplasm (black arrows).

3. Discussion

Around 90% cases of crystal-storing histiocytosis (CSH) are associated with an underlying LP-PCD such as multiple myeloma (MM), lymphoplasmacytic lymphoma (LPL), and monoclonal gammopathy of undetermined significance (MGUS) [1, 2]. Overproduction of kappa light chain protein, abnormalities in specific stored paraprotein sequences, and resistance to intralysosomal degradation have been proposed as possible mechanisms of accumulation and crystallization of immunoglobulins in the cytoplasm of histiocytes [3, 4].

Approximately 8.8% of CSH cases are seen in association with a variety of benign disorders. Conditions with hyperactivated immune system such as rheumatoid arthritis, Fanconi syndrome, Crohn's disease, eosinophilic colitis, and mastocytosis; infections like *H. pylori*; and drugs like clozafamine have been reported in patients with CSH without an underlying LP-PCD [2, 3]. In these cases, materials different from immunoglobulins have been described, including clofazimine-induced CSH, Charcot–Leyden crystal-associated CSH, and CSH associated with hereditary cystinosis [2] (Table 1).

Besides the composition of the crystals, CSH can be classified as localized CSH (L-CSH), involving only one organ or site such as lung, pleura, stomach, kidney, bone marrow, thyroid, thymus, and parotid gland [3, 4], and generalized CSH (G-CSH), involving two or more distant organs or sites. [3]. According to Dogan et al., only 8% of localized CSH cases have been detected in the gastrointestinal tract. In fact, just 3 cases of colonic CSH have been described in the literature so far [3, 8], seen in association with eosinophilic colitis, MGUS, and lymphoma. We present here, colonic-only Charcot–Leyden crystals (CLC) CSH, possibly related to the patient's history of strongyloidiasis with associated peripheral eosinophilia.

Charcot–Leyden crystals have hexagonal and bipyramidal forms [11]. They are compounds of galectin-10 (Gal-10), a member of the family of S-type lectin proteins [12]. Gal-10 is a major constituent of eosinophils, estimated to be around 7–10% of total cellular proteins. A higher percentage is usually a sign of eosinophilic inflammation [12]. This protein is insoluble at neutral pH, remarkably resistant to various enzymes, and exhibits a tendency to form non-covalent aggregates [12]. Activated eosinophils trigger a nonapoptotic extracellular trap cell death called *ETosis*, where Gal-10 is homogeneously redistributed in the cytoplasm, followed by intracellular CLC formation. Subsequently, the eosinophil plasma membrane ruptures, releasing chromatin and vesicles together with CLC [12]. Additionally, pathogens and parasites may also induce eosinophilic apoptosis triggering a massive eosinophilic release of Gal-10, thereby resulting in extracellular CLC formation

Table 1: Nonimmunoglobulin CSH reported in literature.

Source	Sex/age	Patient history/underlying disease	Organ(s) involved by CSH	Type of crystal	Symptoms/ indication for workup	Disease status at last follow-up
Sukpanichnant [5]	M/32 y	Leprosy	SI and LN	Clofazimine crystals	Chronic abdominal pain	Died 2 months after diagnosis; had an acute onset of dyspnea
Gebrail [6]	M/23 y	Hereditary cystinosis	Cornea, conjunctiva, BM	Cystine crystals	Pancytopenia	Not described
Pais [7]	F/44 y	Leprosy	Intra-abdominal LN, omentum, and peritoneum	Clofazimine crystals	Mild abdominal pain	Complete remission
Lewis [8]	F/78 y	Eosinophilic colitis	Colon	Charcot–Leyden crystals	Chronic abdominal pain and diarrhea	Not described
Singh [9]	M/19 y	Leprosy	Duodenum and jejunum	Clofazimine crystals	Acute abdominal pain	Complete remission
Szeto [10]	F/68 y	Disseminated *M. abscessus*, clofazimine enteropathy	Terminal ileum	Clofazimine crystals	Abdominal pain, diarrhea, weight loss, and hematochezia	Complete remission
Present case	M/55 y	Strongyloidiasis	Proximal ascending colon	Charcot–Leyden crystals	Epigastric pain	—

F, female; M, male; y, years; SI, small intestine; BM, bone marrow; LN, lymph nodes.

[11, 12]. It has been demonstrated both in vitro and in vivo that macrophages/histiocytes are able to engulf CLC and Gal-10 to form additional CLCs in the phagosomes of macrophages, leading to CLC CSH [11, 12].

Strongyloidiasis is a disease caused by a nematode *Strongyloides stercoralis.* Clinical manifestations can range from asymptomatic eosinophilia to gastrointestinal symptoms, such as upper abdominal pain, diarrhea, anorexia, nausea, and vomiting. In addition, patients can develop cutaneous or pulmonary symptoms [13]. *Strongyloides* causes direct eosinophilic infiltrate in the colonic mucosa [14], and as a result, CLC deposits could be expected even in the absence of colorectal symptoms, as was seen in our patient. *H. pylori* have been described as a cause of CSH in the stomach [15]. Therefore, it could potentially be a differential etiology for our patients with colonic CSH. However, the colonic location of CSH, the presence of eosinophilic infiltrate in the colonic polyp biopsy, peripheral eosinophilia, and the positive IgG anti-*Strongyloides* antibody make *H. pylori* an unlikely etiology of our patients with CSH [14].

CSH has been reported as a first manifestation or a subclinical stage of underlying neoplasms such as thymic lymphoma, multiple myeloma, or lymphoreticular malignancy [1, 15]. As such, an initial negative evaluation for an LP-PCD does not obviate the need for a close follow-up in patients diagnosed with either immunoglobulin or nonimmunoglobulin CSH.

In conclusion, CSH is an uncommon phenomenon of aggregation of crystals within the histiocytic cytoplasm, which are usually made up of immunoglobulins. Nonimmunoglobulin CSH is extremely rare and is usually associated with benign conditions. We report here a Charcot–Leyden colonic-only CSH associated with *Strongyloides* infection in the absence of LP-PCD.

Disclosure

Manuel Beltran and Sharad Khurana are co-first authors.

Authors' Contributions

Manuel Beltran and Sharad Khurana contributed equally to this work.

References

[1] M. Joo, J. E. Kwak, S. H. Chang et al., "Localized gastric crystal-storing histiocytosis," *Histopathology*, vol. 51, no. 1, pp. 116–118, 2007.

[2] S. Dogan, L. Barnes, and W. P. Cruz-Vetrano, "Crystal-storing histiocytosis: Report of a case, review of the literature (80 cases) and a proposed classification," *Head and Neck Pathology*, vol. 6, no. 1, pp. 111–120, 2012.

[3] R. Kanagal-Shamanna, Z. Y. Xu-Monette, R. N. Miranda et al., "Crystal-storing histiocytosis: A clinicopathological study of 13 cases," *Histopathology*, vol. 68, no. 4, pp. 482–491, 2016.

[4] Y. Fujita, H. Oikawa, Y. Toya et al., "Gastric crystal-storing histiocytosis without any underlying disorders: report of a

case," *Human Pathology: Case Reports*, vol. 14, pp. 73–77, 2018.

[5] S. Sukpanichnant, N. S. Hargrove, U. Kachintorn et al., "Clofazimine-induced crystal-storing histiocytosis producing chronic abdominal pain in a leprosy patient," *The American Journal of Surgical Pathology*, vol. 24, no. 1, pp. 129–135, 2000.

[6] F. Gebrail, M. Knapp, G. Perrotta, and H. Cualing, "Crystalline histiocytosis in hereditary cystinosis," *Archives of Pathology & Laboratory Medicine*, vol. 126, no. 9, 1135 pages, 2002.

[7] A. V. Pais, S. Pereira, I. Garg, J. Stephen, M. Antony, and Y. K. Inchara, "Intra-abdominal, crystal-storing histiocytosis due to clofazimine in a patient with lepromatous leprosy and concurrent carcinoma of the colon," *Leprosy Review*, vol. 75, no. 2, pp. 171–176, 2004.

[8] J. T. Lewis, J. N. Candelora, R. B. Hogan, F. R. Briggs, and S. C. Abraham, "Crystal-storing histiocytosis due to massive accumulation of Charcot-Leyden crystals: A unique association producing colonic polyposis in a 78-year-old woman with eosinophilic colitis," *The American Journal of Surgical Pathology*, vol. 31, no. 3, pp. 481–485, 2007.

[9] H. Singh, K. Azad, and K. Kaur, "Clofazimine-induced enteropathy in a patient of leprosy," *Indian Jounal of Pharmacology*, vol. 45, no. 2, pp. 197-198, 2013.

[10] W. Szeto, M. T. Garcia-Buitrago, L. Abbo, J. D. Rosenblatt, B. Moshiree, and M. I. Morris, "Clofazimine enteropathy: A rare and underrecognized complication of mycobacterial therapy," *Open Forum Infectious Diseases*, vol. 3, no. 3, pp. 1–4, 2016.

[11] J. Su, "A brief history of charcot-leyden crystal protein/galectin-10 research," *Molecules*, vol. 23, no. 11, p. 2931, 2018.

[12] S. Ueki, Y. Miyabe, Y. Yohei et al., "Charcot-leyden crystals in eosinophilic Inflammation : active cytolysis leads to crystal formation," *Current Allergy and Asthma Reports*, vol. 19, no. 8, 2019.

[13] M. Montes, C. Sawhney, and N. Barros, "Strongyloides stercoralis: there but not seen," *Current Opinion in Infectious Diseases*, vol. 23, no. 5, pp. 500–504, 2010.

[14] A. A. Alfadda, M. A. Storr, and E. A. Shaffer, "Eosinophilic colitis: Epidemiology, clinical features, and current management," *Therapeutic Advances in Gastroenterology*, vol. 4, no. 5, pp. 301–309, 2011.

[15] M. Joo, "Rare gastric lesions Associated with helicobacter pylori infection: A histopathological review," *Journal of Pathology and Translational Medicine*, vol. 51, no. 4, pp. 341–351, 2017.

32

EF Bart's Disease with Coinheritance of Gγ-XmnI and Aγ-Globin Polymorphisms: A Case of Nontransfusion-Dependant Thalassemia

Kane M. Laks,[1] Cara Hirner,[1] Barbara Gruner,[1] Jared Coberly,[2] Katsiaryna Laziuk,[2] and Bindu Kanathezhath Sathi[1,3]

[1]*Department of Pediatrics, University of Missouri School of Medicine, Columbia, MO, USA*
[2]*Department of Pathological Sciences, University of Missouri School of Medicine, Columbia, MO, USA*
[3]*Pediatric Hematology Oncology, Valley Children's Hospital, Madera, CA, USA*

Correspondence should be addressed to Bindu Kanathezhath Sathi; bsathi@valleychildrens.org

Academic Editor: Kostas Konstantopoulos

EF Bart's disease is a rare form of nontransfusion-dependant thalassemia (NTDT) due to the coinheritance of homozygous hemoglobin E (β^E/β^E) genotype with hemoglobin H disease. These individuals are routinely found to have thalassemia intermedia with moderate anemia, increased hemoglobin Bart's and hemoglobin F on electrophoresis. The contribution of hemoglobin F-inducing polymorphisms in this disease has not been described previously. Here, we describe the hematological profile in a young child with coinheritance of Gγ-XmnI and Aγ-globin gene polymorphisms in EF Bart's disease. Interestingly, in this rare form of NTDT, normal HbF and elevated HbA2 were noted.

1. Introduction

The hemoglobin (Hb) tetramer consists of 2 α-globin chains and 2 β-globin chains. β-Thalassemia results from reduced (β^+) or absent (β^0) synthesis of the β-globin chains, with 3 possible phenotypes consisting of clinically asymptomatic β-thalassemia carriers (heterozygotes), transfusion-dependent anemia in thalassemia major, and a wide range of genotypes and clinical features of nontransfusion-dependant thalassemia (NTDT) [1, 2]. The $\alpha\alpha$-thalassemia consists of α^+-thalassemias, with only one of the linked pair of $\alpha\alpha$ genes deleted ($-\alpha/\alpha\alpha$), and α^0-thalassemias, with both genes deleted ($-/\alpha\alpha$) [3–5]. While α^+-thalassemia heterozygotes are clinically asymptomatic, α^0-thalassemia heterozygotes and α^+-thalassemia homozygotes exhibit $\alpha\alpha$-thalassemia trait, with similar features as β-thalassemia trait. HbH disease results from a 3-gene deletion, occurring when both α^+-thalassemia and α^0-thalassemia ($-\alpha$/--) are inherited [6, 7]. HbE is a mildly unstable β-hemoglobin variant, with heterozygotes displaying minimal morphological red blood cell abnormalities and with homozygotes exhibiting significant morphological abnormalities and mild anemia, similar to heterozygous β-thalassemia. HbE commonly co-occurs with forms of β-thalassemia and $\alpha\alpha$-thalassemia, given that all 3 hemoglobinopathies are common in Asia [8–10].

EF Bart's disease (HbH/EE) results from interaction of $\alpha\alpha$-thalassemia (--/-α or --/$\alpha^{cs}\alpha$) mutation with homozygous HbEE (β^E/β^E) or (β^E/β^0), with a clinical phenotype of thalassemia intermedia [10]. The hemoglobin profile consists of HbE and often highly elevated levels of HbF, with the remainder being Hb Bart's [11]. Phenotype consists of mild-to-moderate anemia requiring intermittent transfusion therapy, similar to HbH disease [10]. The cases of EF Bart's disease reported to date have not been examined for the presence of the Aγ-globin gene polymorphism, recently discovered and shown in β-thalassemia syndromes to activate the Aγ-globin gene, with a consequent induction of HbF expression manifesting as a milder phenotype and lower likelihood of requiring transfusions [12]. Frequently found to co-occur with the Aγ-globin gene polymorphism is the XmnI polymorphism which enhances HbF during the mild but chronic erythropoietic stress exhibited in carriers of β-thalassemia [12, 13]. Although these polymorphisms have been shown to induce HbF in β^0-thalassemia syndromes, their contribution in $\alpha\alpha$-thalassemia syndromes, or complex heterozygous thalassemia syndromes, is relatively unknown [12, 14, 15]. Here, we describe coexistent Aγ-globin $G>A$ polymorphism and Gγ-XmnI polymorphism in the setting of EF Bart's disease resulting in nontransfusion-dependant thalassemia with elevated HbA2.

2. Methods

This case report was approved by the institutional review board of University of Missouri, Columbia, MO, USA. Parental consent was obtained for this report. α-Gene sequencing was conducted by direct mutation analysis, with α-globin locus deletions and Hb Constant Spring point mutations being identified by multiplex ligation-dependent probe amplification assay. In order to map the approximate location of DNA deletions, fifteen probes hybridizing throughout the α-globin locus were utilized, from the HS40 promoter region through the 3′HVR region. A PCR-based assay was also used, detecting the presence of α–3.7 and α–4.2 deletion [16].

Steps of β-gene sequencing began with the extraction of genomic deoxyribonucleic acid (DNA) from whole blood, followed by the amplification of HBB gene by polymerase chain reaction (PCR), then purification, and sequencing of the PCR product in both directions with fluorescent dye-terminator chemistry. An automated sequencer was used to separate sequencing products, with trace files being analyzed for variations in all exons and introns other than IVS-II-82 through IVS-II-650, 5′untranslated region (UTR), 3′UTR, and the promoter region. Routine studies were then correlated with the results to identify unusual β-globin variants [17].

The γ-globin full gene sequencing consisted of total genomic DNA being extracted from the sample, followed by full γ-globin genes being amplified by PCR in separate reactions, and then Sanger sequencing. A combination of automated calls and manual inspection was used to review the sequence data (test code: WGSEQ, Mayo Laboratories) [18].

3. Results

The index case was a 2-year-old female of Filipino descent who presented to our hematology clinic with microcytic anemia. Growth parameters and iron indices were normal in this child. Both sister and brother of the index case were previously treated at our clinic for anemia occurring from thalassemia (Table 1). The child had mild hepatosplenomegaly, and there was no evidence of thalassemic facies. Hematological indices (Table 1), peripheral blood smear (Figure 1(a)), and Hb electrophoresis (Figure 1(b)) were obtained.

A strong family history of α-thalassemia and HbE disease was present (Table 1). The mother had α-thalassemia trait with 2 α-globin gene deletion in the cis position, Southeast Asian (SEA) variant (α genotype, $^{SEA}/\alpha\alpha$), and HbE trait (β genotype, β/β^E), with microcytic anemia. The father had α-thalassemia trait with a single α-globin gene deletion and heterozygosity for Hb Constant Spring (CS) (α genotype, $\alpha^{3.7}/\alpha^{CS}\alpha$), as well as HbE trait (β genotype, β/β^E), with microcytic anemia. The brother had HbH disease with 2 α-globin gene deletion in the cis position, SEA variant, and an α-gene deletion on the trans allele (α genotype, $^{SEA}/\text{-}\alpha^{3.7}$, and β genotype, β/β). The sister was a compound heterozygote with α genotype, $-^{SEA}/\alpha^{CS}\alpha$, and β genotype, β/β^E (HbH-CS/*E* trait).

3.1. Genotyping Results. α-Gene sequencing revealed 3 α-genes deleted, a single α-gene in the –3.7 kb on one chromosome, and 2 genes in the other chromosome (α genotype$-^{SEA}/-\alpha^{3.7}$).

β-Gene sequencing revealed HBB had β 26, GAG > AAG, Glu > Lys, resulting in homozygous *E* mutation (β genotype, β^E/β^E).

γ-Globin full gene sequencing revealed that, in chromosome 11, HBG1 A gamma, 5′ UTR + 25, $G>A$, was identified in heterozygous status with resultant Aγ ($G>A$) polymorphism. Additionally, in the gene HBG2, Gγ, promoter-158, $C>T$ polymorphism was detected with heterozygous state for XmnI polymorphism. DNA sequencing did not reveal the presence of these polymorphisms in the brother or sister.

4. Discussion

HbE/β-thalassemia with α^0-thalassemia/α^+-thalassemia (HbH disease) results in NTDT thalassemia syndrome called EF Bart's disease [11]. This disease is usually characterized by hypochromic microcytic red blood cells with variable severities, but is generally milder than homozygous β^0-thalassemia. Although these patients are not routinely transfusion-dependent, they may need intermittent transfusion during episodes of increased hemolysis triggered by infection or conditions of increased oxidative.

Stress [19] red cell transfusion therapy may also be required during periods of severe anemia, pregnancy, growth delay, exercise intolerance, and poor school performance [19].

The hemoglobin range in EF Bart's disease has been described to be around 7.4 ± 1.6 g/dL, but our patient has consistently shown a higher steady-state hemoglobin levels than previously reported in the literature [11, 20].

Further complexity can be added to the clinical picture of compound heterozygous thalassemia syndromes by inducers of HbF, which are often protective. For example, the recently described Aγ-globin gene polymorphism, a $G>A$ polymorphism present at position +25 of the Aγ-globin genes, was detected in our case. This is part of a sequence recognized by DNA-binding protein complexes including LYAR (Ly-1 antibody reactive clone), a transcription factor

Table 1: Steady-state hematological indices of index case and family members.

Age	Proband 1 mo	3 mo	1 yr	2 yr	3 yr	Brother	Sister	Mother	Father
α-Genotype			$-^{SEA}/-\alpha^{3.7}$			$-^{SEA}/-\alpha^{3.7}$	$-^{SEA}/\alpha^{CS}\alpha$	$-^{SEA}/\alpha\alpha$	$-\alpha^{3.7}/\alpha^{CS}\alpha$
β-Genotype			β^{E}/β^{E}			β/β	β/β^{E}	β/β^{E}	β/β^{E}
Hb (g/dl)	10.1	8.1	8.9	9.2	9.4	9.1	7.4	12.3	11.5
RBC (10^{12}/l)	4.60	5.04	6.29	6.40	6.56	5.91	5.10	6.16	5.12
Hct (%)	32.5	24.6	25.6	28.3	29.0	30.9	27.7	39.1	36.7
MCV (fl)	70.7	48.8	40.7	44.2	44.2	52.3	54.3	63.5	71.7
MCH (pg)	22.0	16.1	14.1	14.4	14.3	15.4	14.5	20.0	22.5
MCHC (g/dl)	31.1	32.9	34.8	32.5	32.4	29.4	26.7	31.5	31.3
Retic (%)	1.11		0.38	0.72	0.37	1.47	7.50	0.97	1.30
HbF (%)	64.1	47	7.6	2.2	1.5	0.0	0.0	0.0	0.0
HbA2 (%)		3.3		8.0	8.0	1.4	2.3	3.7	2.8
HbE (%)		43.3		89.7	90.5	0.0	12.6	17.2	17.2
Hb Bart's (%)		6.4				0.0	0.6	0.0	0.0
HbH (%)						4.4			
HbCS (%)							2.7		
S. iron (mcg/dl)							102		
S. ferritin (ng/ml)					83.3	62.7	498		

Abbreviations: Hb = hemoglobin; Hb CS = hemoglobin Constant Spring; RBC = red blood cell; Hct = hematocrit; MCV = mean corpuscular volume; MCH = mean corpuscular hemoglobin; MCHC = mean corpuscular hemoglobin concentration; retic = reticulocyte; mo = month; yr = year.

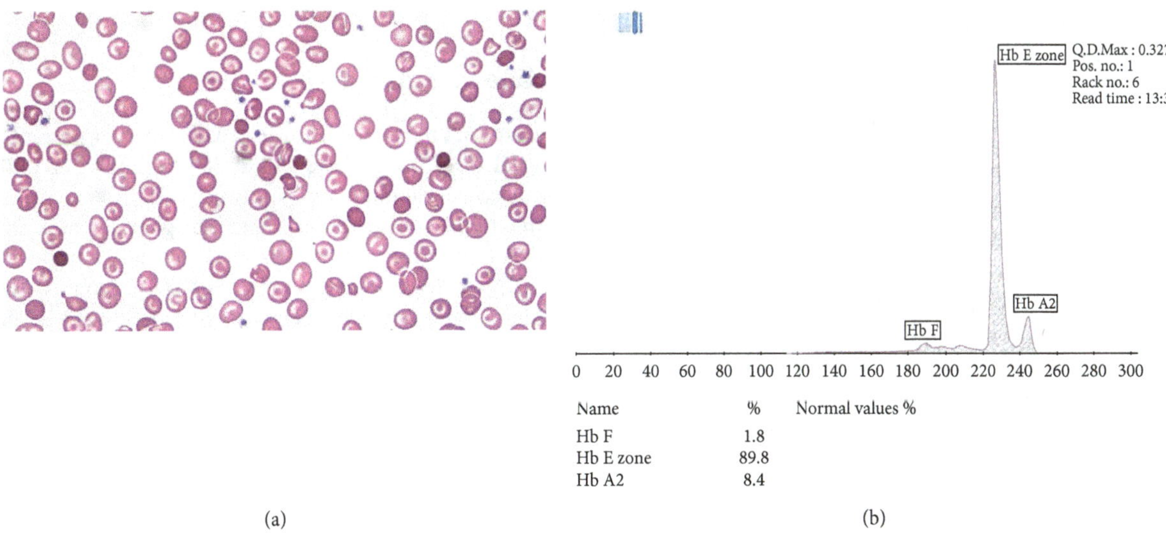

Figure 1: (a) Photomicrographs of Wright-stained peripheral blood film showing microcytosis and hypochromasia. There are multiple-target red blood cells and rare spherocytes and teardrop cells (Wright stain, 1000x). (b) Capillary hemoglobin electrophoresis pattern demonstrating homozygote hemoglobin E (HbE) variant and elevated hemoglobin A2 (HbA2) with the absence of hemoglobin A1 (HbA1) in the peripheral blood sample.

that binds the γ-globin gene and silences it, repressing HbF expression. Conversely, the Aγ-globin gene polymorphism alters the binding activity of LYAR and activates the Aγ-globin gene, inducing HbF expression with a milder phenotype and lower likelihood of requiring transfusions [12, 20]. This polymorphism and the resultant increase in HbF levels are thus considered to be protective in thalassemia syndromes.

Also detected in our case is the XmnI polymorphism, the most common polymorphism associated with HbF induction [21, 22]. Presence of this polymorphism enhances expression of HbF during erythropoietic stress, notably including the mild but chronic erythropoietic stress exhibited in carriers of β-thalassemia, who are thus protected when they express these point mutations [13]. Although heterozygous in our case, the presence of homozygous Gγ-XmnI polymorphism has been reported in another patient with Hb Lepore-EF Bart's disease, where the patient was found to have a milder phenotype of disease [20]. There is very little compensatory HbF increase in these patients. Also, HbH is usually not detectable due to the excessive $\beta^{E}{}_{4}$ globin chains, which do not form tetramers. Previous studies have shown that the Aγ-globin gene polymorphism frequently occurs in complete linkage disequilibrium with the Gγ-XmnI mutation in β-thalassemia, resulting in these two polymorphisms known to increase HbF production occurring together [12].

HbE is the major hemoglobin detected in EF Bart's, with variable levels of Hb Bart's and HbF. Elevated Hb Bart's was detectable on routine hemoglobin electrophoresis in our patient, while HbF was within normal limits. Comigration of HbE to HbA2 zone in routine high-performance liquid chromatography can pose a problem in these cases. We were able to quantify HbE and HbA2 levels via capillary electrophoresis, avoiding the comigration that occurs in cellulose acetate agar and citrate agar electrophoresis. Our patient's HbE was highly elevated at 90%, and interestingly, unlike the cases previously reported with EF Bart's disease, this child showed an elevated HbA2 which was the second dominant hemoglobin and normal levels of HbF for age [11]. A diagnostic dilemma was present due to the abnormal hemoglobin electrophoretic pattern in this child, and detailed DNA sequencing analysis was required to confirm the diagnosis.

Compared to EF Bart's disease or Constant Spring EE Bart's disease, our patient showed a milder phenotype with mild anemia. Contrary to the previous report of 2 patients from Thailand, there was no elevation in HbF in this patient [11]. The mild anemia noted in our child could be due to the coexistence of both α-thalassemia and homozygous HbEE (β^E/β^E) disease which will result in restoration of some degree balance between the α- and β-globin chains.

The α-globin/non-α-globin mRNA ratio has been demonstrated to be a good indicator of disease severity in most of the thalassemia syndromes [23]. The α-globin/non-α-globin mRNA ratio is widely variable in β-thalassemia/HbE patients, with no consistent difference between mild and severe phenotypes [24]. HbE is the result of *G* to *A* mutation in codon 26 of the HBB gene which leads to activation of a cryptic 5′ splice site in codon 25 leading to a reduction in correctly spliced β^E-globin mRNA with resultant β^+ thalassemia [24]. One of the factors that correlate with clinical severity has been found to be the ratio between correctly and aberrantly spliced β^E mRNA in β-thalassemia/HbE disease [24]. The level of mRNA transcript alone will not explain the clinical severity. Other factors involved in transcription, translation, and posttranslational modification of the globin chain, proteolytic capacity of red blood cells, and cellular levels of HbF, ultimately, contributes to the severity of hemoglobin *E* disease [25].

Coinheritance of α^0-thalassemia elevates HbA2 level in homozygous hemoglobin *E* disease [26]. A significant higher expression of Hb A2 has been noted in Hb EE/α^0-thalassemia compared to Hb EE without coexistent α^0-thalassemia. This is likely due to more effective binding of δ-globin chain to α-globin chain to form Hb A2 ($\alpha_2\delta_2$) in conditions of limited availability of α-globin chains as in α^0-thalassemia [26]. The relative elevation in HbA2 in this child could also be due to the survival advantage of the red blood cells with higher δ expression in the presence of abnormal β^E tetramers [25]. Thus, elevation in HbA2 has been found to be a useful marker to differentiate hemoglobin EE disease with and without alpha thalassemia [26].

The interaction of Aγ-globin gene and Gγ-XmnI polymorphisms in complex heterozygous hemoglobinopathies is not fully known, but we speculate this to be protective based on the clinical severity of the disease in this child. Unlike the cases described previously [11], there was no evidence of Hb Bart's in this patient as she grew older, indicating reduced formation of γ_4 tetramers [10, 11].

5. Conclusion

Our patient is 3 years of age and has been transfusion independent to date. This case also presented us with diagnostic challenge due to abnormal hemoglobin electrophoretic pattern, and the variant haemoglobins were confirmed on capillary electrophoresis. Detailed molecular analysis is required in these cases to delineate the complete genotype. Current management of these individuals is supportive with only intermittent need for transfusion. Splenectomy is not routinely indicated or recommended in these patients. The role of erythroid maturation agents, such as luspatercept or sotatercept [19], in complete amelioration of anemia is unknown at this time and must be undertaken only on a clinical trial basis in these complex heterozygous hemoglobinopathies [27].

Acknowledgments

The authors thank Ashutosh Lal, MD, for his input into this clinical case. The authors would like to thank Shalini Sathi for her editorial input and Vazmitsel, MD, for obtaining the hemoglobin electrophoresis and peripheral smear images and for assisting with writing the legends. Bindu Kanathezhath Sathi was supported by the Missouri State Grant for Senior Services and Children with Inherited Blood Disorders (AOC17380120), Leda Sears Trust Fund, at University of Missouri.

References

[1] D. J. Weatherall, "The thalassemias," *Seminars in Hematology*, vol. 4, no. 1, pp. 72–91, 1967.

[2] A. Cao and R. Galanello, "Beta-thalassemia," *Genetics in Medicine*, vol. 12, no. 2, pp. 61–76, 2010.

[3] D. R. Higgs and D. J. Weatherall, "Alpha-thalassemia," *Current Topics in Hematology*, vol. 4, pp. 37–97, 1983.

[4] D. J. Weatherall, "Relationship of hemoglobin bart's and H to alpha thalassemia," *Annals of the New York Academy of Sciences*, vol. 119, pp. 463–473, 1964.

[5] E. P. Vichinsky, "Clinical manifestations of alpha-thalassemia," *Cold Spring Harbor Perspectives in Medicine*, vol. 3, no. 5, Article ID a011742, 2013.

[6] E. Vichinsky, "Advances in the treatment of alpha-thalassemia," *Blood Reviews*, vol. 26, pp. S31–S34, 2012.

[7] A. Lal, M. L. Goldrich, D. A. Haines, M. Azimi, S. T. Singer, and E. P. Vichinsky, "Heterogeneity of hemoglobin H disease in childhood," *New England Journal of Medicine*, vol. 364, no. 8, pp. 710–718, 2011.

[8] E. Vichinsky, "Hemoglobin e syndromes," *Hematology*, vol. 2007, no. 1, pp. 79–83, 2007.

[9] D. C. Rees, L. Styles, E. P. Vichinsky, J. B. Clegg, and D. J. Weatherall, "The hemoglobin E syndromes," *Annals of the New York Academy of Sciences*, vol. 850, pp. 334–343, 1998.

[10] S. Fucharoen and D. J. Weatherall, "The hemoglobin E thalassemias," *Cold Spring Harb Perspectives in Medicine*, vol. 2, no. 8, 2012.

[11] S. Fucharoen, P. Winichagoon, V. Thonglairuam, and P. Wasi, "EF Bart's disease: interaction of the abnormal alpha-and beta-globin genes," *European Journal of Haematology*, vol. 40, no. 1, pp. 75–78, 1988.

[12] G. Breveglieri, N. Bianchi, L. C. Cosenza et al., "An Agamma-globin G->A gene polymorphism associated with beta (0) 39 thalassemia globin gene and high fetal hemoglobin production," *BMC Medical Genetics*, vol. 18, no. 1, p. 93, 2017.

[13] A. Amato, M. P. Cappabianca, M. Perri et al., "Interpreting elevated fetal hemoglobin in pathology and health at the basic laboratory level: new and known γ- gene mutations associated with hereditary persistence of fetal hemoglobin," *International Journal of Laboratory Hematology*, vol. 36, no. 1, pp. 13–19, 2014.

[14] I. S. Chinelato, G. C. D. S. Carrocini, and C. R. Bonini-Domingos, "XmnI polymorphism frequency in heterozygote beta thalassemia subjects and its relation to fetal hemoglobin levels," *Revista Brasileira de Hematologia e Hemoterapia*, vol. 33, no. 6, p. 483, 2011.

[15] T. K. T. Nguyen, P. Joly, C. Bardel, M. Moulsma, N. Bonello-Palot, and A. Francina, "The XmnI Gγ polymorphism influences hemoglobin F synthesis contrary to BCL11A and HBS1L-MYB SNPs in a cohort of 57 β-thalassemia intermedia patients," *Blood Cells, Molecules, and Diseases*, vol. 45, no. 2, pp. 124–127, 2010.

[16] J. P. Schouten, C. J. McElgunn, R. Waaijer et al., "Relative quantification of 40 nucleic acid sequences by multiplex ligation-dependent probe amplification," *Nucleic Acids Research*, vol. 30, no. 12, p. e57, 2002.

[17] P. L. Reddy and L. J. Bowie, "Sequence-based diagnosis of hemoglobinopathies in the clinical laboratory," *Clinics in Laboratory Medicine*, vol. 17, no. 1, pp. 85–96, 1997.

[18] J. Cui, C. Baysdorfer, M. Azimi, E. P. Vichinsky, and C. C. Hoppe, "Identification of three novel Hb F variants: Hb F-hayward [Gγ1(NA1)Gly⟶Asp, GGT > GAT], Hb F-chori-I [AγT16(A13)Gly⟶Asp, GGC > GAC] and Hb F-Chori-II [AγI29(B11)Gly⟶Glu, GGA > GAA]," *Hemoglobin*, vol. 36, no. 3, pp. 305–309, 2012.

[19] A. T. Taher and M. D. Cappellini, "Management of non-transfusion-dependent thalassemia: a practical guide," *Drugs*, vol. 74, no. 15, pp. 1719–1729, 2014.

[20] A. Chaibunruang, G. Fucharoen, A. Jetsrisuparb, and S. Fucharoen, "Hemoglobin Lepore EF bart's disease: a molecular, hematological, and diagnostic aspects," *Annals of Hematology*, vol. 90, no. 11, pp. 1337–1340, 2011.

[21] P. Charoenkwan, P. Teerachaimahit, and T. Sanguansermsri, "The correlation of α-globin gene mutations and theXmnI polymorphism with clinical severity of Hb E/β-Thalassemia," *Hemoglobin*, vol. 38, no. 5, pp. 335–338, 2014.

[22] T. Tatu, W. Sritong, and T. Sa-Nguansermsri, "The associations of SEA-alpha thalassemia 1, XmnI-Ggamma polymorphism and beta-globin gene mutations with the clinical severity of beta-thalassemia syndrome in northern Thailand," *Journal of the Medical Association of Thailand = Chotmaihet Thangphaet*, vol. 97, no. 3, pp. 300–307, 2014.

[23] K. Srinoun, S. Svasti, W. Chumworathayee et al., "Imbalanced globin chain synthesis determines erythroid cell pathology in thalassemic mice," *Haematologica*, vol. 94, no. 9, pp. 1211–1219, 2009.

[24] A. Tubsuwan, T. Munkongdee, N. Jearawiriyapaisarn et al., "Molecular analysis of globin gene expression in different thalassaemia disorders: individual variation of βE pre-mRNA splicing determine disease severity," *British Journal of Haematology*, vol. 154, no. 5, pp. 635–643, 2011.

[25] S. L. Thein, "Genetic modifiers of the β-haemoglobinopathies," *British Journal of Haematology*, vol. 141, no. 3, pp. 357–366, 2008.

[26] K. Singha, H. Srivorakun, G. Fucharoen, and S. Fucharoen, "Co-inheritance of α0 -thalassemia elevates Hb A2 level in homozygous Hb E: diagnostic implications," *International Journal of Laboratory Hematology*, vol. 39, no. 5, pp. 508–512, 2017.

[27] V. Viprakasit, P. Tyan, S. Rodmai et al., "Identification and key management of non-transfusion-dependent thalassaemia patients: not a rare but potentially under-recognised condition," *Orphanet Journal of Rare Diseases*, vol. 9, p. 131, 2014.

33

A Case of Severe COVID-19 in a Patient with Acute Graft-versus-Host Disease after Haploidentical Transplantation

Dan Han [1] **Yuqian Sun,** [2] **Rong Xie,** [1] **Xiaojian Zhu** [3] **and Zhaodong Zhong** [1]

[1] *Department of Hematology, Union Hospital, Tongji Medical College, Huazhong University of Science and Technology, Wuhan 430022, China*

[2] *Peking University Institute of Hematology, Peking University People's Hospital, Beijing Key Laboratory of Hematopoietic Stem Cell Transplantation, Beijing 100044, China*

[3] *Department of Hematology, Tongji Hospital, Tongji Medical College, Huazhong University of Science and Technology, Wuhan 430030, China*

Academic Editor: Tatsuharu Ohno

We report a case of coronavirus disease 2019 (COVID-19) after haploidentical transplantation with acute graft-versus-host disease (aGVHD). COVID-19 and aGVHD were improved under treatment with arbidol, remdesivir, methylprednisolone, and ruxolitinib. However, eventually, the patient died of septic shock and multiple organ failure. It was concluded that the disease condition of this COVID-19 patient after transplantation was serious, complex, and variable, with poor prognosis.

1. Introduction

Coronavirus disease 2019 (COVID-19) is a respiratory disease caused by severe acute respiratory syndrome coronavirus 2 (SARS-CoV-2). SARS-CoV-2 is highly contagious, and the population is generally susceptible to it. In China, the incidence of COVID-19 in the general population is 5.76/100 000, of which 81% are mild, 14% are severe, and 5% are critical cases; the mortality is 2.3% [1]. In addition, nearly 60% of infected individuals are asymptomatic [2].

Allogeneic haematopoietic stem cell transplantation (allo-HSCT) is an effective treatment for haematological malignancy. However, the risk of respiratory tract infection is higher because of the persistent immunodeficient state after transplantation. Graft-versus-host disease (GVHD) is an immune disease caused by graft-versus-host reaction, which is a serious complication and the main cause of death in allo-HSCT. We diagnosed and treated a COVID-19 patient with aGVHD after haploidentical transplantation.

2. Case Presentation

A 20-year-old male patient was admitted to the hospital for "cough and expectoration for 3 days". He had a history of acute B lymphoblastic leukemia and received peripheral blood stem cell transplantation one year ago. Three days prior, skin biopsy of his left upper arm mass confirmed extramedullary recurrence. Laboratory test results are shown in Table 1. Chest CT (Figures 1(a) and 1(b)) showed bilateral scattered high-density shadows and ground-glass opacities in the lungs. Day 3 (on the third day of admission): he received chemotherapy with cytarabine, decitabine, and etoposide. Day 9: transfusions of G-CSF-mobilized peripheral mononuclear cells from the previous donor were used. And he was given ruxolitinib (5 mg, qd) orally to prevent aGVHD. Day 24: the patient began to have a fever, accompanied by cough and expectoration. Chest CT (Figures 1(e) and 1(f)) showed bilateral patchy shadows and filamentous shadows in the lungs, and ground-glass opacity

TABLE 1: Laboratory test results of the patient during hospitalization.

Measure	Reference range	Day 2 baseline	Day 24	Day 27	Day 28	Day 32	Day 37	Day 39
WBC ($\times 10^9$/L)	3.5–9.5	7.45	3.54	5.94	5.22	6.33	13.99	12
NEUT (%)	40%–75%	54.9	89.5	69	62.4	70	85.9	85.5
NEUT ($\times 10^9$/L)	1.8–6.3	4.09	2.46	4.1	3.26	4.43	12.02	10.26
LYM (%)	20%–50%	32.2	26	22.9	25.7	18.4	7.3	12.4
LYM ($\times 10^9$/L)	1.1–3.2	2.4	0.92	1.36	1.34	1.16	1.02	1.49
Hb (g/L)	130–175	117	94	86	97	127	129	125
PLT ($\times 10^9$/L)	125–350	159	149	347	427	302	153	118
D-dimer (mg/L)	0–0.5	0.62	—	1.65	2.13	1.73	—	6.69
FIB (g/L)	2–4	5.15	—	4.17	4.86	4.4	3,2	4.96
PT (s)	11–16	13.5	—	14.6	14.3	12.2	14.7	64.7
APTT (s)	27–45	53.1	—	49.3	56.9	41.7	36.9	57.9
ALT (U/L)	5–40	36	23	51	215	150	53	376
AST (U/L)	8–40	30	20	37	190	86	25	375
ALB (g/L)	33–55	34.7	39.4	36.2	39.4	22	26.2	23.4
T-bil (umol/L)	3–20	5.3	4.4	3.9	7	11.4	15.3	12.1
D-bil (umol/L)	1.7–6.8	0	2.2	2	4.5	6.7	7.8	8.1
BUN (mmol/L)	2.9–8.2	5.96	3.84	5.84	6.68	9.98	16.71	31.3
SCr (umol/L)	57–111	73	79.5	72.2	74.5	58.8	112.1	266.8
K^+ (mmol/L)	3.5–5.3	3.72	4.17	4.25	5.85	3.92	4.01	5.09
Na^+ (mmol/L)	137–147	139	136.9	133.8	130.6	129.2	140.4	133
CRP (mg/L)	<8	28.7	32.7	13.9	60.8	79.78	36.7	93.36
PCT (ng/mL)	<0.05	<0.13	0.37	0.52	10.18	1.48	—	47.87
IL-2 (pg/mL)	0.1–4.1	—	—	—	—	—	—	2.01
IL-4 (pg/mL)	0.1–3.2	—	—	—	—	—	—	1.07
IL-6 (pg/mL)	0.1–2.9	—	—	—	—	—	—	443.46
IL-10 (pg/mL)	0.1–5	—	—	—	—	—	—	4.39
TNF-α	0.1–23	—	—	—	—	—	—	1.2
IFN-γ	0.1–18	—	—	—	—	—	—	0.94

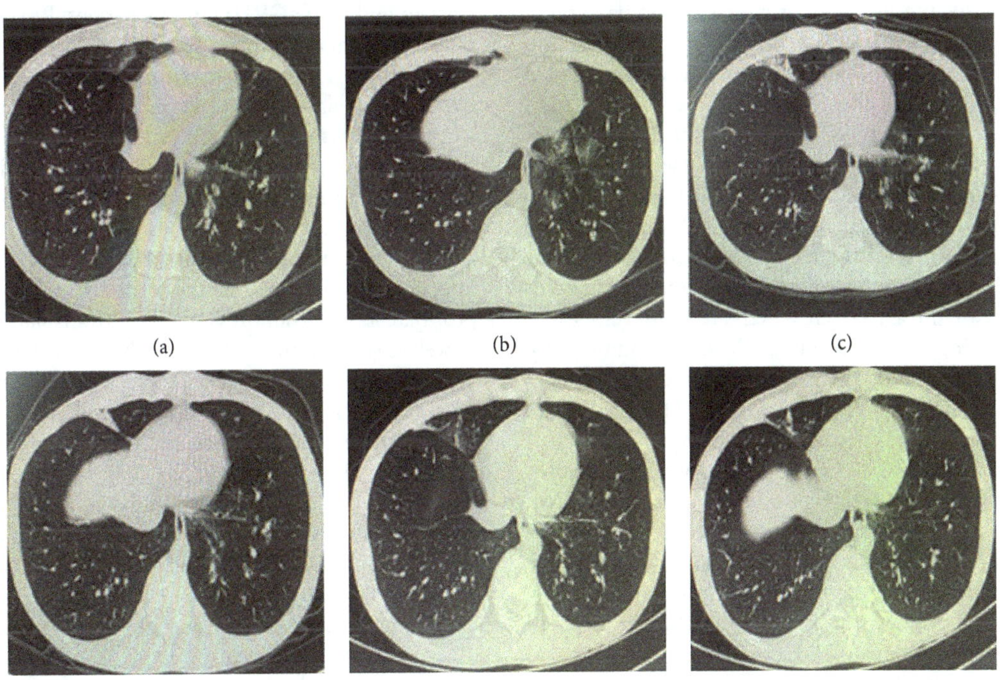

FIGURE 1: Chest imaging results of the patient during hospitalization. (a, b) (Day 2) Scattered bilateral high-density shadows and ground-glass opacities in the lungs. (c, d) (Day 12) Blurred and patchy shadows scattered in the upper and middle lobes of the right lung and the lower lobe of both lungs. (e, f) (Day 24) Bilateral patchy shadows and filamentous shadows in the lungs, and ground-glass opacity in the lower lobes was slightly increased.

of the lower lobes was increased. From the perspective of lung CT, the pulmonary infection of the patient was more serious than before, and combined with the epidemic situation of COVID-19 in China at that time, SARS-CoV-2 infection was considered. Day 27: the SARS-CoV-2 nucleic acid test was positive, and he was transferred to a COVID-19-designated hospital.

Day 28: the patient still had fever, shortness of breath, cough, and expectoration. His temperature was 38.7°C, blood pressure was 100/60 mmHg, heart rate was 106 beats per minute, respiratory rate was 23 breaths per minute, and oxygen saturation was 98% (nasal catheter oxygen inhalation 3 L/min). Bilateral wet rales could be heard in the lungs. The patient was given oxygen via nasal cannula, and drug treatment included arbidol (0.2 g, tid), mucosolvan (30 mg, qd), and magnesium isoglycyrrhizinate (100 mg, qd). Day 31: he developed facial and limb rashes (covering 50% of body surface area) and diarrhoea (approximately 1100 mL/d). Degree II-III aGVHD of the skin and gastrointestinal tract was considered because he had received haematopoietic stem cell infusions 20 days prior and stopped taking ruxolitinib on his own after the transfer. Considering that SARS-CoV-2 was highly contagious and had a high risk of infection during invasive operation, colonoscopy and skin biopsy were not performed. He was given ruxolitinib (5 mg, qd) orally again and methylprednisolone (20 mg, qd) intravenously (because he had fever in the early morning, he had been treated with 10 mg dexamethasone temporarily; therefore, we only used 20 mg methylprednisolone at the beginning). Day 32: SARS-CoV-2 nucleic acid test was still positive. Thus, arbidol was stopped, and he participated in the clinical trial of remdesivir. It was given at 200 mg intravenously on the first day and at 100 mg over the following 9 days. Methylprednisolone was increased to 40 mg qd. Day 34: his temperature fluctuated at 38–39°C. Blood bacterial and fungal cultures were negative, but C-reactive protein (CRP) increased to 119.10 mg/L. Meropenem (1 g, tid) was used to resist bacterial infection, and methylprednisolone was increased to 40 mg bid. Day 37: his aGVHD achieved partial remission (PR), and CRP had decreased to 36.70 mg/L. Then, he was transferred to the respiratory ICU ward for the unified management of patients in the remdesivir clinical trial. He was treated with remdesivir (100 mg, qd), cefoperazone sodium/sulbactam sodium (3 g, tid), linezolid (0.6 g, bid), methylprednisolone (40 mg, qd), and thymalfasin (1.6 mg/d). Day 38: his blood pressure dropped rapidly, and his neutrophil count was 11.96×10^9/L, lymphocyte count was 1.45×10^9/L (Figure 2), and procalcitonin was 47.87 ng/mL. Septic shock was considered. Noradrenaline was given immediately, and respiratory support was strengthened (nasal catheter oxygen inhalation was switched to high-flow oxygen inhalation through the nose). Day 39: he developed liver and kidney function injury and coagulation dysfunction. Day 41: he died of septic shock and multiple organ failure.

3. Discussion

When transplant recipients are infected with SARS-CoV-2, due to immune deficiency or delayed recovery of immune function, the virulence of the virus is stronger, and the viral clearance time is longer [3]. Therefore, posttransplant COVID-19 patients should actively receive antiviral therapy.

The pathogenic mechanism of SARS-CoV-2 has not been fully elucidated. Cao Bin found that there are higher levels of inflammatory cytokines in the plasma of critical COVID-19 patients than in noncritical patients, suggesting that cytokine storm is associated with the occurrence and severity of COVID-19 [4]. Therefore, anti-inflammatory therapy may play an important role in the treatment of COVID-19.

Corticosteroids are the most commonly used anti-inflammatory drugs, but their use has been controversial. Corticosteroids can inhibit excessive inflammatory responses and reduce the bodily damage caused by the inflammatory cytokine storm, but they can also prolong the viral clearance time and increase the risk of secondary infection. However, excessive inflammation and pulmonary damage caused by inflammatory cytokines may cause rapid deterioration due to the disease in critical COVID-19 patients. Compared to patients who only have COVID-19, this patient also had aGVHD; therefore, corticosteroids were used more actively.

In addition to corticosteroids, some immunomodulatory drugs are gradually undergoing trial usage. Ruxolitinib is a selective Janus kinase (JAK) 1/2 inhibitor that has been approved for use by the FDA in the treatment of steroid-refractory aGVHD after allogeneic haematopoietic stem cell transplantation [5]. Given that traditional immunosuppressants, such as calcineurin inhibitors, may increase the risk of infection and tumour recurrence, we used ruxolitinib to prevent and treat aGVHD in this patient. Ruxolitinib can not only prevent aGVHD but also retain the graft-versus-leukemia effect [6]. In addition, ruxolitinib also has an anti-inflammatory effect and has been applied to inflammatory cytokine storm and haemophagocytic syndrome [7]. For this patient, there was no severe respiratory distress in the initial stage of SARS-CoV-2 infection. In the later stage, the disease condition became complicated and serious due to aGVHD, but PR of aGVHD was achieved within a week, and the pulmonary infection was also quickly controlled. This suggests that appropriate immunosuppression in posttransplantation patients, as well as ruxolitinib combined with corticosteroid therapy for aGVHD, may help to alleviate and combat the excessive inflammatory cytokine storm caused by SARS-CoV-2.

The patient deteriorated rapidly after being transferred to another department, which may be related to the following factors: (1) Excessive inflammatory response, immune deficiency, and the use of corticosteroids led to low immune function and kept the patient under constant threat of various pathogens. (2) The ability of SARS-CoV-2 to infect the mucous membrane of the respiratory tract and digestive tract is very prominent [8, 9], and GVHD also easily attacks multiple organs and the vascular endothelium [10, 11]. The destruction of these natural physical and immune barriers greatly increases the risk of infection and mortality. (3) Premature reduction of corticosteroids and the application of immunomodulators after the patient was transferred to the pneumology department may have

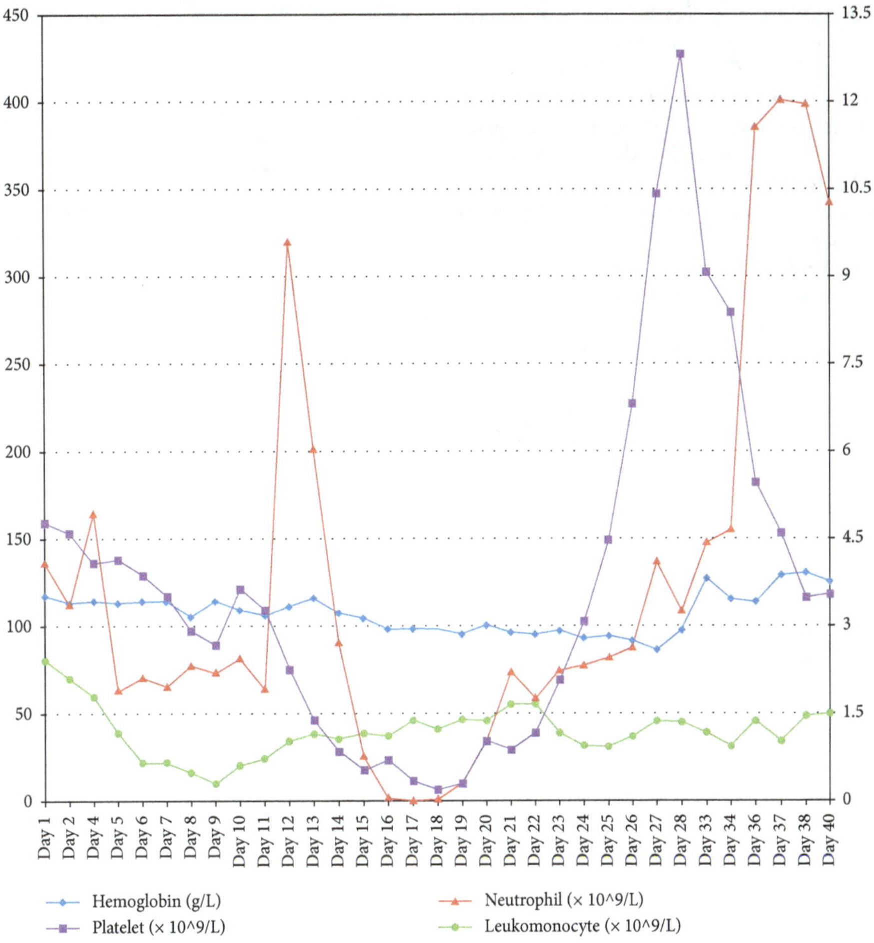

FIGURE 2: Changes of blood routine of the patient during hospitalization.

stimulated the intensity of the inflammatory reaction or the degree of autoimmune attack, resulting in the rapid deterioration of the disease. (4) When the intestinal and respiratory mucous membranes are destroyed or repaired incompletely, the production of ectopic or drug-resistant bacteria in the intestinal tract can easily lead to septic shock.

4. Conclusion

The disease condition of this COVID-19 patient was serious, complex, and variable due to aGVHD. However, there was no uncontrollable trend in progressive deterioration in the early stage, reflecting the importance of the balance between viral pathogenicity, moderate immune response, supportive therapy, and new small molecule drugs with anti-inflammatory and anti-GVHD effects. However, this patient eventually died of septic shock and multiple organ failure, suggesting that it is easy for new complications to arise in the treatment process of COVID-19 with aGVHD. Even if the disease improves, clinicians should be aware of changes in the disease and strengthen the prevention and treatment of infection to avoid life-threatening accidents or the deterioration of the disease.

Consent

No written consent has been obtained from the patient as there is no patient identifiable data included in this casereport.

Disclosure

Dan Han, Yuqian Sun, and Rong Xie are co-first authors.

Authors' Contributions

Dan Han, Yuqian Sun, and Rong Xie contributed equally to the study.

References

[1] Z. Wu and J. M. McGoogan, "Characteristics of and important lessons from the coronavirus disease 2019 (COVID-19) outbreak in China," *The Journal of the American Medical Association*, vol. 323, no. 13, pp. 1239–1242, 2020.

[2] A. Pan, L. Liu, C. Wang et al., "Association of public health interventions with the epidemiology of the COVID-19 out-

break in wuhan, China," *The Journal of the American Medical Association*, vol. 323, no. 19, pp. 1915–1923, 2020.

[3] C.-R. Ju, Q.-Y. Lian, J.-H. Zhang et al., "Recommended prophylactic and management strategies for severe acute respiratory syndrome coronavirus 2 infection in transplant recipients," *Chronic Diseases and Translational Medicine*, vol. 6, no. 2, pp. 87–97, 2020.

[4] C. Huang, Y. Wang, X. Li et al., "Clinical features of patients infected with 2019 novel coronavirus in Wuhan, China," *The Lancet*, vol. 395, no. 10223, pp. 497–506, 2020.

[5] D. Przepiorka, L. Luo, S. Subramaniam et al., "FDA approval summary: ruxolitinib for treatment of steroid-refractory acute graft-versus-host disease," *The Oncologist*, vol. 25, no. 2, pp. e328–e334, 2020.

[6] C. Carniti, S. Gimondi, A. Vendramin et al., "Pharmacologic inhibition of JAK1/JAK2 signaling reduces experimental murine acute GVHD while preserving GVT effects," *Clinical Cancer Research*, vol. 21, no. 16, pp. 3740–3749, 2015.

[7] L. Chen, Y. You, W. J. Zhang et al., "Applicationofruxolitinib in hemophagocytic syndrome," *Linchuang Xueyexue Zazhi (Chinese)*, vol. 31, no. 2, pp. 219–221, 2018.

[8] H. Zhang, H.-B. Li, J.-R. Lyu et al., "Specific ACE2 expression in small intestinal enterocytes may cause gastrointestinal symptoms and injury after 2019-nCoV infection," *International Journal of Infectious Diseases*, vol. 96, pp. 19–24, 2020.

[9] X. Zou, K. Chen, J. Zou, P. Han, J. Hao, and Z. Han, "Single-cell RNA-seq data analysis on the receptor ACE2 expression reveals the potential risk of different human organs vulnerable to 2019-nCoV infection," *Frontiers of Medicine*, vol. 14, no. 2, pp. 185–192, 2020.

[10] L. M. Ball, R. M. Egeler, and R. M. Egeler, "Acute GvHD: pathogenesis and classification," *Bone Marrow Transplantation*, vol. 41, no. S2, pp. S58–S64, 2008.

[11] G. B. McDonald, "How I treat acute graft-versus-host disease of the gastrointestinal tract and the liver," *Blood*, vol. 127, no. 12, pp. 1544–1550, 2016.

34

Triplet Therapy with PD-1 Blockade, Histone Deacetylase Inhibitor and DNA Methyltransferase Inhibitor Achieves Radiological Response in Refractory Double-Expressor Diffuse Large B-cell Lymphoma with 17p Deletion

Runhui Zheng,[1] Xiaobo Chen,[2] Chunyan Wang,[1] Pengfei Qin,[1] Huo Tan,[1] and Xiaodan Luo[1]

[1]*Department of Hematology, First Affiliated Hospital, Guangzhou Medical University, Guangzhou 510230, China*
[2]*Guangzhou Institute of Respiratory Health, Guangzhou Medical University, Guangzhou 510120, China*

Correspondence should be addressed to Xiaodan Luo; xdluo@gzhmu.edu.cn

Academic Editor: Sudhir Tauro

Double-expressor diffuse large B-cell lymphoma (DLBCL) with *17p* deletion is an aggressive and refractory disease. Immune checkpoint blockade and epigenetic drugs have been widely used, but the efficacy of different combined applications varied. We report a case with "double-expressor" DLBCL treated with a combined regimen which consisted of programmed cell death protein 1 (PD-1) inhibitor, DNA methyltransferase inhibitor (DNMTi), and histone deacetylase inhibitor (HDACi). A 50-year-old man presented with a 6-month history of hoarseness, and 10 days of progressive shortness of breath was diagnosed of DLBCL, stage IV. The patient failed to respond to the 1st line (R-EPOCH: rituximab, etoposide, vincristine, cyclophosphamide, doxorubicin, and dexamethasone), 2nd line (R-EPOCH + lenalidomide + ibrutinib), and a 3rd line chemotherapy combined with PD-1 inhibitor (sintilimab), decitabine, and GDP (gemcitabine, DDP, and dexamethasone). Surprisingly, patient's condition was improved after treatment with PD-1 inhibitor in combination with DNMTi/HDACi. Restaging PET revealed dramatically radiological response.

1. Background

Diffuse large B-cell lymphoma (DLBCL) is the most common type of non-Hodgkin lymphoma (NHL) [1, 2]. Approximately 60% of DLBCL patients achieve complete remission (CR) with standard R-CHOP (rituximab with cyclophosphamide, doxorubicin, vincristine, and prednisolone) chemotherapy [3]. However, 30–40% are refractory to therapy or later relapse (R/R cases), especially those with *17p* deletion and/or *TP53* mutation and high-grade B-cell lymphoma with *MYC* and *BCL2* or *BCL6* translocation [2, 4, 5]. Programmed cell death protein 1 (PD-1) is a key immune checkpoint receptor that is frequently expressed on tumor-infiltrating T cells in B-cell lymphomas [6]. In recent years, although therapeutic blockade of PD-1/PD-L1 has shown potential clinical activity in several types of NHL, the efficiency in DLBCL was not as satisfactory as in Classical Hodgkin lymphoma (cHL) [2, 4, 7–10]. The diversity of clinical responses to monotherapy with PD-1/PD-L1 inhibitors is in part explained by genetic heterogeneity and the diversity of signal pathways involved in the development of B-NHL [8, 11]. Therefore, a combinational regimen of PD-1/PD-L1 inhibitors with other synergistic drugs is needed. Here, we report a case in which PD-1 inhibitor in combination with DNA methyltransferase inhibitor (DNMTi) and histone deacetylase inhibitor (HDACi) was administered to a patient diagnosed of refractory "double-expressor" DLBCL with *17p* deletion.

2. Case Presentation

A 50-year-old man presented with a 6-month history of hoarseness and 10 days of progressive shortness of breath. Fiberoptic bronchoscopy revealed intratracheal mass in right main bronchi with complete right mainstem bronchus occlusion (Figure 1(a)). Transbronchial biopsy showed a diffuse proliferation of atypical medium- to large-sized lymphoid cells which were positive for CD20, BCL6 (70%), BCL2 (95%), MUM1 (partial), CD79a, PD-L1 (22C3, 25%), PD-L1 (28–8, 25%), TP53, and c-Myc (40%). They are negative for CD3, CD5, and CD10. The Ki67 proliferative fraction is 80%+ (Figure 2). Fluorescence in situ hybridization (FISH) results demonstrated the presence of *17p* deletion and *BCL-2* rearrangement, while c-Myc translocation was negative. Initial fluorodeoxyglucose positron emission tomography (FDG-PET) revealed left hilum and mediastinal mass (41 × 87 × 76 mm, FDG uptake 20.6) with compression of the pulmonary artery, lower tracheal segment, bilateral main bronchi, and superior vena cava (Figure 1(b)). Vocal cords were involved, and there was a small pericardial effusion. Bone marrow and cerebrospinal fluid are negative for lymphoma. Gene mutation by "Next-generation" sequencing showed *STAT6*, *EZH2*, *TP53*, *KMT2D*, *BCL6*, and *CREBBP* mutation. These findings were consistent with DLBCL, stage IV. The patient was started urgently on dose-adjusted R-EPOCH therapy (rituximab, etoposide, vincristine, cyclophosphamide, doxorubicin, and dexamethasone) since DLBCL patients with poor prognosis treated with R-CHOP usually had shorter remission according to our clinical observations. It is also reported that DA-EPOCH-R produced durable remission in patients with aggressive B-cell lymphomas [12, 13], so we did not risk choosing R-CHOP. A chest computed tomography (CT) scan showed no sign of improvement. In a phase II study from MD Anderson Cancer Center of using rituximab, lenalidomide, and ibrutinib lead in prior to combination with chemotherapy for patients with newly diagnosed DLBCL, the CR rate was 96%. The regimen also has promising activity in R/R Non-Germinal Center B-cell-like DLBCL [14]. Therefore, R2-CHOP-I therapy (rituximab, lenalidomide, ibrutinib, vincristine, cyclophosphamide, doxorubicin, and dexamethasone) was administered as 2nd line. However, the patient developed respiratory distress soon, and a tracheal stent was implanted into the completely occluded bronchus (Figure 1(c)). A repeat PET showed progressive disease. In view of the patient's clinical status with rapidly progressing respiratory distress, a combination regimen with PD-1 inhibitor (Sintilimab, 10 ml: 100 mg), DNMTi (Decitabine, 10 mg), and GDP (gemcitabine, DDP and dexamethasone) was given as 3rd line. Follow-up CT scan showed only a slight improvement (much less than 50%) of bronchus occlusion without the shrinkage of the hilum and mediastinal mass.

For 4th line, a triple combination of decitabine, sintilimab plus HDACi (Chidamide, 5 mg) were administered (decitabine 10 mg i. v. d1-5, Sintilimab 200 mg, i. v., d1, Chidamide 20 mg p. o. twice a week). Chidamide, which inhibits class I HDACs 1, 2, 3, as well as class II HDAC 10, is the first oral subtype-selective histone deacetylase inhibitor approved in China. It was rapidly absorbed after oral administration and exhibited an elimination half-life in plasma of 17–18 hrs. The recommended dose for lymphomas was 10 mg twice per week for 4 consecutive weeks in a 6-week cycle [15, 16]. Right after the 4th line treatment, a significant clinical improvement was noted. Bilateral bronchus was clear, and restaging PET 2 weeks later revealed over 90% shrinkage of hilum and mediastinal mass (16 × 15 mm, FDG uptake 8.0, PET-CT score 5) and significant improvement of bronchus occlusion (Figures 1(d) and 1(e)). The patient achieved partial remission (PR), and a total of 3 cycles of this combination therapy were given. The patient had only myelosuppression presented with absolute neutrophil count $<1.5 \times 10^9$/L and platelets $<80 \times 10^9$/L which lasted for less than a week. The PR duration was about 40 days until a repeat PET-CT showed PD (41 × 33 mm, FDG uptake 18.4, PET-CT score 5). Then, venetoclax was used due to BCL-2 rearrangement, in combination with Chidamide, Sintilimab, and radiotherapy (50 Gy). Decrease in lesion size and FDG uptake were observed (15 × 13 mm, FDG uptake 1.9, PET-CT score 4). However, PET-CT revealed new metastatic foci (10 × 10 mm, FDG uptake 3.4, PET-CT score 5) on the right cardiodiaphragmatic angle 1 month after radiotherapy. Fortunately, the patient had a twin brother as transplant donor and syngeneic stem cell transplantation was performed about 6 months after diagnosis and CR was confirmed by a repeat PET-CT +35 d posttransplant. The patient is alive without lymphoma, and thymosin alpha-1 and recombinant human interleukin-2 are used to induce GVL. Treatment timescales are shown in Table 1, and response assessment was made according to the Lugano classification [17].

3. Discussion

Immune checkpoint blockade has been considered an important breakthrough in cancer treatment. The field of clinical trials in DLBCL associated with immune checkpoint blockade such as PD-1/PD-L1 inhibitor is being actively studied. Unlike cHL, the clinical response to monotherapy with PD-1/PD-L1 blockade in R/R DLBCL was not confirmed [2, 4, 7–9]. Results in a phase I trial of nivolumab monotherapy were promising with a response rate of 36% in R/R DLBCL. Clinical trials of different PD-1/PD-L1 inhibitors are ongoing, and a subset of patients experienced progressive disease after a short response [18]. Therefore, there is an urgent need to designate an effective PD-1/PD-L1 inhibitor-based combination regimen for R/R DLBCL.

This "double-expressor" DLBCL with *17p* deletion failed the 1st line chemotherapy and presented with increase in overall tumor burden both in lesion size and FDG uptake after 2nd line chemotherapy. It is difficult to identify whether these responses were "tumor flare" or true disease progression since lenalidomide and ibrutinib were used in the 2nd line treatment. "Tumor flare" has been observed in patients treated with immunomodulatory drugs [19], but aggressive lymphoma is different from solid tumor or

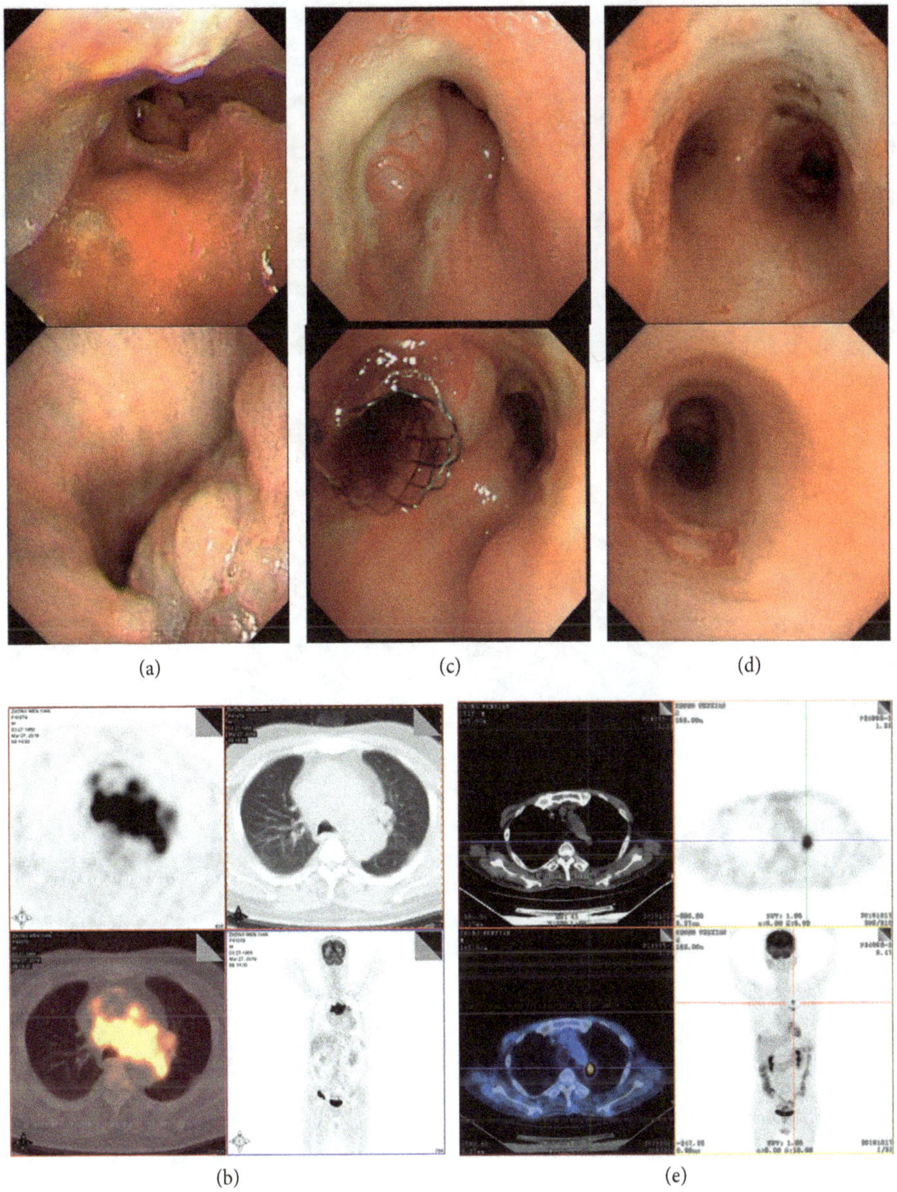

Figure 1: Fiberoptic bronchoscopy and PET/CT images. (a) Fiberoptic bronchoscopy revealed intratracheal mass in right main bronchi with complete right mainstem bronchus occlusion before treatment. (b) PET/CT image showing left hilum and mediastinal mass ($41 \times 87 \times 76$ mm, FDG uptake 20.6) with compression of the pulmonary artery, lower tracheal segment, bilateral main bronchi, and superior vena cava. (c) Right mainstem bronchus was completely occluded, and a tracheal stent was implanted. (d) Bronchus occlusion was significantly improved after treatment with PD-1 inhibitor and DNMTi/HDACi. (e) Restaging PET image showing dramatically shrinkage of hilum and mediastinal mass (16×15 mm, FDG uptake 8.0) after a triple combination treatment of DNMTi/HDACi plus PD-1 inhibitor.

chronic lymphocytic leukemia possibly presented with self-limited lymphocytosis or increase in the size of lymph nodes. Increased FDG uptake with a concomitant increase in lesion size was consistent with what was found by fiberoptic bronchoscopy in this case. Thus, the Lugano classification was used to assess lymphoma response rather than the lymphoma response to immunomodulatory therapy criteria (LYRIC) [19]. The most important reason to change the regimen was that the rapid progression of mass could result in suffocating and death. The PD-1 inhibitor was chosen since PD-L1 was positive in 25% of tumor cells. Rapid progression of disease did not allow us to choose monotherapy of PD-1 inhibitor because of the low response rates and lack of durability. On one hand, it is reported that PD-L1 expression on tumor cells in DLBCL was shown to be associated with poor prognosis in DLBCL in most clinical data [7, 20]. One the other hand, resistant DLBCL has been identified to simultaneously utilize multiple pathways that could compensate for the one provided by PD1 blockade. The PD-1/PD-L1 signal pathway turns down the activation of the immune response, and PD-1 blockade only modestly improved T cells proliferation and cytokine production but was insufficient to restore the antitumor activity [21]. By targeting multiple pathways, which in addition to PD1,

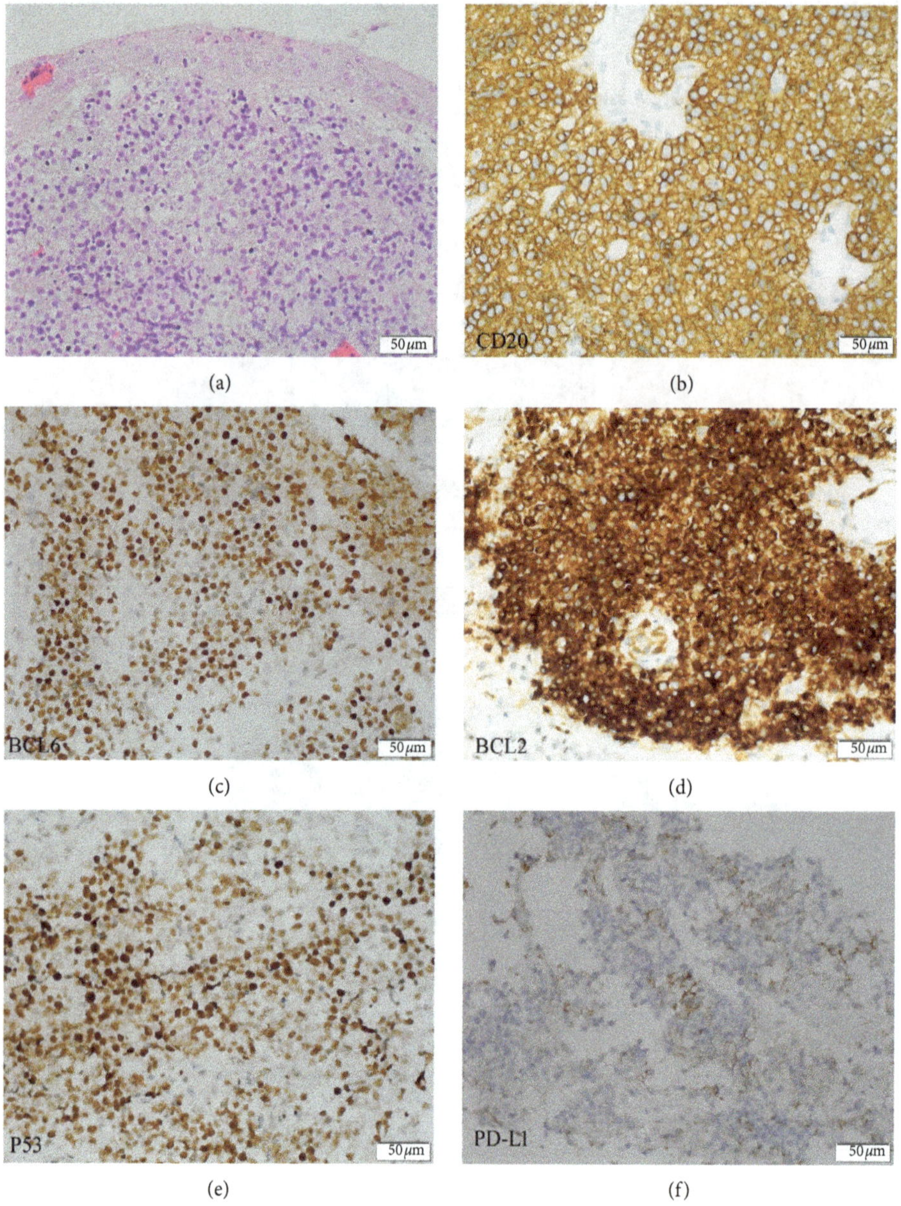

FIGURE 2: Immunohistochemical characteristics of tumor cells. (a) Transbronchial biopsy of the mediastinal mass (H&E staining) showing a diffuse proliferation of atypical medium- to large-sized lymphoid cells. (b) CD20-positive neoplastic cells from mediastinal biopsy aspirate. (c) BCL6-positive neoplastic cells (70%) from mediastinal biopsy aspirate. (d) BCL2-positive neoplastic cells (95%) from mediastinal biopsy aspirate. (e) P53-positive neoplastic cells from mediastinal biopsy aspirate. (f) PD-L1-positive neoplastic cells from mediastinal biopsy aspirate.

combination regimen may overcome the resistance to anti-PD1 therapy.

Multiple components of DLBCL microenvironment are affected by epigenetic regulators such as HDACis or DNMTi [22]. In this report, *STAT6, EZH2, TP53, KMT2D, BCL6,* and *CREBBP* mutations are mostly associated with epigenetic dysregulation. After decitabine was added to the treatment, the patient showed a slight improvement rather than progression for the first time. Moreover, mutation of *CREBBP* encoding proteins with established roles in histone acetylation often results in impaired *p53* activation while also promoting the oncogenic effects of *BCL-6* [23]. HDACis as epigenetic modulators could reduce PD-L1 and PD-L2 expression rapidly on tumor cells, upregulate the immune response, and alter the drug resistance [22, 24]. Therefore, a triple combination of DNMTi/HDACi plus PD-1 inhibitor was performed, and the therapy led to a significant radiological response. *EZH2* mutation was also found in this case. It is reported that the EZH2 inhibitor demonstrated an enhanced clinical activity in DLBCL, so EZH2 inhibition could be a promising strategy [25].

Despite this triplet therapy provided very good partial metabolic response which lasted for 40 days, the patient had progressive disease inevitably even after radiotherapy was performed. However, over 50% shrinkage of lesion size and

TABLE 1: Treatment timescales.

	Start time	Therapy	Number of cycles	Time for repeat CT/PET	Effect
1st	2019/7/19	R-EPOCH: rituximab, etoposide, vincristine, cyclophosphamide, doxorubicin, and dexamethasone	1	2019/8/8 (CT)	Stable disease
2nd	2019/8/15	R-EPOCH + lenalidomide (25 mg d1-7) + ibrutinib (420 mg once a day)	1	2019/9/4 (PET)	Progressive metabolic disease
3rd	2019/9/5	GDP (gemcitabine, DDP, and dexamethasone) + Sintilimab (200 mg d1) + Decitabine (10 mg d1-5)	1	2019/9/17 (CT)	Stable disease
4th	2019/9/29			2019/10/17 (PET)	Partial metabolic response and >90% shrinkage of mass
	2019/10/22	Sintilimab (200 mg, iv. d1) + Decitabine (10 mg, iv, d1-5) + Chidamide (20 mg, po, twice a week)	3.		
	2019/11/12			2019/11/26 (PET)	Progressive metabolic disease
5th	2019/11/29	Radiotherapy (50 Gy) + Sintilimab (200 mg d1) + Chidamide (20 mg twice a week) + venetoclax	1	2020-2-5 (PET)	Progressive metabolic disease
	2020/2/10	Syngeneic stem cell transplantation		2020-3-25 (PET)	Complete metabolic response

CT, computed tomography; PET, positron emission tomography. Response assessment was made according to the Lugano classification [17]: Stable disease: <50% decrease from baseline in SPD of up to 6 dominant, measurable nodes, and extranodal sites; no criteria for progressive disease are met. Progressive metabolic disease: PET-CT Score 4 or 5 with an increase in intensity of uptake from baseline and/or new foci consistent with lymphoma at interim or end-of-treatment assessment. Partial metabolic response: PET-CT score 4 or 5 with reduced uptake compared with baseline and residual mass(es) of any size. Complete metabolic response: score 1, 2, or 3 with or without a residual mass on 5 PET-CT score.

decreased FDG uptake were observed after radiotherapy. Though the presence of bulky disease remains a significant predictor of disease recurrence, radiotherapy as bridging strategy for stem cell transplantation played an important role in reducing tumor burden.

4. Conclusions

The combination of epigenetic-modulating agents with immune checkpoint blockade provides exciting avenue for future research. This case suggests that PD-1 blockade in combination with DNMTi/HDACi can be encouraging in refractory DLBCL. Further research is warranted to evaluate this novel therapeutic regimen.

Abbreviations

CR: Complete remission
cHL: Classical Hodgkin lymphoma
DLBCL: Diffuse large B-cell lymphoma
DNMTi: DNA methyltransferase inhibitor
FISH: Fluorescence in situ hybridization
GDP: Gemcitabine, DDP, and dexamethasone
HDACi: Histone deacetylase inhibitor
PD-1: Programmed cell death protein 1
PET: Positron emission tomography
PMBCL: Primary mediastinal B-cell lymphoma
NHL: Non-Hodgkin lymphoma
R-CHOP: Rituximab with cyclophosphamide, doxorubicin, vincristine, and prednisolone
R-EPOCH: Rituximab, etoposide, vincristine, cyclophosphamide, doxorubicin, and dexamethasone
R/R: Relapse or refractory.

Consent

Written informed consent was obtained from the patient for publication of this case report and accompanying images.

Authors' Contributions

Runhui Zheng assembled, analyzed, and interpreted the patient data regarding the hematological disease; Xiaodan Luo assembled and analyzed the patient data and wrote the manuscript; Xiaobo Chen performed fiberoptic bronchoscopy and provided related high-resolution images; Chunyan Wang and Pengfei Qin assisted with data analysis and edited the manuscript; Huo Tan assisted with data analysis and edited the manuscript. All authors read and approved the final manuscript. Xiaodan Luo and Runhui Zheng equally contributed to this work.

Acknowledgments

The authors would like to acknowledge Juhong Jiang in the Pathology Department for histological interpretation of lymphoid tissue and providing high-resolution images. This work was supported by grant from the Guangdong Province Natural Science Foundation (2018A030313661).

References

[1] N. Sukswai, K. Lyapichev, J. D. Khoury, and L. J. Medeiros, "Diffuse large B-cell lymphoma variants: an update," *Pathology*, vol. 52, no. 1, pp. 53–67, 2019.

[2] J. L. Crombie and P. Armand, "Diffuse large B-cell lymphoma

and high-grade B-cell lymphoma," *Hematology/Oncology Clinics of North America*, vol. 33, no. 4, pp. 575–585, 2019.

[3] P. Feugier, A. Van Hoof, C. Sebban et al., "Long-term results of the R-CHOP study in the treatment of elderly patients with diffuse large B-cell lymphoma: a study by the groupe d'Etude des Lymphomes de l'Adulte," *Journal of Clinical Oncology*, vol. 23, no. 18, pp. 4117–4126, 2005.

[4] M. Pascual, M. Mena-Varas, E. F. Robles et al., "PD-1/PD-L1 immune checkpoint and p53 loss facilitate tumor progression in activated B-cell diffuse large B-cell lymphomas," *Blood*, vol. 133, no. 22, pp. 2401–2412, 2019.

[5] M. Crump, S. S. Neelapu, U. Farooq et al., "Outcomes in refractory diffuse large B-cell lymphoma: results from the international SCHOLAR-1 study," *Blood*, vol. 130, no. 16, pp. 1800–1808, 2017.

[6] C. Y. Ok and K. H. Young, "Checkpoint inhibitors in hematological malignancies," *Journal of Hematology & Oncology*, vol. 10, no. 1, p. 103, 2017.

[7] Z. Y. Xu-Monette, J. Zhou, and K. H. Young, "PD-1 expression and clinical PD-1 blockade in B-cell lymphomas," *Blood*, vol. 131, no. 1, pp. 68–83, 2018.

[8] L. M. Juárez-Salcedo, J. Sandoval-Sus, L. Sokol, J. C. Chavez, and S. Dalia, "The role of anti-PD-1 and anti-PD-L1 agents in the treatment of diffuse large B-cell lymphoma: the future is now," *Critical Reviews in Oncology/Hematology*, vol. 113, pp. 52–62, 2017.

[9] M. K. Song, B. B. Park, and J. Uhm, "Understanding immune evasion and therapeutic targeting associated with PD-1/PD-L1 pathway in diffuse large B-cell lymphoma," *International Journal of Molecular Sciences*, vol. 20, no. 6, 2019.

[10] X. Zhang, L. Chen, Y. Zhao, H. Yin, H. Ma, and M. He, "Safety and efficacy in relapsed or refractory classic hodgkin's lymphoma treated with PD-1 inhibitors: a meta-analysis of 9 prospective clinical trials," *BioMed Research International*, vol. 2019, Article ID 9283860, 13 pages, 2019.

[11] S. Kruger, M. Ilmer, S. Kobold et al., "Advances in cancer immunotherapy 2019 - latest trends," *Journal of Experimental & Clinical Cancer Research*, vol. 38, no. 1, p. 268, 2019.

[12] W. H. Wilson, S.-H. Jung, P. Porcu et al., "A Cancer and Leukemia Group B multi-center study of DA-EPOCH-rituximab in untreated diffuse large B-cell lymphoma with analysis of outcome by molecular subtype," *Haematologica*, vol. 97, no. 5, pp. 758–765, 2012.

[13] K. Dunleavy, M. A. Fanale, J. S. Abramson et al., "Dose-adjusted EPOCH-R (etoposide, prednisone, vincristine, cyclophosphamide, doxorubicin, and rituximab) in untreated aggressive diffuse large B-cell lymphoma with MYC rearrangement: a prospective, multicentre, single-arm phase 2 study," *The Lancet Haematology*, vol. 5, no. 12, pp. e609–e617, 2018.

[14] A. Goy, R. Ramchandren, N. Ghosh et al., "Ibrutinib plus lenalidomide and rituximab has promising activity in relapsed/refractory non-germinal center B-cell-like DLBCL," *Blood*, vol. 134, no. 13, pp. 1024–1036, 2019.

[15] M. Dong, Z.-Q. Ning, P.-Y. Xing et al., "Phase I study of chidamide (CS055/HBI-8000), a new histone deacetylase inhibitor, in patients with advanced solid tumors and lymphomas," *Cancer Chemotherapy and Pharmacology*, vol. 69, no. 6, pp. 1413–1422, 2012.

[16] Y. Shi, B. Jia, W. Xu et al., "Chidamide in relapsed or refractory peripheral T cell lymphoma: a multicenter real-world study in China," *Journal of Hematology & Oncology*, vol. 10, no. 1, p. 69, 2017.

[17] B. D. Cheson, R. I. Fisher, S. F. Barrington et al., "Recommendations for initial evaluation, staging, and response assessment of Hodgkin and non-Hodgkin lymphoma: the Lugano classification," *Journal of Clinical Oncology*, vol. 32, no. 27, pp. 3059–3067, 2014.

[18] A. M. Lesokhin, S. M. Ansell, P. Armand et al., "Nivolumab in patients with relapsed or refractory hematologic malignancy: preliminary results of a phase Ib study," *Journal of Clinical Oncology*, vol. 34, no. 23, pp. 2698–2704, 2016.

[19] B. D. Cheson, S. Ansell, L. Schwartz et al., "Refinement of the Lugano Classification lymphoma response criteria in the era of immunomodulatory therapy," *Blood*, vol. 128, no. 21, pp. 2489–2496, 2016.

[20] J. Kiyasu, H. Miyoshi, A. Hirata et al., "Expression of programmed cell death ligand 1 is associated with poor overall survival in patients with diffuse large B-cell lymphoma," *Blood*, vol. 126, no. 19, pp. 2193–2201, 2015.

[21] J. S. O'Donnell, G. V. Long, R. A. Scolyer, M. W. L. Teng, and M. J. Smyth, "Resistance to PD1/PDL1 checkpoint inhibition," *Cancer Treatment Reviews*, vol. 52, pp. 71–81, 2017.

[22] D. Banik, S. Moufarrij, and A. Villagra, "Immunoepigenetics combination therapies: an overview of the role of HDACs in cancer immunotherapy," *International Journal of Molecular Sciences*, vol. 20, no. 9, 2019.

[23] L. Pasqualucci, D. Dominguez-Sola, A. Chiarenza et al., "Inactivating mutations of acetyltransferase genes in B-cell lymphoma," *Nature*, vol. 471, no. 7337, pp. 189–195, 2011.

[24] X. Wang, B. C. Waschke, R. A. Woolaver et al., "Histone deacetylase inhibition sensitizes PD1 blockade-resistant B-cell lymphomas," *Cancer Immunology Research*, vol. 7, no. 8, pp. 1318–1331, 2019.

[25] J. K. Lue and J. E. Amengual, "Emerging EZH2 inhibitors and their application in lymphoma," *Current Hematologic Malignancy Reports*, vol. 13, no. 5, pp. 369–382, 2018.

35

A Rare CD4–CD8+ Adult T-Cell Leukemia/Lymphoma with Unique Molecular Mutations: A Case Report with Literature Review

Jui Choudhuri,[1,2] Leah Geiser Roberts,[3] Yan Zhang,[2,4] Yanhua Wang,[1,2] and Yanan Fang[1,2]

[1]*Department of Pathology, Montefiore Medical Center, Bronx, New York City 10467, NY, USA*
[2]*Albert Einstein College of Medicine, Pelham PKWY South Bronx, New York City 10467, NY, USA*
[3]*Liberty University College of Osteopathic Medicine (LUCOM), Lynchburg, VA, USA*
[4]*Jacobi Medical Center and NCB Hospital, Bronx, New York City 10467, NY, USA*

Correspondence should be addressed to Yanan Fang; yfang@montefiore.org

Academic Editor: Kiyotaka Kawauchi

Adult T-cell leukemia/lymphoma (ATLL) is a mature T-cell neoplasm caused by infection of the human T-cell lymphotropic virus type 1 (HTLV-1). Most ATLL cases are CD4-positive and CD8-negative. Though rare, there are a few dual negative (CD4–CD8–), dual positive (CD4+CD8+), and CD4–CD8+ cases reported in literature. ATLL is associated with HTLV-1 infection, but HTLV-1 alone cannot cause the malignant transformation of infected T cells. Additional genetic and/or epigenetic events are required for the development of the disease. Here, we report an unusual CD4–CD8+ATLL in a 76-year-old male with a unique molecular genetic profile. Molecular studies revealed alterations in 10 genes. Three of them are predicted to be pathogenic by the computational models, including the frameshift change in ZFHX4 and missense mutations in RHOA and POT1. The specific mutations of POT1 (c.281A > G; p.Q94R), RHOA (c.47G > A; p.C16Y), and ZFHX4 (c.2871delC; p.F958Sfs*31) have never been previously reported in ATLL to the best of our knowledge. The clinical significance of other genetic alterations is unknown. Further research is warranted to correlate this patient's molecular findings with other ATLL cases. Correlation specifically with other cases of CD8+ ATLL could prove to be useful in understanding the pathogenesis of this rare variant of an already rare form of leukemia/lymphoma.

1. Introduction

Adult T-cell leukemia/lymphoma (ATLL) is a rare and aggressive T-cell neoplasm associated with the human T-cell lymphotropic virus type 1 (HTLV-1) infection [1]. Most ATLL cases involve proliferation of CD4+CD25+ T cells and have been strongly associated with HTLV-1, which preferentially infects CD4+ T cells and leads to clonal expansion. These are typically mature T cells, expressing CD2 and CD5, often negative/dim for CD7, with downregulation of CD3 and T-cell receptor- (TCR-) beta [1]. While ATLL is characteristically the expansion of CD4+CD8–CD25+ T cells, there are occasional cases reported in literature of dual negative (CD4–CD8–), dual positive (CD4+CD8+), and CD4–CD8+ ATLL [2–5]. These unusual ATLL cases have been reported to be more aggressive and with a worse prognosis [2–4].

ATLL is a rare entity in Europe and North America, and it is much more common in populations with endemic HTLV-1 infection such as in southern Japan, sub-Saharan Africa, the Caribbean Basin, and South America [1]. In nonendemic regions, infection and subsequent ATLL can be found most commonly in areas high in immigrant populations. In United States, the incidence of ATLL is approximately 0.05 per 100,000 [6]. The virus can spread via vertical transmission, sexual intercourse, transfusion of contaminated cellular blood products, and use of needles contaminated with the virus (e.g., sharing needles in IVDU) [1]. The mean age of diagnosis of ATLL is approximately 60 years and with no sexual predominance [6]. Familial clustering has been seen, suggesting a possible component of genetic predisposition. Patients can have varied clinical presentation of the disease. The disease is typically subdivided into four clinical presentations: smoldering (indolent), chronic, lymphoma, and acute form [7]. Lymphoma and acute forms are associated with worst prognosis [1].

Studies have been performed trying to find distinct molecular genetic profiles that would predispose a carrier to develop ATLL, but discrete and consistent mutations have not been fully established, and there is still a wide spectrum of mutations being studied. The most common genetic mutations found in ATLL are p16 (30–70% cases) and p53 (10–50% cases) although they are nonspecific [8]. Studies have shown that chromosomal abnormalities are frequent and increase with aggressiveness of the disease. Recent molecular studies have shed a light on the molecular basis of the leukemogenesis of ATLL [9, 10]. We present a rare case of ATLL with a CD4–CD8+ phenotype and the molecular findings associated with it.

2. Case Presentation

The case is a 76-year-old male who had moved to the United States from Jamaica, one of the Caribbean islands, five years prior to presenting at a medical facility for unintentional weight loss and night sweats over 3 months and was found to have generalized lymphadenopathy. The patient reported no history of trauma, recent travel, fever, chills, nausea, or vomiting. Past medical history was significant for type 2 diabetes mellitus, hypertension, and remote history of prostate cancer. The initial blood profile showed anemia with a hemoglobin level of 6.7 g/dL and mild thrombocytopenia with a platelet count of 125×10^9/L. White blood cell count was $9.0 \times 10^3/\mu$L with differential count as follows: neutrophils, 89%; lymphocytes, 7%; and monocytes, 3%. Lactate dehydrogenase (LDH) was mildly elevated, and calcium level was within the reference range. A computed tomography (CT) showed diffuse hilar and inguinal lymphadenopathy. Flow cytometry of peripheral blood was negative for involvement by non-Hodgkin B- or T-cell lymphoma. An initial fine needle aspiration cytology was paucicellular with some large atypical cells concerning for lymphoma.

A biopsy was performed on a left cervical lymph node. Flow cytometry showed a population of atypical T cells which were positive for CD2, CD7 (dim), and CD8, while negative for surface CD3, CD5, and CD4 (reference commercial laboratory 1, Figure 1). The hematoxylin and eosin staining of the lymph node revealed complete effacement of the lymph node architecture and replaced by sheets of pleomorphic atypical medium-to-large lymphocytes (Figure 2). The atypical lymphocytes exhibited irregular nuclear contour, condensed chromatin, and distinct nucleoli. By immunohistochemical staining (Figure 2), the atypical lymphocytes were positive for CD3, CD8, and CD25; variably positive for CD2, CD7, and TIA-1; and negative for CD4, CD5, CD20, CD34, TdT, EBER, and CD30. Ki67 demonstrated a high proliferation index (>90%).

Given the suspicion for ATLL, HTLV-1 serology was performed and found to be reactive. HTLV-1 viral sequence was detected in the lymphoma by polymerase chain reaction (PCR) and fluorogenic probe specific for HTLV-1 pol (reference laboratory 2) consistent with the diagnosis of ATLL. Clonal pattern of T-cell receptor gene rearrangement was also detected. Bone marrow biopsy was negative for lymphoma involvement. The patient received six cycles of cyclophosphamide, doxorubicin hydrochloride, Oncovin, and prednisone (CHOP) and intrathecal methotrexate resulting in apparent remission. Six months later, the patient presented with enlarged lymph nodes/facial swelling, and imaging/biopsy result confirmed relapse. The patient received salvage ifosfamide, carboplatin, and etoposide (ICE) therapy. However, there was worsening disease evident on the CT scan, and the patient eventually expired.

Further genetic testing (outside reference laboratory 3) on the lymph node biopsy had revealed ten genomic alterations: DIS3 (c.387-6A > G), ESR1 (c.148G > A; p.A50T), PIK3R1 (c.1205T > C; p.V402A), MYD88 (c.43G > A; p.A15T), PLCG1 (c.1021G > A; p.G341R), POT1 (c.281A > G; p.Q94R), PTEN (c.851A > G; p.E284G), RHOA (c.47G > A; p.C16Y), SAMHD1 (c.184C > T; p.P62S), and ZFHX4 (c.2871delC; p.F958Sfs*31). Three mutations identified in DIS3, ESR1, and PIK3R1 were most likely germline alterations given that they were also identified in the peripheral blood sample as well which was not involved by ATLL (on flow cytometry), and the allele frequency was approximately 50%. Three mutations identified in our patient were predicted to be pathogenic including RHOA, ZFHX4, and POT1 genes. The remaining genetic alterations in this case have neither been reported before nor been predicted to be pathogenic using computational models (computational model used by the reference company and/or https://cancer.sanger.ac.uk/cosmic). Thus, those genetic alterations remain of unclear clinical significance at this point.

3. Discussion

We report an unusual case of CD4–CD8+ ATLL with unique genetic alterations. Rare cases of CD4–CD8+ have been reported previously [3, 5, 11]. In the study of 107 ATLL cases, Kamihira et al. found the incidence of the CD4–CD8+ to be 4%, while 81% for conventional phenotype CD4+CD8– and 7% each for the dual positive (CD4+CD8+) and dual negative (CD4-CD8-) cases [5]. It is not yet clear whether these CD8+ ATLL cases are due to the infection and transformation of CD8+ T cells directly or modified expression of CD8+ on the CD4+ T cells [12].

ATLL is a mature T-cell neoplasm closely associated with the HTLV-1 infection. The HTLV-1 genome includes the *Gag*, *Pol*, and *Env* genes, and it also includes several regulatory proteins such as Tax and the helix basic-loop zipper protein (HBZ). Tax is known to play a crucial role in initial transformation of cells but is not considered to be a necessary protein for ongoing transformation and progression of established ATLL as it is often found to be absent later down the disease course [13]. While the HBZ RNA promotes proliferation of ATLL cells and plays an important role in the later stages of infection and maintenance of ATLL [10], it has been noted that the onset of ATLL generally occurs

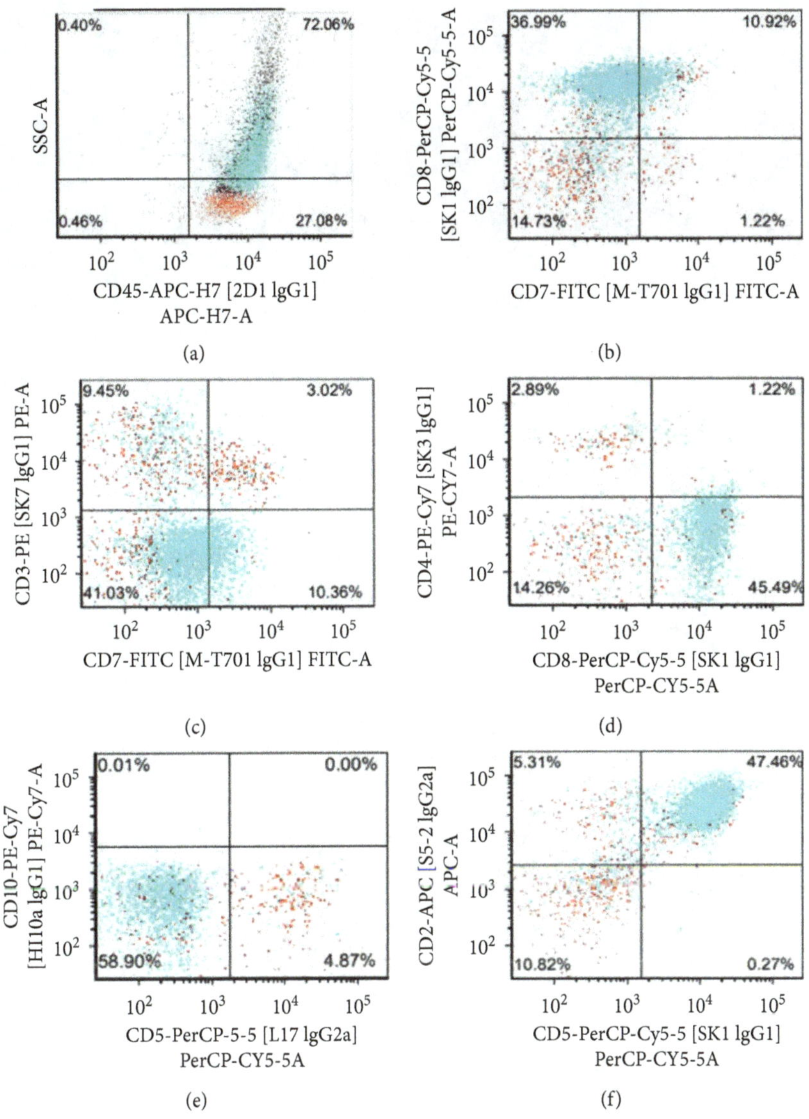

Figure 1: Flow cytometry of the lymph node showing atypical T cells positive for CD2, CD7 (dim), and CD8, with negative surface CD3, CD4, and CD5.

following a latency period of approximately 30–50 years after initial HTLV-1 infection, suggesting HTLV-1 viral factors alone are not sufficient for malignant transformation of infected T cells. Other than HTLV-1 viral factors and proteins, additional genetic and/or epigenetic events play a major role in the development of disease. Environmental factors have also been implicated given varying mean age of onset based on geographic location as well as familial clustering [14].

Studies have shown that the mutation rate for ATLL is higher as compared to other malignancies with an average of 2.3 mutations per mega base in coding regions [10]. In ATLL pathogenesis, additional genetic mutations are needed for tumorigenesis other than viral products. Some of the genes involved include p53, CCR4, NOTCH1, and CDKN2A [9, 15]. Recent large-scale integrated molecular studies have identified a number of genes and signaling pathways involved in ATLL [9]. In particular, many genetic alterations were found affecting the TCR/NF-$\kappa\beta$ pathway and other T-cell-related pathways. For example, the most commonly identified activating mutations include PLCG1, PRKCB, CARD11, VAV1, IRF4, and FYN. Although some involved genes in our case have been reported to be mutated in ATLL or other tumors previously, these specific point mutations and frameshift change have not been reported in ATLL before. Among all the genetic alterations, three of them are predicted to be pathogenic: RHOA, ZFHX4, and POT1.

RHOA is a key regulator in T-cell receptor-/NF-kB signaling pathway and contributes to cytoskeletal regulation, cellular proliferation, and oncogenic transformation. RHOA mutations have been found in ATLL, angioimmunoblastic T-cell lymphoma (AITL), and peripheral T-cell lymphoma with T-follicular helper phenotype, as well as other solid tumors. The mutations in ATLL appear to have unique distribution compared to other T-cell lymphomas and solid tumors [16]. RHOA mutations associated with ATLL are

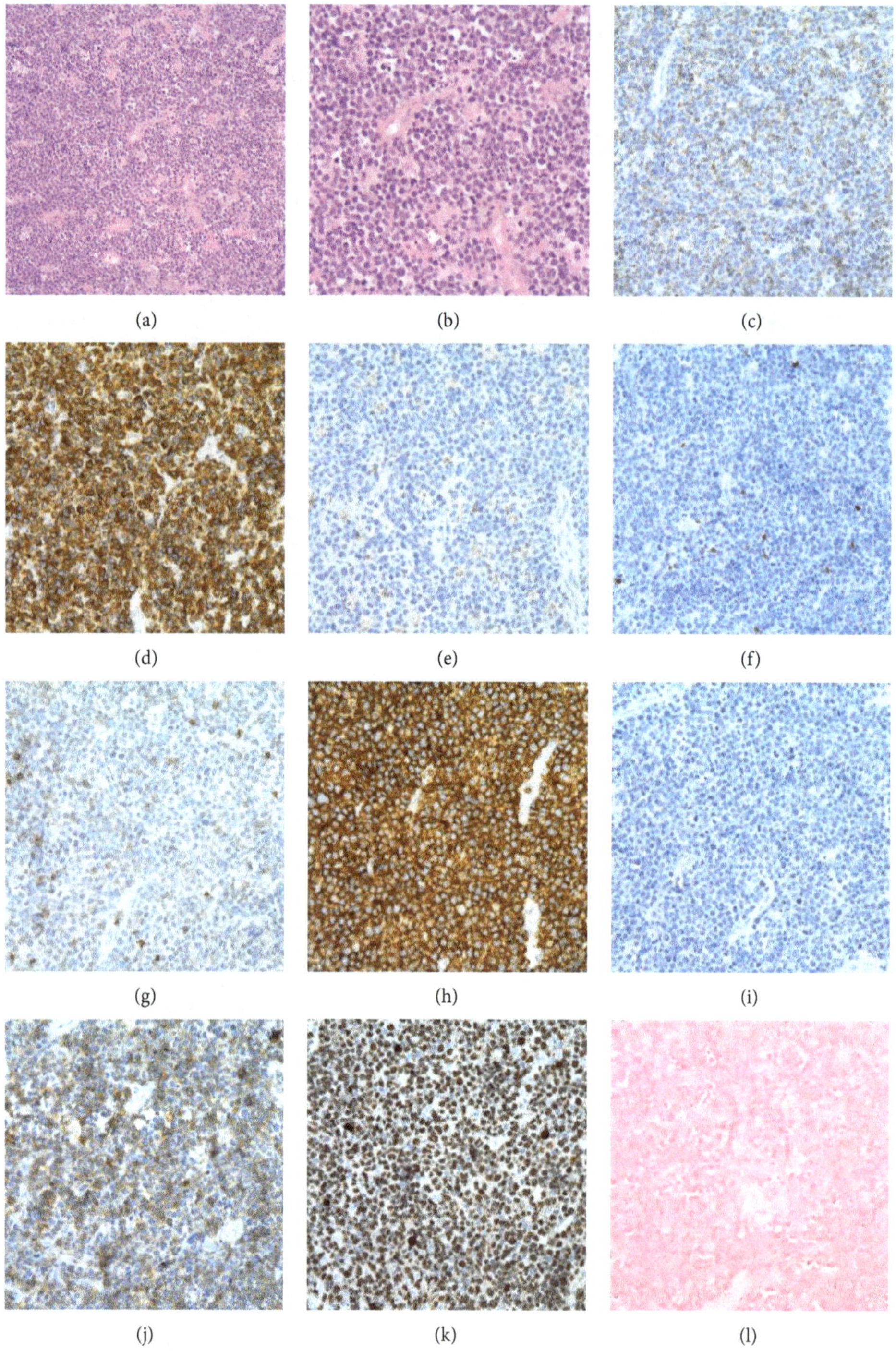

FIGURE 2: Biopsy of the left cervical lymph node. Hematoxylin and eosin (a, b), immunohistochemistry staining (c–j), and in situ hybridization (l). (a, b) H&E sections showing sheets of pleomorphic atypical medium-to-large lymphocytes. (c) CD2. (d) CD3. (e) CD4. (f) CD5. (g) CD7. (h) CD8. (i) CD20. (j) CD25. (k) Ki67. (l) Epstein–Barr virus- (EBV-) encoded RNAs (EBER) (original magnification, ×200 (a, c–l) and ×400 (b)).

mostly focused around the GTP-binding pocket with greater variance in the discrete mutational hotspots (Cys16, Gly17, and Ala161) [16]. The mutation can be either loss of function or gain of function although both are thought to be involved in ATLL leukemogenesis [16]. By analyzing 12 cases, Nagata et al. also found that different RHOA mutations appear to be associated with distinct immunophenotype and T-cell subsets [16]. The patient in this case did have a missense mutation involving the cysteine at the 16th location, which is one of the above mentioned discrete mutational hotspots associated with ATLL. The patient does not, however, present with the most common mutation (Cys16Arg) [16]. The mutation (c.47G > A; p.C16Y) identified in our patient was reported in a case of acute myeloid leukemia and predicted to be pathogenic based on computational models [17]. The unique mutation may be associated with his rare CD4−CD8+ immunophenotype.

ZFHX4, a member of nucleosome remodeling and deacetylase (NuRD) family, is involved in DNA damage-repair pathway [18]. ZFHX4 mutations have previously been reported in various cancers including multiple myeloma, glioblastoma, and esophageal cancer but not in ATLL. ZFHX4 mutations have been found associated with poorer prognosis in various cancers [18–20]. The molecular pathogenesis of ZFHX4 is not well understood. Limited study showed that knockdown of the ZFHX4 gene led to decreased migration and invasiveness in esophageal squamous cancer cells in vitro [19]. The frameshift mutation of ZFHX4 (c.2871delC; p.F958Sfs*31) in this case has never been reported but is expected to be pathogenic.

POT1 mutations are associated with a variety of different malignancies as well [21, 22]. POT1 binds and protects telomeres; loss of this makes the host genome vulnerable to degradation and fusion which ultimately leaves the genome unstable. Mutations in POT1 induce genomic instability through dysfunctional telomeres [21]. Genomic instability puts the cell at risk for genetic alterations that can lead to malignant transformation. The mutation identified (c.281A > G; p.Q94R) has been reported in chronic lymphocytic leukemia but has not been reported in ATLL yet [21, 23]. This mutation is also predicted to be pathogenic by the computational model [24].

Among other genetic alterations identified in this case, three of them (DIS3, ESR1, and PIK3R1) are most likely germline alterations. The remaining four genetic alterations in PTEN, MYD88, PLCG1, and SAMHD1 have never been reported, and the clinical significance is unknown, which does not exclude the possible contribution to the disease. Among these genes, PLCG1 is a key molecule involved in T-cell receptor- (TCR-) nuclear factor- (NF-) κB signaling, and its activating mutations have been commonly found in ATLL cases (36%) [9]. PTEN-mediated PI3K/AKT pathway activation is also involved in ATLL leukemogenesis [25]. MYD88 plays an important role in the pathogenesis of B-cell lymphomas and other tumors [26]. However, the missense mutations detected in this case including PLCG1 (c.1021G > A; p.G341R), PTEN (c.851A > G; p.E284G), and MYD88 (c.43G > A; p.A15T) have neither been reported in any tumor nor been predicted to be pathogenic by the computational models.

4. Conclusion

Given the current available data, RHOA, POT1, and ZFHX4 are the most likely culprits involved in this patient's leukemogenesis, based on the various databases and literature reviews. However, the significance of the others is not excluded. It is possible that other identified mutations are involved in the progression of this patient's HTLV-1 infection to CD4−CD8+ ATLL. More investigation and research are warranted for specially studying ATLL in different geographical regions. However, it is challenging given the extremely small sample size of unusual phenotypic cases such as ours, CD4−CD8+ ATLL. The overall prognosis of ATLL continues to be poor and with a high relapse rate despite aggressive chemotherapy. Further advances in the molecular aspects might be a clue to the therapeutic course for this disease.

References

[1] E. Matutes, "Adult T-cell leukaemia/lymphoma," *Journal of Clinical Pathology*, vol. 60, no. 12, pp. 1373–1377, 2007.

[2] K. Tamura, T. Unoki, K. Sagawa et al., "Clinical features of OKT4+/OKT8+ adult T-cell leukemia," *Leukemia Research*, vol. 9, no. 11, pp. 1353–1359, 1985.

[3] I. Lorand-Metze and M. S. Pombo-de-Oliveira, "Adult T-cell leukemia (ATL) with an unusual immunophenotype and a high cellular proliferation rate," *Leukemia & Lymphoma*, vol. 22, no. 5-6, pp. 523–526, 1996.

[4] M. S. Pombo De Oliveira, P. Loureiro, A. Bittencourt et al., "Geographic diversity of adult t-cell leukemia/lymphoma in Brazil," *International Journal of Cancer*, vol. 83, no. 3, pp. 291–298, 1999.

[5] S. Kamihira, H. Sohda, S. Atogami et al., "Phenotypic diversity and prognosis of adult T-cell leukemia," *Leukemia Research*, vol. 16, no. 5, pp. 435–441, 1992.

[6] N. Mehta-Shah, L. Ratner, and S. M. Horwitz, "Adult T-cell leukemia/lymphoma," *Journal of Oncology Practice*, vol. 13, no. 8, pp. 487–492, 2017.

[7] M. Shimoyama, "Diagnostic criteria and classification of clinical subtypes of adult T-cell leukaemia-lymphoma," *British Journal of Haematology*, vol. 79, no. 3, pp. 428–437, 1991.

[8] Y. Hatta and H. Koeffler, "Role of tumor suppressor genes in the development of adult T cell leukemia/lymphoma (ATLL)," *Leukemia*, vol. 16, no. 6, pp. 1069–1085, 2002.

[9] K. Kataoka, Y. Nagata, A. Kitanaka et al., "Integrated molecular analysis of adult T cell leukemia/lymphoma," *Nature Genetics*, vol. 47, no. 11, pp. 1304–1315, 2015.

[10] Y. Kogure and K. Kataoka, "Genetic alterations in adult T-cell leukemia/lymphoma," *Cancer Science*, vol. 108, no. 9, pp. 1719–1725, 2017.

[11] T. Amagasaki, Y. Tomonaga, Y. Yamada et al., "Adult T-cell leukemia with an unusual phenotype, Leu-2a positive and Leu-3a negative," *Blut*, vol. 50, no. 4, pp. 209–211, 1985.

[12] S. Raza, S. Naik, V. P. Kancharla, F. Tafera, and M. R. Kalavar, "Dual-positive (CD4+/CD8+) acute adult T-cell leukemia/lymphoma associated with complex karyotype and refractory hypercalcemia: case report and literature review," *Case Reports in Oncology*, vol. 3, no. 3, pp. 489–494, 2010.

[13] L. H. Ioachim and L. J. Medeiros, *Ioachim's Lymph Node Pathology*p. 680, 4th edition, Lippincott Williams & Wilkins (LWW), Philadelphia, PA, USA, 2009.

[14] T. Watanabe, "Adult T-cell leukemia: molecular basis for clonal expansion and transformation of HTLV-1-infected T cells," *Blood*, vol. 129, no. 9, pp. 1071–1081, 2017.

[15] M. Matsuoka and K.-T. Jeang, "Human T-cell leukaemia virus type 1 (HTLV-1) infectivity and cellular transformation," *Nature Reviews Cancer*, vol. 7, no. 4, pp. 270–280, 2007.

[16] Y. Nagata, K. Kontani, T. Enami et al., "Variegated RHOA mutations in adult T-cell leukemia/lymphoma," *Blood*, vol. 127, no. 5, pp. 596–604, 2016.

[17] RHOA, "COSMIC: The catalogue of somatic mutations in

cancer," 2020, https://cancer.sanger.ac.uk/cosmic/mutation/overview?id=118446369.

[18] B. A. Walker, E. M. Boyle, C. P. Wardell et al., "Mutational spectrum, copy number changes, and outcome: results of a sequencing study of patients with newly diagnosed myeloma," *Journal of Clinical Oncology*, vol. 33, no. 33, pp. 3911–3920, 2015.

[19] T. Qing, S. Zhu, C. Suo, L. Zhang, Y. Zheng, and L. Shi, "Somatic mutations in ZFHX4 gene are associated with poor overall survival of Chinese esophageal squamous cell carcinoma patients," *Scientific Reports*, vol. 7, no. 1, p. 4951, 2017.

[20] Y. Chudnovsky, D. Kim, S. Zheng et al., "ZFHX4 interacts with the NuRD core member CHD4 and regulates the glioblastoma tumor-initiating cell state," *Cell Reports*, vol. 6, no. 2, pp. 313–324, 2014.

[21] S. Chang, "Cancer chromosomes going to POT1," *Nature Genetics*, vol. 45, no. 5, pp. 473–475, 2013.

[22] O. Calvete, P. Garcia-Pavia, F. Domínguez et al., "The wide spectrum of POT1 gene variants correlates with multiple cancer types," *European Journal of Human Genetics*, vol. 25, no. 11, pp. 1278–1281, 2017.

[23] A. J. Ramsay, V. Quesada, M. Foronda et al., "POT1 mutations cause telomere dysfunction in chronic lymphocytic leukemia," *Nature Genetics*, vol. 45, no. 5, pp. 526–530, 2013.

[24] POT1, "COSMIC: Catalogue of somatic mutations in cancer," 2020, https://cancer.sanger.ac.uk/cosmic/mutation/overview?id=105799806.

[25] S. Nakahata, T. Ichikawa, Y. Saito et al., "NDRG2 plays a pivotal role in ATLL leukaemogenesis by regulating the PTEN-mediated PI3K/AKT signalling pathway," *Retrovirology*, vol. 11, no. 1, p. 87, 2014.

[26] NIH, "U.S. national library of medicine," 2020, https://medlineplus.gov/genetics/gene/myd88/#conditions.

36

Burkitt-Like Lymphoma with 11q Aberration: A Case Report and Review of a Rare Entity

Sepideh N. Asadbeigi and Chelsey D. Deel

Department of Pathology, University of Oklahoma Health Sciences Center, Oklahoma, USA

Correspondence should be addressed to Chelsey D. Deel; chelsey-deel@ouhsc.edu

Academic Editor: Håkon Reikvam

Burkitt-like lymphoma with 11q aberration is a rare diagnostic entity commonly occurring in children and young adults with a nodal presentation. This entity shares many similar morphologic and immunophenotypic features with conventional Burkitt lymphoma and other aggressive B-cell lymphomas, making its recognition challenging. However, the presence of its characteristic 11q gain/loss pattern is helpful in the diagnosis. We report a case of Burkitt-like lymphoma presenting as a right neck mass in a 17-year-old female patient that demonstrated no improvement with antibiotic therapy. The neoplasm displayed a diffuse proliferation of intermediate-sized atypical lymphoid cells with prominent nucleoli in a background of apoptotic debris, morphologically raising concern for conventional Burkitt lymphoma. Subsequent immunohistochemical and cytogenetic studies established the most likely diagnosis of Burkitt-like lymphoma with 11q aberration. Though rare, Burkitt-like lymphoma exhibits significant morphologic overlap with other high-grade B-cell lymphomas, making it an important entity to consider on the differential diagnosis of these lesions.

1. Introduction

Burkitt lymphoma (BL) is a well-defined aggressive B-cell lymphoma with rearrangements characteristically involving MYC and the immunoglobulin (IG) heavy (t(8;14)) or, more rarely, light chain loci (t(2;8) and t(8;22)) [1, 2]. The term Burkitt-like lymphoma with 11q (BLL-11q) aberration has emerged as a new provisional diagnostic entity in the Revised 4th Edition of the World Health Organization (WHO) Classification of Tumors of Hematopoietic and Lymphoid Tissues to describe cases morphologically resembling BL that have unique clinical, cytogenetic, and molecular features [3]. Initially reported by Poirel and colleagues in 2009 [4], this lymphoma is a rare and aggressive lymphoid neoplasm which is defined by the genetic hallmark of its 11q-gain/loss pattern. BLL-11q morphologically resembles Burkitt lymphoma (i.e., "starry sky" pattern and high proliferative rate) and has a similar immunophenotype (CD10+, BCL-6+, BCL-2(-), and Ki-67 approaching 100%) [1, 2, 5]. However, this lymphoma lacks *MYC* rearrangements and carries an 11q-arm aberration with proximal gains and telomeric losses [2]. Because of its resemblance to other aggressive B-cell lymphomas such as Burkitt lymphoma and unique associated clinical/prognostic features, Burkitt-like lymphoma with 11q aberration remains an important diagnostic entity for consideration in these lesions.

2. Case Report

A 17-year-old previously healthy female presented to the outpatient surgery clinic for evaluation of a right neck mass, present for eight months and demonstrating no improvement with multiple rounds of antibiotic therapy. The patient had no relevant personal or family history of malignancy and denied B symptoms. Physical examination identified a large right substernocleidomastoid nontender and immobile mass. A computed tomography (CT) scan in January 2019 revealed an enlarged lymph node within the right jugular digastric region (3.0 cm in greatest dimension), causing mass effect on the jugular vein. A repeat CT scan performed in

August 2019 demonstrated interval increase in the size of the lymph node (7.3 × 5.6 × 3.5 cm). The patient was subsequently referred for surgical biopsy of the mass.

Frozen section assessment of the cervical mass was suggestive of Burkitt lymphoma. Microscopic examination of the resected tissue showed a diffuse proliferation of intermediate-sized atypical lymphoid cells with prominent nucleoli in a background of apoptotic debris. By immunohistochemistry, the high-grade cells were positive for CD20, CD10, BCL-6, and MYC and negative for BCL-2, TdT, CD30, CD56, and MUM-1. Ki-67 highlighted a high proliferative index (Figure 1). Flow cytometry identified 86% of events as lymphocytes, a majority of which were B cells expressing CD45 (bright), CD20, CD19, CD10, CD22, CD38 (moderate-bright), FMC-7, CD23 (dim partial), and kappa light chain (Figure 2). No expression of CD56 was identified. Based on morphology, a differential diagnosis of Burkitt lymphoma, diffuse large B-cell lymphoma, and high-grade B-cell lymphoma was entertained.

Fluorescence in situ hybridization (FISH) testing with break-apart probes specific for rearrangements of the *BCL6* gene, *MYC* gene, *BCL2* gene, and t(8;14) did not show any abnormal rearrangements. Conventional cytogenetics identified two abnormal cell lines. The first abnormal cell line had a modal number of 46 chromosomes, including one normal *X* chromosome and attachment of unknown material to another *X* chromosome at p22.1 as well as chromosome 11 at q23. The second abnormal cell line had unknown material attached to 4q31.3 in addition to the anomalies detected in the first cell line. A staging bone marrow biopsy demonstrated no evidence of involvement by lymphoma. Overall, the clinical presentation, morphology, and concurrent ancillary studies make Burkitt-like lymphoma with 11q aberration the most likely diagnosis.

A positron emission tomography (PET) scan identified hypermetabolic activity (SUV 34.1) in the primary right level 2A cervical mass (5.8 × 4.1 cm) as well as a left level 2A lymph node (1.6 × 1.1 cm, SUV 2.4) (Figure 3). The patient received treatment per ANHL 1131 group B protocol, including induction chemotherapy with cyclophosphamide, vincristine, prednisone, doxorubicin, and methotrexate (COPADM) and consolidation chemotherapy with cytarabine and methotrexate (CYM). The patient also received intrathecal methotrexate and hydrocortisone therapy. Follow-up CT scans showed a continuous significant reduction in the tumor size compared to prior analysis. A posttreatment PET/CT scan demonstrated a marked interval decrease in size and hypermetabolism of the right cervical mass, compatible with a near complete response. The patient is being followed per post chemotherapy protocol, and, to date, there is no evidence of new disease or recurrence.

3. Discussion

3.1. Clinical Features. Burkitt-like lymphoma with 11q aberration (BLL-11q) is a rare, aggressive lymphoid neoplasm, accounting for less than 10% of all Burkitt lymphoma cases in most series [2, 6]. Interestingly, its incidence may be enriched in the posttransplant setting, with one article reporting BLL-11q in 43% of posttransplant Burkitt lymphomas and 60% of EBV-negative posttransplant Burkitt lymphomas [7]. Though only a limited number of cases have been reported, several unique clinical features have emerged as helpful diagnostic considerations. BLL-11q mostly affects children and adults younger than age 40 with a male predominance, though cases have been reported in patients up to 82 years old [2, 6–9]. Compared to conventional Burkitt lymphoma, BLL-11q usually has a nodal presentation, often with a single bulky tumor, along with some localized lymphadenopathy [5, 10–12]. The most commonly involved regions are the head and neck and abdominal lymph nodes [10]. Bone marrow or cerebrospinal fluid (CSF) involvement is not typically seen in these cases, though bone marrow involvement has been reported [11]. Rare cases have also been reported in the posttransplant setting, though its role in other immunodeficient states remains unknown [7]. Patients with BLL-11q are usually HIV and EBV negative [13].

3.2. Microscopic Features. By morphology, Burkitt-like lymphoma with 11q aberration shares similar features with Burkitt lymphoma, validating the utility of keeping this rare entity on the differential diagnosis of these lesions. Sections show a diffuse proliferation of intermediate-to-large sized cells with round nuclei, small nucleoli, and basophilic cytoplasm accompanied by frequent mitotic figures and apoptotic bodies [9–12]. Sporadically, a follicular or nodular pattern can be observed. The presence of tingible-body macrophages can impart a "starry sky" pattern typically seen in BL. In comparison with BL, however, BLL-11q can demonstrate more cytologic pleomorphism and reduced numbers of macrophages and apoptotic bodies, raising the differential of diffuse large B-cell lymphoma and high-grade B-cell lymphoma [2, 10, 14].

3.3. Ancillary Studies

3.3.1. Immunohistochemistry. Providing additional diagnostic complexity, the immunohistochemistry of BL-11q mirrors that of conventional, *MYC*-positive BL with a germinal center (GC) phenotype. All cases show positive expression of CD20, CD10, and BCL-6 with negative expression of MUM1/IRF4 [14]. Most cases in the literature also demonstrate a very high Ki-67 proliferation index (greater than 95%) and negativity for BCL-2, both features that can be seen in BL [10]. To provide assistance in distinguishing between these two entities, several studies have evaluated additional immunohistochemical markers. LMO2 is a marker of germinal center origin that is expressed in germinal center-derived lymphomas as well as acute B-lymphoblastic leukemia and acute myeloid leukemia. Interestingly, LMO2 protein expression is usually downregulated in conventional, *MYC*-positive Burkitt lymphoma. In contrast, positive LMO2 expression can be seen in up to 70% of BLL-11q cases, potentially serving as a useful marker to distinguish between these entities [6].

Additionally, the intensity of *MYC* protein expression appears to differ between these two entities, with

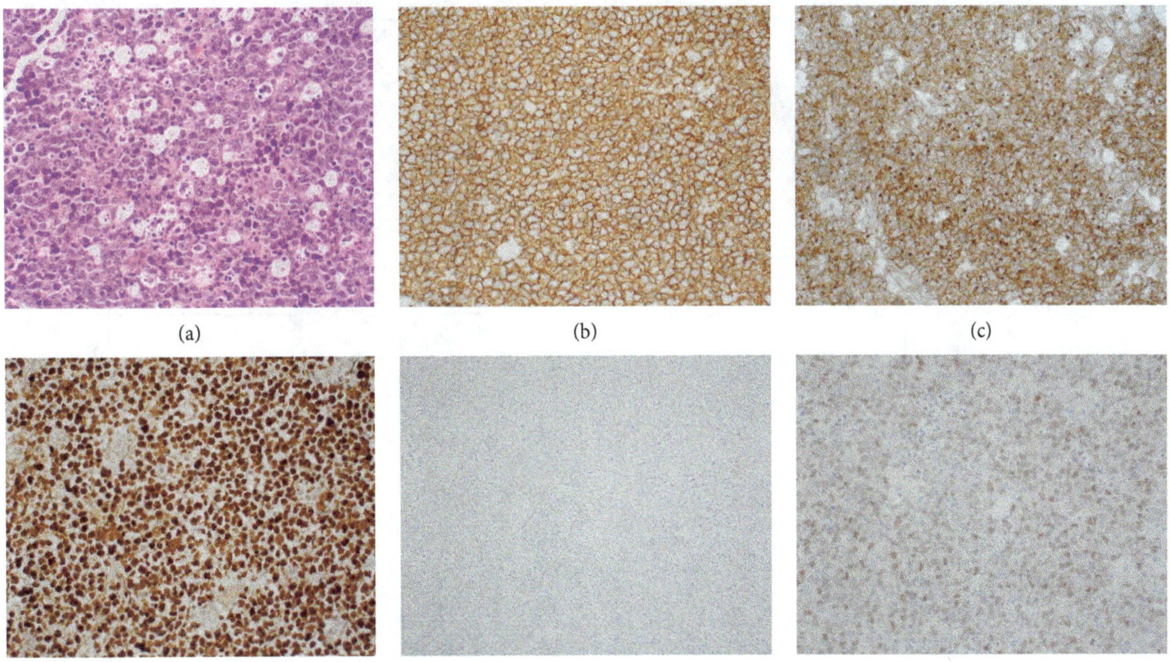

FIGURE 1: Neck mass in a 17-year-old female. (a) Sections show a diffuse proliferation of intermediate-sized atypical cells with prominent nucleoli in a background of apoptotic debris and numerous tingible-body macrophages (hematoxylin-eosin, original magnification 40x). The tumor cells are positive for (b) CD20 (original magnification 40x), (c) CD10 (original magnification 40x), and (d) BCL-6 (original magnification 40x) and negative for (e) CD56 (original magnification 20x). The tumor cells show weak *MYC* expression (f) (original magnification 40x).

conventional BL displaying uniform, bright expression while BLL-11q may show weak, focal *MYC* expression [10]. Rymkiewicz et al. [14] mentioned additional potential immunohistochemical markers, such as CD43, CD44, and CD56, that may provide limited utility.

3.3.2. Flow Cytometry. Flow cytometry analysis shows an antigen expression pattern that is, for the most part, similar to Burkitt lymphoma. The neoplastic cells are usually positive for CD45, pan-B-cell markers (CD19, CD20, and CD22), and CD10 with negative expression for CD5 and CD23. Rymkiewicz et al. investigated a comprehensive flow-cytometry-based profile of Burkitt-like lymphoma with 11q aberration that yielded potentially distinguishing results. In their evaluation, BLL-11q had less frequent diminished expression of CD45 and less frequent CD38^{higher} expression, compared to conventional Burkitt lymphoma. Additionally, CD16/CD56 expression was seen in 60% of BLL-11q lymphomas and in none of *MYC*-positive BL [14].

3.3.3. Cytogenetics. The realm of cytogenetic analysis reveals the most distinguishing feature of Burkitt-like lymphoma with 11q aberration, namely, the 11q aberration. In most studies, conventional cytogenetics and FISH analysis demonstrate a lack of *MYC* (8q24) rearrangements, including the conventional t(8;14), as well as rearrangements in *BCL2* or *BCL6*. All cases demonstrate an abnormality of the 11q arm, with the prototypical abnormality showing high level gains including 11q23.2-23.3 and telomeric losses of 11q24.1-qter. Additionally, compared to conventional BL, BLL-11q cases are more likely to demonstrate complex karyotypes [2, 10, 14]. Gonzalez-Farre et al. reported additional differences from Burkitt lymphoma, namely, the presence of 5q21.3-q32 gains and 6q12.1-q21 losses in BLL-11q and the absence of 1q gains typically seen in BL.9. Despite its utility, two studies state that the 11q aberration pattern is not specifically associated with BLL-11q but may be seen in a subset of cases of *MYC*-positive BL and high-grade B-cell lymphoma (HGBL), NOS [2, 10]. Additionally, gains/amplifications of 11q22-11q24 can be seen in 8–15% of diffuse large B-cell lymphoma (DLBCL) and GC-derived *IRF4*-translocation-positive lymphomas [2]. Therefore, assessment of morphology and immunophenotype remains paramount for recognition of this rare entity.

3.3.4. Molecular Pathology. In BLL-11q, duplication and deletion of the 11q23 and 11q24-qter regions, respectively, simultaneously upregulate and downregulate different sets of genes [2, 11, 13]. Through comparison of gene expression profiles, Salaverria et al. identified two candidate genes involved in the proliferation of the tumor cells: *PAFAH1B2* and *ETS1*. *PAFAH1B2*, which was also upregulated at the protein level, appears to be selectively upregulated in BLL-11q cases, confirming its role as an oncogene in lymphomagenesis. In the region of loss at 11q24-qter, mutations in

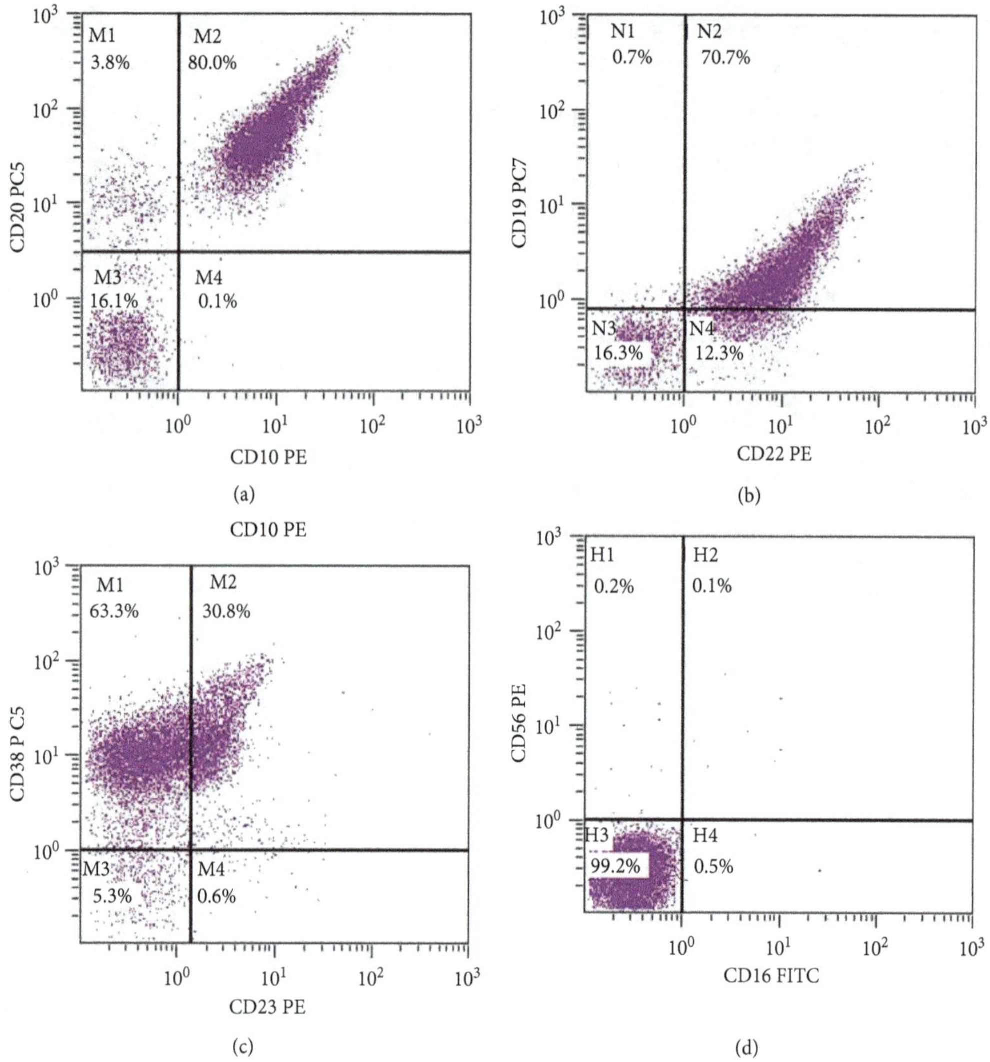

FIGURE 2: Flow cytometry from a neck mass in a 17-year-old female demonstrating neoplastic (a) CD20-positive B-cells with CD10 co-expression. The neoplastic cells demonstrate positive expression for (b) CD19, CD22, and (c) CD38 with (d) no CD16 or CD56 expression.

ETS1, a tumor suppressor gene, were identified [2]. A subsequent study echoed these findings, identifying recurrent mutations in *BTG2*, *DDX3X*, *ETS1*, *EP300*, and *GNA13*. Notably, all cases lacked the typical Burkitt lymphoma mutations in the *ID3*, *TCF3*, or *CCND3* genes [10].

3.4. Differential Diagnosis. Based on the histologic patterns described above, BLL-11q can mimic a variety of lymphomas. Differential diagnostic considerations for BLL-11q include conventional Burkitt lymphoma, diffuse large B-cell lymphoma, and high-grade B-cell lymphoma (HGBL) [8, 9, 13].

The main differential diagnosis for BLL-11q is conventional, *MYC*-positive Burkitt lymphoma, an entity with which it shares similar morphologic and immunophenotypic features [1, 2]. BL occurs in three distinct clinical settings: endemic, sporadic, and immunodeficiency-associated. These three types exhibit different levels of EBV positivity (predominantly seen in the endemic type) [15, 16], a feature not seen in cases of BLL-11q which are uniformly EBV-negative [13, 14]. Additional distinguishing clinical features of BL include its wider age range, more common extranodal presentation, and more frequent occurrence of bone marrow and CSF involvement [13]. The morphology of BL is well defined, classically displaying a diffuse proliferation of medium-sized lymphocytes with abundant mitotic figures and tingible-body macrophages, imparting the "starry sky pattern" [13, 16]. BLL-11q shares many of these morphologic features; however, it can exhibit more prominent cytologic pleomorphism [10].

The immunophenotype of these two entities is similar, composed of neoplastic B cells with a GC phenotype, negative BCL-2 expression, and a markedly increased Ki-67 proliferative index (approaching 100%) [2, 10]. As mentioned above, markers such as LMO2 and MYC have been proposed as diagnostic stains to separate BL and BLL-11q, with BLL-11q demonstrating positivity for LMO2 and weaker, more focal *MYC* expression [6]. Flow cytometry analysis demonstrates a similar immunophenotype between

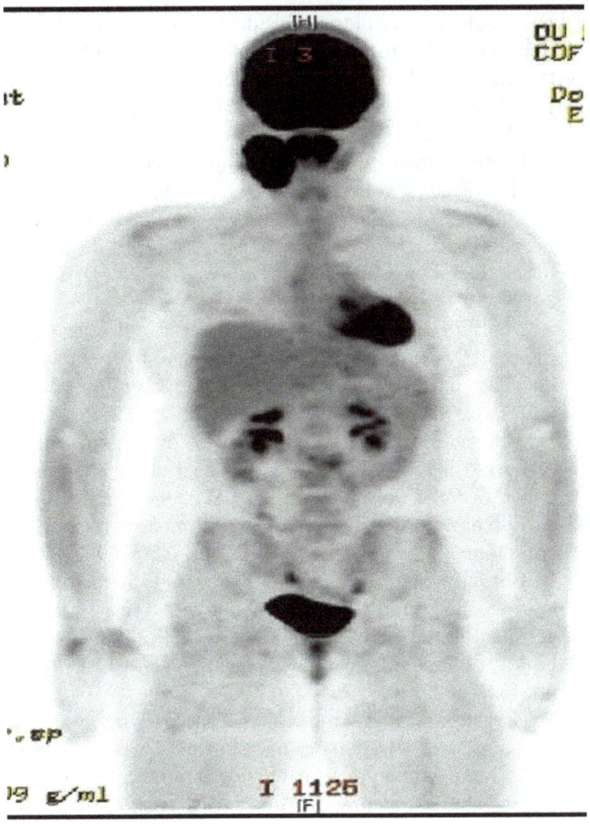

FIGURE 3: PET scan from a 17-year-old female showing a large FDG-avid right cervical mass, compatible with primary malignancy. No FDG-avid malignancy is identified elsewhere in the body.

BL and BLL-11q, with one article highlighting less frequent diminished expression of CD45 and less frequent CD38^{higher} expression in BLL-11q, compared to conventional Burkitt lymphoma [14].

Cytogenetic and FISH analyses allow more definitive classification. More than 90% of BL cases show rearrangements of the *MYC* oncogene, located on chromosome 8. Usually, this rearrangement involves the immunoglobulin heavy chain locus on chromosome 14; however, in up to 20–25% of cases, *MYC* rearranges with the kappa (chromosome 2) or lambda (chromosome 22) light chain loci [1]. Though a subset of conventional Burkitt lymphoma cases can have the defined 11q aberration, these cases nonetheless have the *MYC* rearrangement. BLL-11q, in contrast, demonstrates no *MYC* rearrangements and also lacks additional cytogenetic features reminiscent of BL (1q gains). Thus, cases with suspected Burkitt lymphoma by morphology and immunophenotype that lack *MYC* rearrangements should be worked up for BLL-11q. As mentioned before, molecular analysis is dissimilar in these two entities, demonstrating recurrent mutations in *BTG2*, *DDX3X*, *ETS1*, *EP300*, and *GNA13* for BLL-11q and mutations in the *ID3*, *TCF3*, *and CCND3* genes for BL [10, 11].

Diffuse large B-cell lymphoma (DLBCL) is another diagnostic consideration in this context. Typically occurring in older adults, DLBCL can nonetheless exhibit heterogeneous morphology that may overlap with cases of BLL-11q. Clinically, these patients exhibit nodal or extranodal presentation that can be localized or widespread. Essentially a diagnosis of exclusion, the immunohistochemical profile of DLBCL is positive for pan-B-cell markers (CD19, CD20, and CD22) with variable expression of CD10, BCL-6, and MUM-1, depending on the cell of origin [13, 17]. BCL-2 can be negative in some cases; however, diffuse positivity helps to distinguish DLBCL from BL and BLL-11q. The cytogenetic profile is similarly heterogeneous, with some cases displaying *MYC* rearrangements and an 11q abnormality seen in 8–15% of cases [2]. Nevertheless, the region of gain extends to the telomere and is not coincident with the minimal observed region of gain in BLL-11q [11].

High-grade B-cell lymphoma, similar to BLL-11q, is a new diagnostic entity in the WHO classification system. Replacing the previous category of B-cell lymphoma, unclassifiable, with features intermediate between diffuse large B-cell lymphoma and Burkitt lymphoma (BCLU), this category encompasses a heterogeneous group of aggressive mature B-cell lymphomas. Clinically, these cases are distinct from BLL-11q, usually presenting as advanced, disseminated disease in elderly patients. The morphology of HGBL can display Burkitt-like features but with more cytologic atypia or blastoid morphology. The immunophenotype, like DLBCL, is variable with positive expression of pan-B-cell markers. This entity is in large part defined by its cytogenetic data. The presence of a *MYC* rearrangement, along with *BCL2* and/or *BCL6* rearrangements, is diagnostic of high-grade B-cell lymphoma with *MYC*, *BCL2*, and/or *BCL6* rearrangements (so-called "double/triple hit" lymphoma). HGBL, NOS is a diagnosis of exclusion used very rarely to denote cases lacking the just mentioned cytogenetic findings but with morphology overlapping between DLBCL and BL. HGBL, NOS can demonstrate a *MYC* rearrangement in 20–35% of cases, and a subset has been identified with an 11q aberration. These cases are important to identify due to their unique prognosis and treatment strategies; however, clinical and cytogenetic data help to distinguish it from Burkitt-like lymphoma with 11q aberration [13, 17].

Interestingly, in their assessment of BLL-11q cases, Gonzalez-Farre et al. identified two cases displaying a follicular growth pattern with an underlying meshwork of follicular dendritic cells, raising the differential diagnosis of large B-cell lymphoma with *IRF4* rearrangement. However, these cases did not express IRF4/MUM1 and exhibited the "starry sky" pattern with frequent mitotic figures, a feature not associated with large B-cell lymphoma with IRF4 rearrangement. In summary, a combination of clinical, morphologic, immunophenotypic, and cytogenetic information is needed to fully evaluate and separate these diagnostic entities [10].

3.5. Treatment and Prognosis. Currently, the treatment of choice for this tumor is variable and depends on the clinical scenario. Rymkiewicz et al. treated their 10 BLL-11q patients with either a modified R-CODOX-M/R-IVAC regimen (rituximab, fractionated cyclophosphamide, vincristine, doxorubicin, and high-dose methotrexate alternating with fractionated ifosfamide, etoposide, and high-dose cytarabine, along with intrathecal methotrexate and cytarabine) or the

GMALL-B-ALL/NHL2002 protocol (rituximab, fractionated cyclophosphamide (or ifosfamide), vincristine, methotrexate, cytarabine, teniposide, and prednisone or doxorubicin). At the last follow-up, 8 of 10 patients were alive (median follow-up = 54 months). Previous cohort studies mentioned in this article suggest that the BLL-11q patients treated with a BL-directed regimen show a similar relapse-free outcome to BL patients. However, BLL-11q patients treated with the conventional DLBCL regimen (R-CHOP) have a higher risk of relapse [14]. Salaverria et al. followed up with their patients for 36 months, and all but one was alive at the last follow-up, suggesting an excellent survival rate for these patients. In general, the five-year overall survival of BLL-11q patients is approximately 80% which is similar to BL. Patients with localized nodal disease appear to show a more favorable outcome after therapy [2]. The treatment of choice in our patient, including induction chemotherapy with cyclophosphamide, vincristine, prednisone, doxorubicin, and methotrexate (COPADM) and consolidation chemotherapy with cytarabine and methotrexate (CYM), was initially introduced for advanced childhood B-cell non-Hodgkin lymphomas and acute lymphoblastic leukemia of the L3 subtype, with similar patient populations being studied in the current ANHL 1131 protocol [18]. This regimen is similar to NCCN-recommended chemotherapy regimens for Burkitt lymphoma, a treatment course that previous articles suggest is preferable to a conventional DLBCL-based regimen [14]. The patient has had a near complete response over the course of treatment.

In conclusion, BLL-11q is a rare and new provisional diagnostic entity with overlapping morphologic and immunophenotypic features with BL. However, unique clinical, cytogenetic, and molecular data can assist in formulating this diagnosis. Therefore, incorporation of multiple ancillary studies may be warranted. Though data remain limited, a supplementary workup for this rare diagnosis is warranted for any case with BL, DLBCL, or HGBCL morphology, germinal center (GC) expression, and a markedly increased proliferative index (>90%), without *MYC* rearrangements. Although there is no definite treatment choice for this lymphoma, an accurate diagnosis is essential in order to choose the most suitable treatment based on the available regimens and clinical trials.

References

[1] B. Pienkowska-Grela, G. Rymkiewicz, B. Grygalewicz et al., "Partial trisomy 11, dup (11) (q23q13), as a defect characterizing lymphomas with burkitt pathomorphology without MYC gene rearrangement," *Medical Oncology*, vol. 28, no. 4, pp. 1589–1595, 2011.

[2] I. Salaverria, I. Martin-Guerrero, R. Wagener et al., "A recurrent 11q aberration pattern characterizes a subset of MYC-negative high-grade B-Cell lymphomas resembling burkitt lymphoma," *Blood*, vol. 123, no. 8, pp. 1187–1198, 2014.

[3] S. H. Swerdlow, E. Campo, N. L. Harris et al., *WHO Classification of Tumours of Haematopoietic and Lymphoid Tissues*, IARC, Lyon, France, 4th edition, 2017.

[4] H. A. Poirel, M. S. Cairo, M. S. Cairo et al., "Specific cytogenetic abnormalities are associated with a significantly inferior outcome in children and adolescents with mature B-cell non-hodgkin's lymphoma: results of the FAB/LMB 96 international study," *Leukemia*, vol. 23, no. 2, pp. 323–331, 2009.

[5] K. M. Strobel, J. N. Crane, K. L. Bradford, Y. Naeini, W. A. May, and V. Y. Chang, "Burkitt-like lymphoma in a pediatric patient with familial adenomatous polyposis," *Cancer Genetics*, vol. 239, pp. 33–35, 2019.

[6] Y. Liu, T. Bian, Y. Zhang et al., "A combination of LMO2 negative and CD38 positive is useful for the diagnosis of burkitt lymphoma," *Diagnostic Pathology*, vol. 14, no. 1, p. 100, 2019.

[7] J. F. Ferreiro, J. Morscio, D. Dierickx et al., "Post-transplant molecularly defined burkitt lymphomas are frequently MYC-negative and characterized by the 11q-gain/loss pattern," *Haematologica*, vol. 100, no. 7, pp. e275–279, 2015.

[8] H. Moshref Razavi and M. Hrynchak, "Unusual presentation of Burkitt-like lymphoma with 11q aberration in an elderly patient," *Blood*, vol. 133, no. 4, p. 381, 2019.

[9] A. Rosenthal and L. Rimsza, "Genomics of aggressive B-cell lymphoma," *Hematology*, vol. 2018, no. 1, pp. 69–74, 2018.

[10] B. Gonzalez-Farre, J. E. Ramis-Zaldivar, J. Salmeron-Villalobos et al., "Burkitt-like lymphoma with 11q aberration: a germinal center-derived lymphoma genetically unrelated to burkitt lymphoma," *Haematologica*, vol. 104, no. 9, pp. 1822–1829, 2019.

[11] B. Grygalewicz, R. Woroniecka, G. Rymkiewicz et al., "The 11q-gain/loss aberration occurs recurrently in MYC-negative Burkitt-like lymphoma with 11q aberration, as well as MYC-positive burkitt lymphoma and MYC-positive high-grade B-cell lymphoma, NOS," *American Journal of Clinical Pathology*, vol. 149, no. 1, pp. 17–28, 2017.

[12] K. Collins, L. Mnayer, and P. Shen, "Burkitt-like lymphoma with 11q aberration," *Clinical Case Reports*, vol. 7, no. 9, pp. 1823-1824, 2019.

[13] A. Szumera-Cieckiewicz, G. Rymkiewicz, B. Grygalewicz et al., "Comprehensive histopathological diagnostics of aggressive B-cell lymphomas based on the updated criteria of the world health organization's 2017 classification," *Polish Journal of Pathology*, vol. 69, no. 1, pp. 1–19, 2018.

[14] G. Rymkiewicz, B. Grygalewicz, M. Chechlinska et al., "A comprehensive flow-cytometry-based immunophenotypic characterization of burkitt-like lymphoma with 11q aberration," *Modern Pathology*, vol. 31, no. 5, pp. 732–743, 2018.

[15] B. Graham and D. T. Lynch, *Cancer, Burkitt Lymphoma*, StatPearls Publishing, Treasure Island, FL, USA, 2019.

[16] L. Rimsza, S. Pittaluga, S. Dirnhofer et al., "The clinicopathologic spectrum of mature aggressive B cell lymphomas," *Virchows Archiv*, vol. 471, no. 4, pp. 453–466, 2017.

[17] K. E. Grimm and D. P. O'Malley, "Aggressive B-cell lymphomas in the 2017 revised WHO classification of tumors of hematopoietic and lymphoid tissues," *Annals of Diagnostic Pathology*, vol. 38, pp. 6–10, 2019.

[18] C. Patte, A. Auperin, J. Michon et al., "The societe francaise d'oncologie Pediatrique LMB89 protocol: highly effective multiagent chemotherapy tailored to the tumor burden and initial response in 561 unselected children with B-cell lymphomas and L3 leukemia," *Blood*, vol. 97, no. 11, pp. 3370–3379, 2001.

37

Paroxysmal Nocturnal Hemoglobinuria with a Distinct Molecular Signature Diagnosed Ten Years after Allogenic Bone Marrow Transplantation for Acute Myeloid Leukemia

Alberto Santagostino,[1] Laura Lombardi,[1] Gerard Dine,[1] Pierre Hirsch,[2] and Srimanta Chandra Misra[1,3]

[1]*Department of Clinical Hematology, Troyes General Hospital, 10000 Troyes, France*
[2]*Sorbonne University, Inserm, Centre de Recherche Saint-Antoine, CRSA, AP-HP, Department of Laboratory Hematology Saint-Antoine Hospital, Paris, France*
[3]*Department of Clinical Hematology, Saint Antoine Hospital, Paris, France*

Correspondence should be addressed to Srimanta Chandra Misra; misras754@gmail.com

Academic Editor: Ramon Tiu

Paroxysmal nocturnal hemoglobinurea (PNH) is a rare disorder of complement regulation due to somatic mutation of PIGA (phosphatidylinositol glycan anchor) gene. We herewith report a case who developed a symptomatic PNH long after an allogenic marrow transplant. Some reasonable arguments concerning the origin of PNH clone have been discussed. The molecular studies revealed presence of JAK2 and TET2 mutations without a BCOR mutation. The literature review has been performed to probe into the complex interplay of autoimmunity and clonal selection and expansion of PNH cells, which occurs early in hematopoietic differentiation. The consequent events such as hypoplastic and/or hemato-oncologic features could further be explained on the basis of next-generation sequencing (NGS) studies. Paroxysmal nocturnal hemoglobinuria (PNH) is a rare clonal disorder of hematopoietic stem cells, characterized by a somatic mutation of the phosphatidylinositol glycan-class A (PIGA). The PIGA gene products are crucial for biosynthesis of glycosylphosphatidylinositol (GPI) anchors, which attaches a number of proteins to the plasma membrane of the cell. Amongst these proteins, the CD55 and CD59 are complement regulatory proteins. The CD55 inhibits C3 convertase whereas the CD59 blocks the membrane attack complex (MAC) by inhibiting the incorporation of C9 to MAC. The loss of complement regulatory protein renders the red cell susceptible to complement-mediated lysis leading to intravascular and extravascular hemolysis. The intravascular hemolysis explains most of the morbid clinical manifestations of the disease. The clinical features of syndrome of PNH are recurrent hemolytic episodes, thrombosis, smooth muscle dystonia, and bone marrow failure; other important complications include renal failure, myelodysplastic syndrome (MDS), and acute myeloid leukemia (AML). The most used therapies were blood transfusions, immunosuppressive, and steroid. Allogeneic stem cell transplantation was also practiced. At present, the therapy of choice is eculizumab (Soliris, Alexion Pharmaceuticals), a humanized monoclonal antibody that blocks activation of the terminal complement at C5. The limiting factor for this therapy is breakthrough hemolysis and the frequent dosing schedule. Ravulizumab (ALXN1210) is the second generation terminal compliment inhibitor which seems to provide a sustained control of hemolysis without breakthrough hemolysis and with a longer dosing interval.

1. Case Report

A 63-year-old man presented in August 2017 with moderate pancytopenia associated with hemolysis [1]. The blood results were Hb 8.5 g/dL, MCV 103 fL, WBC 3.2 × 109/L, platelets 128 × 109/L, reticulocytes 321 × 109/L, LDH 3462 U/L, reduced haptoglobin <0.01 μmol/L, ferritin 461 ng/mL, total bilirubin 4 mg/dL, creatinine 142 g/L, and normal value of folate and vitamin B12. Clinically, he presented fatigue and cholecystitis.

The patient was diagnosed in 2007 as myelodysplastic syndrome with excess blasts (MDS-EB) followed in another centre. In 2009, the patient evolved acute myeloid leukemia (AML) treated with classic induction therapy idarubicin and cytarabine and consolidation therapy followed by allogeneic stem cells transplantation in 2010 with matched unrelated donor (MUD) achieving a complete remission with complete donor chimerism. In November 2016, he presented a moderate anemia (Hb 10 g/dL), treated with darbepoetin alfa. The aspiration was impossible. The bone marrow biopsy specimen was normocellular with dysmyelopoiesis but without blasts. The annual follow-up at the allotransplant centre showed chimerism of donor as 22% in July 2017. In August 2017, the flow cytometric analysis of peripheral blood cells revealed 96.2% of PNH clone type III. Another control of bone marrow biopsy specimen in September 2017 showed erythroblastic hyperplasia without blasts. Therefore, the diagnosis was paroxysmal nocturnal hemoglobinuria (PNH). The patient began therapy with eculizumab, and prior to this treatment, he required 3 transfusions of packed RBCs. The patient was vaccinated against *Neisseria meningitidis* 2 weeks before the start of treatment. Eculizumab therapy began in October 2017 with an induction dose of 600 mg × 2 intravenous (iv) weekly for 4 weeks followed by a single dose of 900 mg (iv) after 7 days, then 900 mg iv every 15 days. Seven months later, the patient continues eculizumab without bleeding or thrombosis signs and with a stable value of hemoglobin (9-10 g/l). He presents a reduction of hemolysis index and a good quality of life. In molecular analysis, we found JAK2 V617 F mutation with an allelic frequency of 44%, and the NGS study revealed a frameshift mutation of TET2 with an allelic frequency of 34%. The patient is very closely followed up for an imminent relapse. During preparation of this manuscript, the patient relapsed with a diagnosis of AML.

2. Discussion

PNH is a rare hemolytic anemia first described in 1882 by Strübing [2] This is a disorder of complement regulation, caused by somatic mutations in the PIGA gene which is 17 kb long with 6 exons and maps to short arm of X chromosome.

The other important disorders of complement regulations are atypical hemolytic uremic syndrome (aHUS), caused by cell surface alternative pathway dysregulation and C3 glomerulopathy (C3G) due to fluid-phase alternative pathway dysregulation The mechanism underlying these dysregulations are diverse, predominantly acquired autoimmune in C3G, somatic mutations in PNH, or an inherited germline mutations in aHUS [3].

The location of PIGA gene in X chromosome explains the ability of the mutation to cause PNH as only one allele is functional in male as well as in female.

The development of PNH involves a multistep process, such as clonal selection and clonal expansion resulting in hypoplastic/aplastic anemia (AA) and sometimes malignant transformation leading to MDS and AML.

Nafa et al. identified 15 different somatic mutations in 12 patients, out of which 10 were caused by frameshift mutations; they postulated that the predominance of frameshift mutation might pave the way for a clonal selection [4].

The clonal selection of PIGA-mutated hematopoietic cells might be immune mediated as PNH has its close association with aplastic anemia (AA). AA may develop during the course of PNH and vice versa (AA/PNH syndrome), both being predisposed to AML and MDS [5].

The complication of clinically relevant PNH has been described in 15% to 25% of the patients with AA treated by immunosuppressive therapy (IST). The clonal hematopoiesis is much higher among patients with aplastic anemia, with high incidence of BCOR and BCORL1 and PIGA mutations, whereas TET2 and JAK2 were infrequently mutated, suggesting a distinct mechanism of clonal selection and thus a complex interplay between immunology and oncogenesis [6]. In our patient, the presence of TET2 and JAK2 without the presence of BCOR is consistent with the fact that the patient never had hypoplastic features. The pathogenesis was driven more towards oncogenetic events.

Moreover, regardless of typical manifestations of PNH, GPI anchor-deficient, "PNH-type" cells are detectable at higher frequencies [7].

There is growing evidence that the expansion of the PNH clone results from T-cell-mediated autoimmune damage to hematopoietic stem cells, with the GPI molecule as target. Indeed, GPI-specific CD8 + T cells, which have been identified in PNH patients, would spare selectively GPI-negative stem cells [8].

However, the mutant PIGA cell clone itself fails to explain a clonal expansion. Hence, there might be a second somatic mutation (second hit) conferring the mutant PIGA cell a proliferative advantage. Inoue et al. [9] were successful in discovering ectopic expression of HMGA2 in the mutant PIGA cell accounting for clonal hematopoiesis.

Later, the deep sequencing by Shen et al. in PNH patients revealed (TET2) zinc finger SUZ12, transcription factor ASXL1, BCL6 corepressor (BCOR), JAK2, and U2 small nuclear RNA auxiliary factor 1 (U2AF1), thus adding the complexity of clonal architecture and growth advantage. They presented data from whole exome sequencing (WES) of clonal (GPI-deficient) and nonclonal cells from PNH patients to examine the mutational history of PNH which depicted 4 different scenarios:

(1) PIGA as the initial ancestral event accompanied by secondary mutations

(2) PIGA as an event secondary to other mutations

(3) PIGA as the lone mutation

(4) PIGA mutation coexisting with other mutations responsible for the development of an MDS clone

However, in some cases, the leukemogenic effects might be driven by mutations such as JAK2, TET2, or STAC3, suggesting that these primary events arose, conveying an initial growth advantage, with a PIGA mutation as a subclone conveying an additional growth advantage [10]. The STAC3 mutation was not studied in our patient; Mochizuki et al. [11] supported the suggestion that GPI-deficient stem cells have a survival advantage in the setting of immune-mediated BM injury or postallotransplant.

We do not know the origin of the PNH clone (donor or patient). This is an open question. We postulate the PNH clone was derived from the patient because our patient presents a reduction of donor chimerism of 22% at the PNH debut but the analysis of donor PNH clone was not performed. In our patient, there are two hypotheses which merit a serious consideration.

Firstly, whether the clonal selection of PIGA-mutated clone is driven by donor T cell irrespective of the origin of the clone. The possibility is quite low as the PNH clone emerged following reduction of chimerism and before the relapse of MDS.

The second possibility is that the patient might be harboring a coexistence of MDS and PNH clone long before the diagnosis of SMD. This second hypothesis might be appropriate in our case.

Some intrinsic immune dysregulation led a clonal selection of both of the clones, which obtained proliferative advantage. This hypothesis is further consolidated by the findings of the high frequency of the driver mutation JAK2 as well as TET2 mutation. In 2007, JAK2 was not systematically searched for, and the implication of TET2 was unknown before 2009.

Hence, the AML diagnosed in 2007 probably arose from a preexisting myeloproliferative/myelodysplastic overlapping syndrome. The present PNH clone was probably driven by the existing MPN/MDS. This intriguing issue questioned long back by Professor Willium Dameshek in 1969 who made a proposal to consider PNH as a candidate disorder of myeloproliferative neoplasm (MPN) [12]. The definite classification of MDS came only in 1982 as an attempt to define different preleukemic conditions, where as in 1950s, Professor Damashek had already made a conceptual construct of MPN.

We conclude that the PNH clone belongs to the receiver which reappeared during loss of chimerism and parallels with the relapse.

References

[1] A. Röth, S. T. Rottinghaus, A. Hill et al., "Ravulizumab (ALXN1210) in patients with paroxysmal nocturnal hemoglobinuria: results of 2 phase 1b/2 studies," *Blood Advances*, vol. 2, no. 17, pp. 2176–2185, 2018.

[2] P. Strübing, "Paroxysmale haemoglobinurie," *DMW-Deutsche Medizinische Wochenschrift*, vol. 8, no. 1, pp. 1–3, 2009.

[3] E. K. S. Wong and D. Kavanagh, "Diseases of complement dysregulation—an overview," *Seminars in Immunopathology*, vol. 40, no. 1, pp. 49–64, 2018.

[4] K. Nafa, M. Bessler, H. Castro-Malaspina, S. Jhanwar, and L. Luzzatto, "The spectrum of somatic mutations in the PIG-A gene in paroxysmal nocturnal hemoglobinuria includes large deletions and small duplications," *Blood Cells, Molecules, and Diseases*, vol. 24, no. 3, pp. 370–384, 1998.

[5] G. Socié, J. Y. Mary, A. de Gramont et al., "Paroxysmal nocturnal haemoglobinuria: long-term follow-up and prognostic factors," *Lancet*, vol. 348, no. 9027, pp. 573–577, 1996.

[6] T. Yoshizato, B. Dumitriu, K. Hosokawa et al., "Somatic mutations and clonal hematopoiesis in aplastic anemia," *New England Journal of Medicine*, vol. 373, no. 1, p. 3547, 2015.

[7] R. A. Brodsky, G. L. Mukhina, S. Li et al., "Improved detection and characterization of paroxysmal nocturnal hemoglobinuria using fluorescent aerolysin," *American Journal of Clinical Pathology*, vol. 114, no. 3, pp. 459–466, 2000.

[8] L. Luzzatto, "Recent advances in the pathogenesis and treatment of paroxysmal nocturnal hemoglobinuria," *F1000Research*, vol. 5, p. 209, 2016.

[9] N. Inoue, T. Izui-Sarumaru, Y. Murakami et al., "Molecular basis of clonal expansion of hematopoiesis in 2 patients with paroxysmal nocturnal hemoglobinuria (PNH)," *Blood*, vol. 108, no. 13, pp. 4232–4236, 2006.

[10] W. Shen, M. J. Clemente, N. Hosono et al., "Deep sequencing reveals stepwise mutation acquisition in paroxysmal nocturnal hemoglobinuria," *Journal of Clinical Investigation*, vol. 124, no. 10, pp. 4529–4538, 2014.

[11] K. Mochizuki, C. Sugimori, Z. Qi et al., "Expansion of donor-derived hematopoietic stemcells with PIGA mutation associated with late graft failure after allogeneic stem cell transplantation," *Blood*, vol. 112, no. 5, pp. 2160–2162, 2008.

[12] W. Dameshek, "Foreword and a proposal for considering paroxysmal nocturnal hemoglobinuria (PNH) as a "candidate" myeloproliferative disorder," *Blood*, vol. 33, no. 2, pp. 263-264, 1969.

38

Acquired Hemophilia A (FVIII Deficiency) Associated with Papillary Thyroid Cancer: Treatment with Recombinant Porcine FVIII

S. Nguyen ,[1,2] P. Teh,[2] J. Zhou,[1,3] E. Y. Chang ,[4,5] and A. von Drygalski [1,3]

[1]*Department of Medicine, University of California San Diego, San Diego, CA, USA*
[2]*Department of Medicine, University of California Riverside, Riverside, CA, USA*
[3]*Department of Molecular Medicine, The Scripps Research Institute, La Jolla, CA, USA*
[4]*Radiology Service, VA San Diego Healthcare System, San Diego, CA, USA*
[5]*Department of Radiology, University of California San Diego, San Diego, CA, USA*

Correspondence should be addressed to S. Nguyen; sonhanguyen29@gmail.com

Academic Editor: Kiyotaka Kawauchi

Acquired hemophilia A (AHA) is a rare autoimmune disorder caused by autoantibodies against Factor VIII (FVIII). It has a high mortality due to bleeding complications. FVIIa-based bypassing agents are the first line of treatment but not always effective. Recombinant porcine (rp) FVIII (Obizur®) was recently approved for rescue treatment but with little evidence-based information regarding efficacy. We report a case of papillary thyroid cancer associated with AHA malignancy that responded to a single dose of rpFVIII after failure to achieve hemostasis with FVIIa-based bypassing products.

1. Case Presentation

A 71-year-old Asian male presented to the UCSD Medical Center with generalized body bruising, intermittent gingival bleeding, hematuria, and epistaxis for one month. His medical history was remarkable for metastatic papillary thyroid cancer, which was diagnosed three years earlier. He underwent total thyroidectomy, radiotherapy, and stereotactic radiosurgery and was receiving ulixertinib (BioMed Valley Discoveries, Kansas, USA), an experimental ERK1/2 kinase inhibitor, on a clinical trial protocol for patients with advanced solid tumors. The patient had no prior personal or family history of bleeding problems and was not on anticoagulation. On presentation in the Emergency Department, the patient reported acute right groin pain after a mechanical fall. His physical examination was significant for diffuse ecchymoses across the abdomen without petechiae or palpable purpura. The right hip demonstrated tenderness upon palpation. Laboratory studies showed a hemoglobin of 11.6 g/dL, normal prothrombin time (PT), prolonged activated partial prothrombin time (aPTT) (107.4 seconds) with 1% FVIII plasma activity, and a FVIII inhibitor titer of 57 Bethesda units (BU). Computed tomography (CT) scan of the abdomen showed a large right iliopsoas hematoma (Figures 1(a) and 1(b)). He was admitted and treated with rhFVIIa at 90 $\mu g \cdot kg^{-1}$ every two hours and red cell transfusions during the next 2 days. However, his hemoglobin continued to drop to 7.7 g/dL. Due to unresponsiveness to rhFVIIa, the patient was switched to FEIBA (75 units/kg, 2-3 times daily) for 2 more days. His hemoglobin continued to drop to 7.4 g/dL despite blood transfusions with increasing iliopsoas bleeding on a subsequent CT scan (Figures 1(c) and 1(d)). At this point, rpFVIII at 100 units/kg was administered (half of the labeled dose), which stopped the bleeding promptly based on clinical assessment (no new signs of bleeding) and hemoglobin stabilization. Also, there was no additional requirement for blood transfusions. FVIII plasma activity shortly after infusion of rpFVIII was not available, but 24 hours later, the plasma activity was higher than predicted based on an assumed 8-hour half-life of exogenous rhFVIII

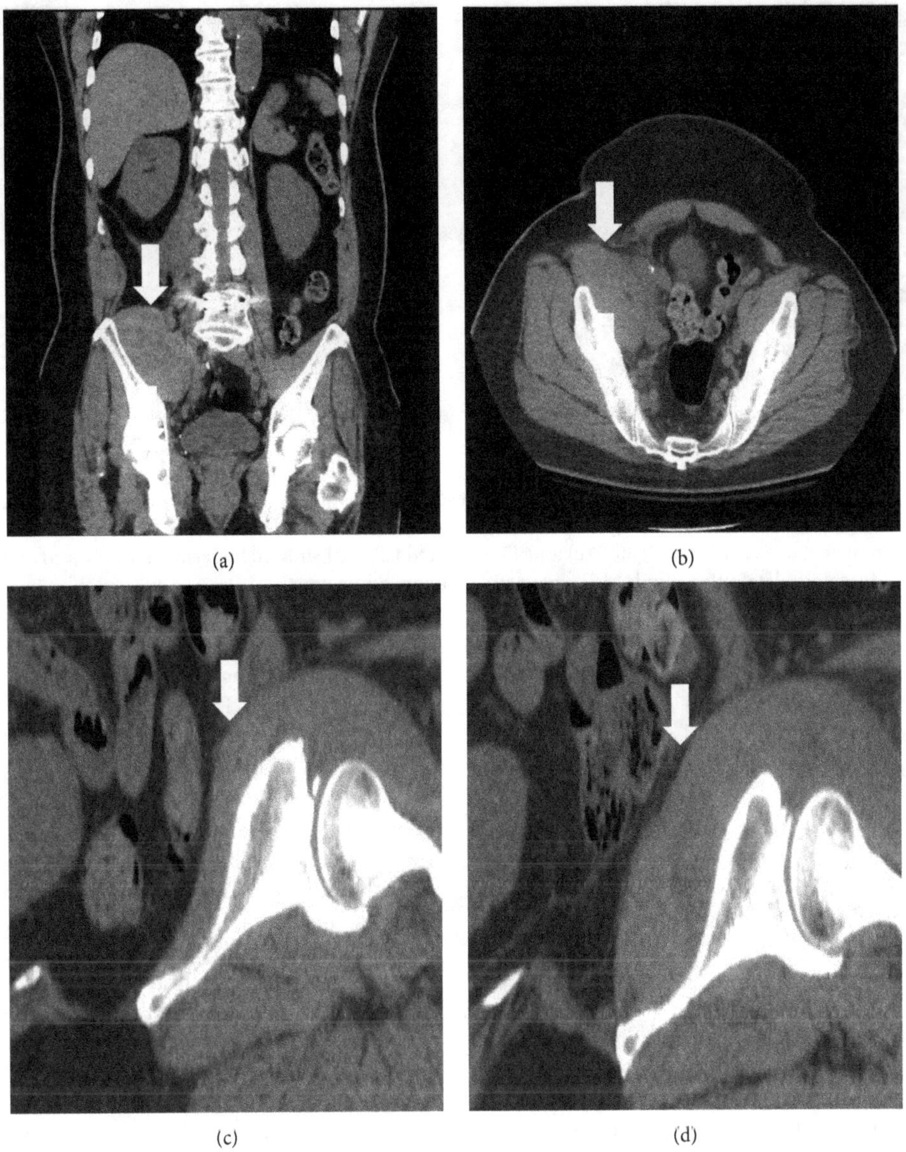

Figure 1: Computed tomography scan of the abdomen and pelvis. Coronal (a) and axial (b) planes show asymmetrically enlarged right iliacus muscle (white arrows), consistent with hematoma. Sagittal plane of the hips: left unaffected hip (c) in comparison to the right hip (d), which showed right psoas muscle bleed after treatment of recombinant human factor VIIa and Factor Eight Inhibitor Bypassing Activity (FEIBA).

(49% actual versus approximately 25% predicted), indicating an appropriate response and low likelihood of cross-reactive antibodies to rpFVIII. The patient was discharged to a skilled nursing facility the next day. High-dose prednisone (approximately 1 mg/kg = 80 mg/daily) was initiated on the first day of hospitalization. After discharge, the patient continued to receive high-dose prednisone for one month, which eradicated the inhibitory FVIII antibody. Thereafter, a slow taper was implemented (reduction by 10 mg/daily per week). Screening of plasma collected prior to administration of rpFVIII confirmed the absence of anti-porcine FVIII antibodies (proprietary test, Shire Pharmaceuticals).

Fifteen weeks later, the patient presented at the UCSD Hemophilia and Thrombosis Treatment Center for right knee pain after a mechanical fall. Laboratory studies showed 116% FVIII activity with a FVIII inhibitor titer of <0.4 U. Point-of-care musculoskeletal ultrasound (POC MSKUS) of the right knee showed semicompressible hypoechoic contents in the suprapatellar, lateral, and medial recesses. Joint aspiration failed to withdraw fluid due to high resistance. These findings were consistent with coagulated blood in the joint space. Conventional MRI to assess other abnormalities did not reveal acute injury and also confirmed absence of an effusion (Figure 2). In conjunction with normal FVIII activity levels, this finding made acute hemarthrosis due to injury and lingering FVIII deficiency less likely although the exact time point of bleeding remained elusive. Also, the normalized FVIII

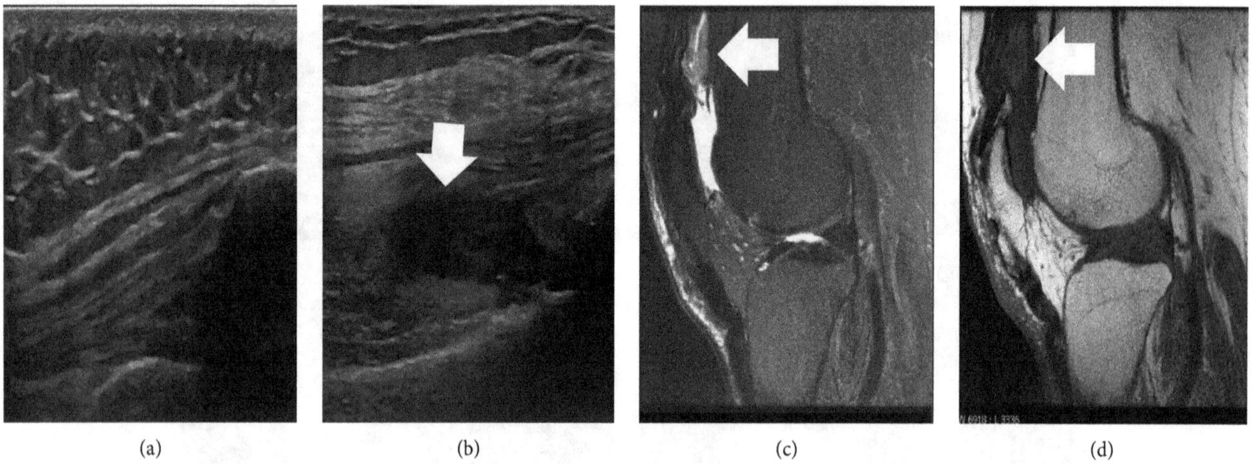

Figure 2: Point-of-care musculoskeletal ultrasound and magnetic resonance imaging of suprapatellar recesses in the knees. Longitudinal MSKUS image (a) of the unaffected knee was compared to the affected knee (b), which showed semicompressible hypoechoic contents (white arrow) in the suprapatellar recess. T2-weighted (c) and T1-weighted (d) MRI showed hyperintense (white arrows), corresponding to blood clots. MSKUS, musculoskeletal ultrasound; MRI, magnetic resonance imaging.

activity level ruled out the development of clinically relevant, cross-reactive anti-porcine FVIII antibodies.

Figure 3 depicts the timeline and course of the patient's management starting at diagnosis until inhibitor eradication.

This case demonstrates that early intervention with rpFVIII in AHA may be a valuable strategy. It also emphasizes the usefulness of POC MSKUS for management of musculoskeletal hemophilic bleeding.

2. Discussion

Acquired hemophilia A (AHA) is a rare and potentially fatal bleeding disorder. It is caused by autoantibodies against circulating coagulation Factor VIII (FVIII), leading to inhibition of Factor VIII binding to von Willebrand factor, activated factor IX, or negatively charged phospholipids [1]. The incidence of AHA ranges between 0.2 and 1.0 cases per one million per year [2]. Its prognosis is poor with a high mortality rate within the first several months after diagnosis (9–27%), due to comorbidities, advanced patient age, location, and severity of bleeding [3–5]. Management is often challenging due to delayed diagnosis with the suboptimal efficacy of FVIIa-based bypassing agents, resulting in fatal bleeding complications [6, 7].

The development of immune-mediated autoantibodies against FVIII in AHA is associated with a range of clinical disorders. Up to 50% of the cases are idiopathic [8, 9]. In the other half of the cases, development of autoantibodies is associated with solid or hematological neoplasms, autoimmune diseases, pregnancy, or medication effects (especially antibiotics and interferon) [10]. However, the mechanisms underlying the development of AHA remain poorly defined.

The management of AHA mainly consists of two components: efforts to achieve prompt hemostasis and autoantibody ("inhibitor") eradication. The treatment for hemostatic control includes the use of plasma-derived or recombinant FVIIa bypassing agents, namely, Factor Eight Inhibitor Bypassing Activity (FEIBA®, Baxter Healthcare Corporation, Deerfield, IL, USA) or recombinant human (rh) FVIIa (Novo Seven; Novo Nordisk A/S, Bagsvaerd, Denmark). Both of these agents achieve hemostasis by generating thrombin in the absence of FVIII at the site of bleeding [11, 12]. However, they differ in their biochemical properties, composition, and pharmacokinetics. While FEIBA has a longer half-life of 4–7 hours, the half-life for rhFVIIa is approximately 2 hours [13, 14]. Neither of these agents have a reliable biomarker that correlates with clinical efficacy, and bleed containment cannot be achieved in all patients [10, 15]. In addition, both agents are associated with the risk of thromboembolic events, especially in patients with AHA who are frequently older and have comorbidities [16–18].

RpFVIII was approved by the Food and Drug Administration in 2014 for rescue treatment of severe bleeding in AHA patients. RpFVIII is a 1448 amino acid heterodimer with a molecular mass of 170 kDa. Its B-domain is partially deleted, allowing functional clotting FVIII while preventing inactivation by circulating human anti-FVIII antibodies. The recommended initial dose of rpFVIII is 200 U/kg. Therapeutic FVIII activity levels are generally achieved with goal FVIII levels >25% and maintained with intermittent rpFVIII administration until bleeding resolves. The advantages of this new therapy included no related serious adverse events, thrombotic events, allergic reactions, or thrombocytopenia in the registration study [10]. In addition, the level of FVIII can be directly monitored to evaluate its efficacy. However, its approval was granted based on a study of only 28 patients with little real-world experience available [19, 20].

From personal experience, it is postulated by hemophilia experts that rpFVIII may be more effective than FVIIa-based bypassing products. If correct, then rpFVIII might be the first agent used, but it is often not. Although rpFVIII shows excellent efficacy, it is rarely considered as the first-line treatment due to cost per dose. The cost of a single dose of

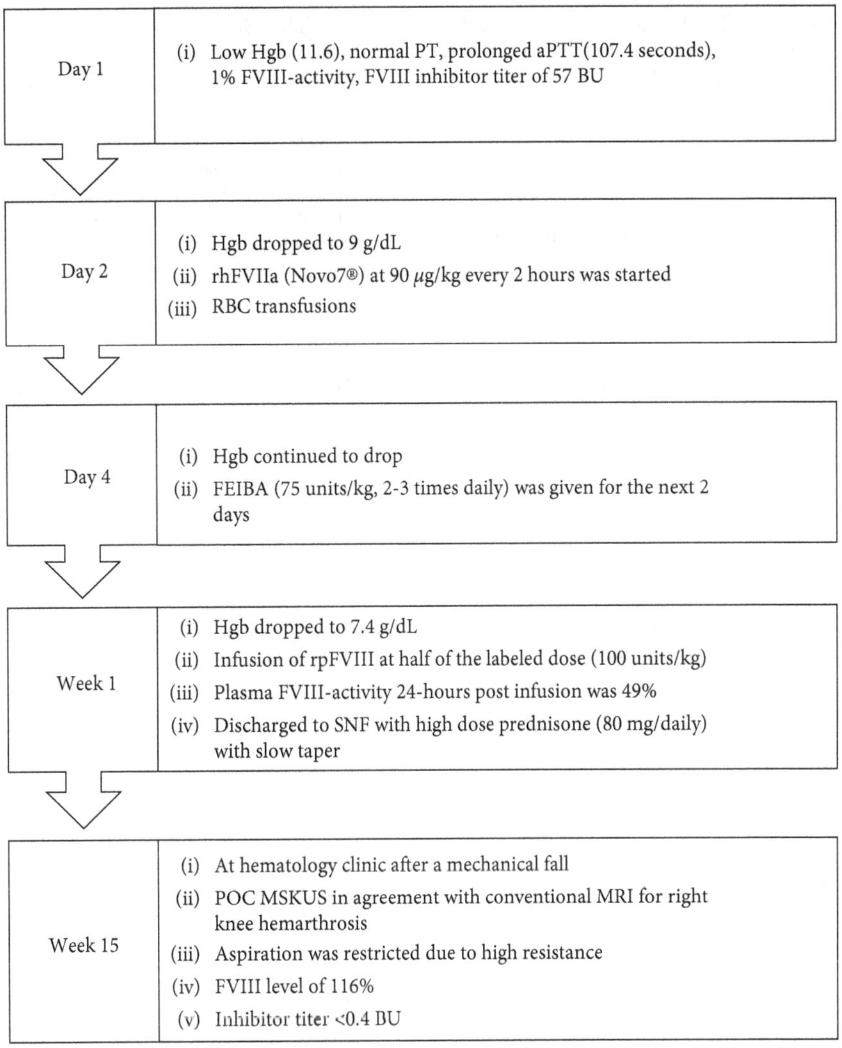

FIGURE 3: Timeline course of hospitalization stay and follow-up at the hematology clinic after a mechanical fall. High-dose corticosteroids were started on day 1 and tapered after one month, once eradication if the anti-FVIII antibody was achieved. Hgb, hemoglobin; PT, prothrombin time; aPTT, activated partial thromboplastin time; FVIII, Factor eight; BU, Bethesda units; rhFVIIa, activated recombinant human factor VII; RBC, red blood cell; FEIBA, Factor Eight Inhibitor Bypassing Activity; SNF, skilled nursing facility; POC MSKUS, point-of-care musculoskeletal ultrasound; MRI, magnetic resonance imaging.

rpFVIII per recommended label (200 U/kg) is approximately 10-fold higher than a single dose of FVIIa-based bypassing products. However, in some reports, restoration of hemostasis was obtained with lower doses of 100 U/kg rpFVIII [21, 22]; which was true in our patient. Based on this experience, we surmise that meaningful pharmacoeconomic savings may have been obtained if rpFVIII had been utilized front-line, not only sparing multiple doses of FVIIa-based bypassing agents but also shortening hospitalization.

Meanwhile, although it is not as common as in congenital hemophilia, hemarthrosis and muscle bleeds can occur in AHA [2]. Therefore, prompt diagnosis is critical to guide efficient medical management. Recently, we reported that the sensitivity of MSKUS to diagnose hemarthrosis surpasses the sensitivity of MRI, which is a widely accepted "reference standard" [23]. Using POC MSKUS allowed accurate and rapid detection of musculoskeletal bleeding in the clinic setting [24–26]. In this case, accurate diagnosis was critical to confidently diagnose the absence of hemarthrosis in the face of normalizing plasma FVIII levels, thereby preventing potentially prothrombotic interventions with hemostatic agents based on clinical perception alone. These observations illustrate the usefulness of POC MSKUS in detecting musculoskeletal bleeding not only in congenital hemophilia but also in AHA.

3. Summary and Conclusions

The patient represents an example of rare AHA, diagnosed in the setting of acute life-threatening bleeding that was successfully managed with a single low dose of rpFVIII after many doses of FVIIa-based bypassing agents. Treatment was followed by successful immune eradication of the inhibitory FVIII antibodies. This case highlights various new aspects in the management of AHA, including the usefulness of POC MSKUS for rapid detection of intra-articular and muscle bleeding. Most importantly though, it highlights the efficacy of rpFVIII, suggesting that front-line use rather than the use as a rescue agent may be a favorable strategy in AHA management.

Consent

Informed written consent was obtained from the patient.

Disclosure

Data collection was approved by the University of California San Diego (UCSD) Human Research Protection Program.

References

[1] D. W. Sborov and G. M. Rodgers, "How I manage patients with acquired haemophilia A," *British Journal of Haematology*, vol. 161, no. 2, pp. 157–165, 2013.

[2] L. N. Boggio and D. Green, "Acquired hemophilia," *Reviews in Clinical and Experimental Hematology*, vol. 5, no. 4, pp. 389–404, 2001.

[3] P. W. Collins, S. Hirsch, T. P. Baglin et al., "Acquired hemophilia A in the United Kingdom: a 2-year national surveillance study by the United Kingdom haemophilia centre doctors' organisation," *Blood*, vol. 109, no. 5, pp. 1870–1877, 2007.

[4] H. Zeitler, G. Goldmann, N. Marquardt, and G. Ulrich-Merzenich, "Long term outcome of patients with acquired haemophilia—a monocentre interim analysis of 82 patients," *Atherosclerosis Supplements*, vol. 14, no. 1, pp. 223–228, 2013.

[5] D. Green and K. Lechner, "A survey of 215 non-hemophilic patients with inhibitors to factor VIII," *Thrombosis and Haemostasis*, vol. 45, no. 3, pp. 200–203, 1981.

[6] P. Knoebl, P. Marco, F. Baudo et al., "Demographic and clinical data in acquired hemophilia A: results from the European Acquired Haemophilia Registry (EACH2)," *Journal of Thrombosis and Haemostasis*, vol. 10, no. 4, pp. 622–631, 2012.

[7] S. Sallah and J. Y. Wan, "Inhibitors against factor VIII in patients with cancer," *Cancer*, vol. 91, no. 6, pp. 1067–1074, 2001.

[8] M. Franchini and P. M. Mannucci, "Acquired haemophilia A: a 2013 update," *Thromb Haemostasis*, vol. 110, no. 12, pp. 1114–1120, 2013.

[9] M. Cugno, R. Gualtierotti, A. Tedeschi, and P. L. Meroni, "Autoantibodies to coagulation factors: from pathophysiology to diagnosis and therapy," *Autoimmunity Reviews*, vol. 13, no. 1, pp. 40–48, 2014.

[10] M. Franchini, G. Castaman, A. Coppola et al., "Acquired inhibitors of clotting factors: AICE recommendations for diagnosis and management," *Blood Transfusion*, vol. 13, no. 3, pp. 498–513, 2015.

[11] P. L. Turecek, K. Varadi, H. Gritsch, and H. P. Schwarz, "FEIBAR: mode of action," *Haemophilia*, vol. 10, no. 2, pp. 3–9, 2004.

[12] M. Hoffman and D. M. Monroe III, "The action of high-dose factor Vlla (FVIIa) in a cell-based model of hemostasis," *Disease-a-Month*, vol. 49, no. 1, pp. 14–21, 2003.

[13] K. Varadi, C. Negrier, E. Berntorp et al., "Monitoring the bioavailability of FEIBA with a thrombin generation assay," *Journal of Thrombosis and Haemostasis*, vol. 1, no. 11, pp. 2374–2380, 2003.

[14] A. Villar, S. Aronis, M. Morfini et al., "Pharmacokinetics of activated recombinant coagulation factor VII (NovoSevenR) in children vs. adults with haemophilia A," *Haemophilia*, vol. 10, no. 4, pp. 352–359, 2004.

[15] J.-Y. Borg, C. Négrier, I. Durieu et al., "FEIBA in the treatment of acquired haemophilia A: results from the prospective multicentre French 'FEIBA dans l'hémophilie A acquise' (FEIBHAC) registry," *Haemophilia*, vol. 21, no. 3, pp. 330–337, 2015.

[16] M. Hoffman and Y. Dargaud, "Mechanisms and monitoring of bypassing agent therapy," *Journal of Thrombosis and Haemostasis*, vol. 10, no. 8, pp. 1478–1485, 2012.

[17] H. J. Ehrlich, M. J. Henzl, and E. D. Gomperts, "Safety of factor VIII inhibitor bypass activity (FEIBAR): 10-year compilation of thrombotic adverse events," *Haemophilia*, vol. 8, no. 2, pp. 83–90, 2002.

[18] K. A. O'Connell, J. J. Wood, R. P. Wise, J. N. Lozier, and M. M. Braun, "Thromboembolic adverse events after use of recombinant human coagulation factor VIIa," *JAMA*, vol. 295, no. 3, pp. 293–298, 2006.

[19] P. W. Collins, E. Chalmers, D. P. Hart et al., "Diagnosis and treatment of factor VIII and IX inhibitors in congenital haemophilia: (4th edition). UK Haemophilia Centre Doctors Organization," *British Journal of Haematology*, vol. 160, no. 2, pp. 153–170, 2013.

[20] A. Huth-Kuhne, F. Baudo, P. Collins et al., "International recommendations on the diagnosis and treatment of patients with acquired hemophilia A," *Haematologica*, vol. 94, no. 4, pp. 566–575, 2009.

[21] M. D. Tarantino, A. Cuker, B. Hardesty, J. C. Roberts, and M. Sholzberg, "Recombinant porcine sequence factor VIII (rpFVIII) for acquired haemophilia A: practical clinical experience of its use in seven patients," *Haemophilia*, vol. 23, no. 1, pp. 25–32, 2017.

[22] M. Stemberger, P. Möhnle, J. Tschöp, L. Ney, M. Spannagl, and M. Reincke, "Successful bleeding control with recombinant porcine factor VIII in reduced loading doses in two patients with acquired haemophilia A and failure of bypassing agent therapy," *Haemophilia*, vol. 22, no. 5, pp. e472–e474, 2016.

[23] S. Nguyen, X. Lu, Y. Ma, J. Du, E. Y. Chang, and A. Von Drygalski, "Musculoskeletal ultrasound for intra-articular bleed detection: a highly sensitive imaging modality compared with conventional magnetic resonance imaging," *Journal of Thrombosis and Haemostasis*, vol. 16, no. 3, pp. 490–499, 2018.

[24] J. A. Aznar, S. Pérez-Alenda, M. Jaca et al., "Home-delivered ultrasound monitoring for home treatment of haemarthrosis in haemophilia A," *Haemophilia*, vol. 21, no. 2, pp. e147–e150, 2015.

[25] F. Baudo, P. Collins, A. Huth-Kuhne et al., "Management of bleeding in acquired hemophilia A: results from the European acquired haemophilia (EACH2) registry," *Blood*, vol. 120, no. 1, pp. 39–46, 2012.

[26] A. Ceponis, I. Wong-Sefidan, C. S. Glass, and A. Von Drygalski, "Rapid musculoskeletal ultrasound for painful episodes in adult haemophilia patients," *Haemophilia*, vol. 19, no. 5, pp. 790–798, 2013.

39

Non-Nodal CD5-Negative Mantle Cell Lymphoma with Secondary TP53 Deletion

Robert K. McCall[1] **Changlee S. Pang,**[2] **and Mark J. Pettenati**[3]

[1]*Molecular Pathology Laboratory Network, Maryville, TN, USA*
[2]*University of Colorado School of Medicine, Aurora, CO, USA*
[3]*Wake Forest Baptist Medical Center, Winston-Salem, NC, USA*

Correspondence should be addressed to Robert K. McCall; mccallrk@gmail.com

Academic Editor: Pier Paolo Piccaluga

Mantle cell lymphoma is a non-Hodgkin lymphoproliferative neoplasm with several clinical and morphologic variants linked, primarily, through genetic derangement of the *cyclin D1* locus. Aberrant phenotypes have been described, though prognostic data in such cohorts are limited due to a paucity of cases. We report a case of mantle cell lymphoma with non-nodal clinical presentation, aberrant loss of CD5 expression, and concomitant cytogenetic deletion of 17p. While non-nodal disease is often associated with an improved prognosis in mantle cell lymphoma, this 67-year-old patient experienced a more challenging clinical course with a poor initial response to chemotherapy. Therefore, this case may represent a type of non-nodal mantle cell lymphoma with a prognosis similar to that of classical cases due to the additional phenotypic and genetic alterations found in this patient.

1. Introduction

Mantle cell lymphoma (MCL) is a distinct lymphoproliferative disorder requiring the combination of morphologic, immunophenotypic, and cytogenetic information for diagnosis. Classically, MCL is characterized by infiltration, either nodular or diffuse, of lymphoid tissue by small-to-medium-sized B-lymphocytes with irregular nuclei and scant cytoplasm [1, 2]. Immunohistochemical staining is typically positive for CD5, CD19, CD20, and CD79b. CD5 is especially helpful in differentiating between MCL and low-grade lymphomas such as follicular lymphoma or marginal zone lymphoma, although, multiple CD5-negative cases of MCL [3–5] have been reported in the past few decades. Derangement of the *cyclin D1 (CCND1)* locus has proved more diagnostically sensitive than CD5 positivity for the identification of MCL [3, 5] with t(11; 14)(q13; q32) representing the most common cytogenetic aberration. A wide range of secondary nonspecific genetic abnormalities has also been shown to occur in cases of MCL [6, 7]. For example, *TP53* mutation/17p deletion portends a poor prognosis according to several studies [8–15]. To complicate matters, morphologic variants of MCL include blastoid, pleomorphic, marginal zone-like, and small cell types. Clinical heterogeneity has also been established with variable involvement of the lymph nodes, spleen, and bone marrow. Non-nodal MCL (a.k.a. mantle cell leukemia) often presents as asymptomatic lymphocytosis with spleen and/or bone marrow infiltration by atypical lymphocytes, similar to chronic lymphocytic leukemia/small lymphocytic lymphoma (CLL/SLL). Interestingly, all previously reported cases of non-nodal MCL [4, 15–17] have been CD5-positive.

We present a rare case of CD5-negative non-nodal MCL with secondary *TP53* mutation/17p deletion and a complicated clinical course.

2. Case Report

A 67-year-old male with a past medical history of basal cell carcinoma, hyperlipidemia, and chronic back pain, secondary to a compression fracture of the T12 vertebra status after vertebroplasty, presented with an infection of the anterior shin in addition to left upper quadrant discomfort. The patient denied fever, chills, night sweats, and weight loss. Physical examination failed to reveal palpable lymphadenopathy or hepatosplenomegaly. Laboratory testing identified a prominent leukocytosis with a white blood cell count (WBC) of 449,000, absolute lymphocyte count (ALC) of 416,400, platelet count of 120,000, and lactate dehydrogenase level of 185 U/L (reference range: 90–250 U/L). The peripheral blood smears showed numerous small-to-medium-sized lymphocytes with relatively round nuclear contours, coarsely clumped chromatin ("soccer ball" pattern), and inconspicuous nucleoli (Figure 1), all of which are features morphologically consistent with chronic lymphocytic leukemia. A PET/CT scan was performed and notable for splenomegaly (18 cm) with mild hypermetabolic activity. Scattered prominent para-aortic lymph nodes were also identified, though not enlarged or hypermetabolic.

The bone marrow biopsy material was B+ fixed, paraffin embedded, and stained with hematoxylin and eosin (H&E). Bone marrow aspirate smears and additional peripheral blood smears were stained with Wright–Giemsa. The majority of lymphocytes on the repeat peripheral blood smears were morphologically consistent with that described for the initial smear (Figure 1); however, a subset of these small lymphocytes contained focal nuclear membrane irregularities with deep nuclear grooves (Figure 1, inset). Additionally, a subpopulation of lymphocytes was noted with cells slightly increased in size and conspicuous-to-distinct, centrally located nucleoli, reminiscent of prolymphocytes. The bone marrow aspirate smears were dominated, 98% of cells, by the heterogenous lymphocyte population reflected in the peripheral blood. Neoplastic transformed cells resembling centroblasts or immunoblasts were not identified in the aspirate material. The bone marrow core biopsy and clot section were hypercellular for patient age (80%), and normal marrow elements were diffusely replaced by monomorphic atypical lymphocytes. The atypical lymphocytes were small in size and contained round to mildly irregular nuclear contours, inconspicuous nucleoli, and scant cytoplasm.

Immunophenotype was established by flow cytometry of the initial peripheral blood sample and immunohistochemistry on the bone marrow core biopsy and clot section (Figure 2). Flow cytometric analysis revealed a monoclonal B-cell population expressing CD19, CD20 (moderate), FMC7, and kappa light chain (moderate to bright). These cells failed to express CD2, CD3, CD4, CD5, CD7, CD8, CD10, CD23, and CD38. Immunohistochemistry highlighted a diffuse population of CD20 (Figure 2(b)), CD79a, and cyclin D1-positive atypical lymphocytes (Figure 2(e)). The same cells were negative for CD5 (Figure 2(c)), CD10, CD23, and SOX11. Ki-67 (MIB1) immunohistochemistry suggested a low proliferation rate (overall 10%, Figure 2(f)).

Cytogenetic studies (band resolution: 460) on the bone marrow aspirate material were interpreted as normal male karyotype with no observable clonal chromosomal abnormalities. Subsequent fluorescent *in situ* hybridization (FISH) revealed cyclin D1/immunoglobulin heavy chain (*CCND1/IgH*) fusion events in 66% of cells analyzed (Figure 3(a)) and

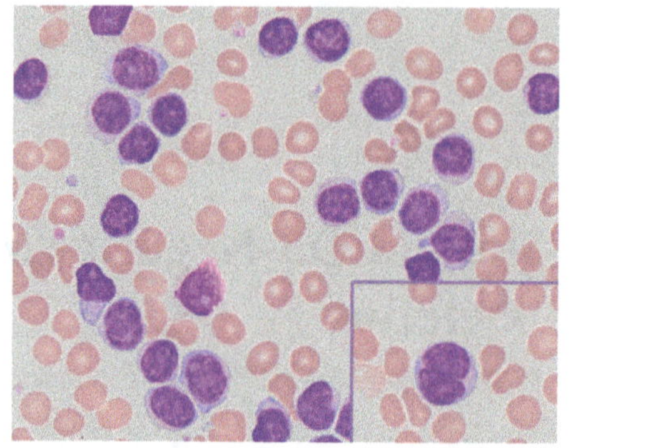

Figure 1: Peripheral blood smear demonstrating CLL/SLL-like morphology of atypical lymphocytes. Inset shows a representative peripheral blood lymphocyte with characteristic nuclear irregularity seen in a subset of B-cells in this case.

deletion of the *TP53* locus (17p-) in 98% of cells analyzed (Figure 3(b)).

Initial treatment of this patient involved leukophoresis (500 cc WBC), allopurinol (300 mg/day), and induction chemotherapy with bendamustine (90 mg/m^2 × 2). Due to an elevated WBC on day 1 of chemotherapy, the patient again underwent leukophoresis. No tumor lysis was observed, and the patient was discharged on day 4 after induction. This initial therapy was followed by four cycles of bendamustine in combination with rituximab (R-bendamustine). Response to treatment was determined via flow cytometric analysis of the patient's peripheral blood, and the therapeutic regimen changed to rituximab, etoposide, prednisone, vincristine, cyclophosphamide, and doxorubicin (R-EPOCH) due to poor results with R-bendamustine. Following four cycles of R-EPOCH, the patient's WBC had improved to 5,100 with an ALC of 800. Bone marrow transplantation was recommended, but declined by the patient. The patient completed two years of rituximab maintenance therapy (375 mg/m^2) and is currently on surveillance with no signs of recurrent disease.

3. Discussion

The neoplastic cells in classical MCL are small-to-medium-sized lymphocytes with irregular nuclear contours and minimal cytoplasm. The immunophenotype is typically CD5, CD19, CD20, CD43, FMC7, surface IgM/IgD, and cyclin D1-positive. CD23 expression may be weakly positive, but is usually negative along with CD10. As the name implies, the putative normal counterpart to the neoplastic lymphocytes is the naïve pregerminal center B-cell occupying the inner mantle zone of the lymphoid follicle [1, 2]. These morphologic and immunophenotypic criteria are not entirely specific to MCL and present a formidable diagnostic dilemma. For this reason, great care should be taken in all possible cases of non-Hodgkin low-grade lymphoma to rule out MCL as the prognosis is significantly different.

Our case highlights the morphologic and immunophenotypic crossover between MCL and other low-grade lymphomas, specifically atypical CLL/SLL. Indeed, the initial

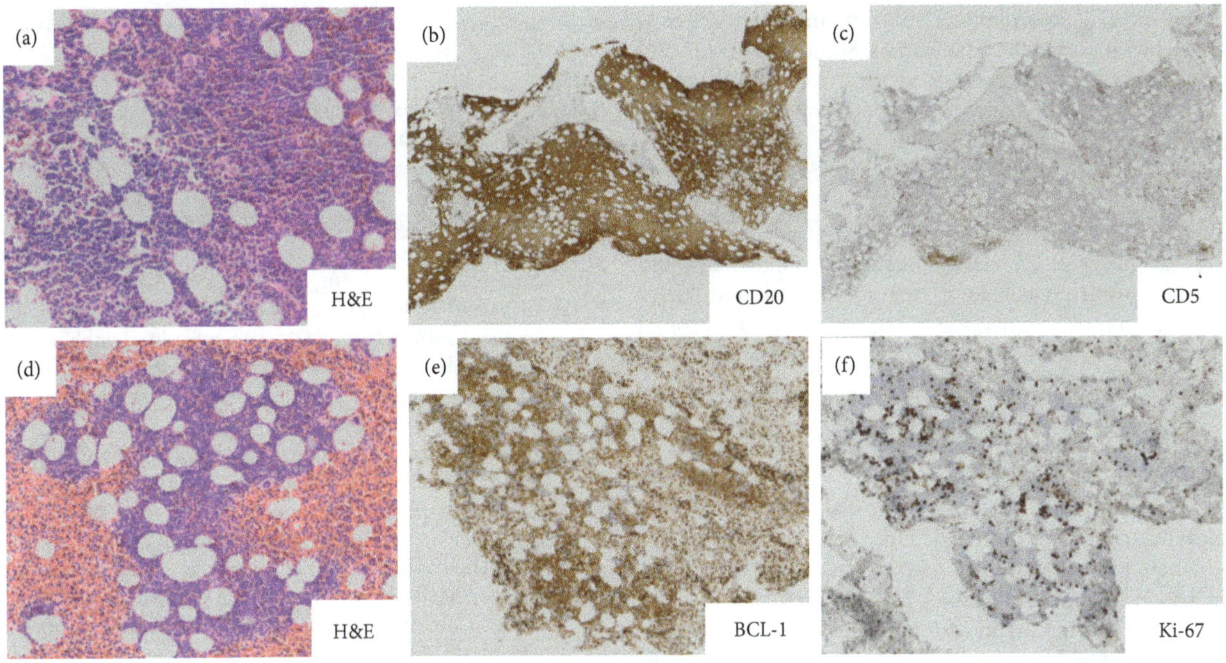

FIGURE 2: (a) H&E, high power view of bone marrow core needle biopsy with diffuse lymphoid infiltrate; (b) CD20 highlights B-cell lineage of lymphoid infiltrate; (c) CD5 expression is not seen in the neoplastic lymphoid population; (d) H&E: intermediate power view of clot section with diffuse lymphoid infiltrate; (e) BCL-1 (cyclin D1) is expressed by the neoplastic lymphoid population; (f) Ki-67 indicates a low proliferation rate in MCL.

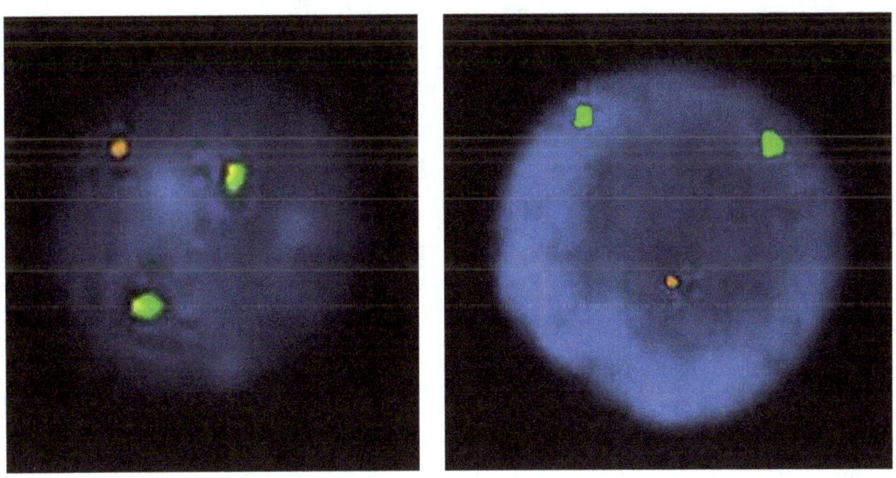

FIGURE 3: Interphase FISH demonstrating (a) t(11; 14) gene rearrangement by dual fusion signal (yellow) and (b) loss of a single copy of 17p (red/orange).

peripheral blood smear in this case was more suggestive of atypical CLL than classical MCL. Given the rarity of non-nodal MCL, the clinical scenario could also easily be interpreted as most compatible with a diagnosis of CLL. While FMC7 positivity and CD23 negativity can occur in atypical CLL [18], the moderate to bright intensity of immunoglobulin light chain expression and moderate CD20 expression in this case served as clues for further investigation and raised the pathologist's suspicion for non-nodal MCL.

The most common cytogenetic aberration in MCL is t(11; 14)(q13; q32) which juxtaposes the *CCNDI* gene on chromosome 11 and the *IgH* gene on chromosome 14. Similar to the morphologic and immunophenotypic findings, this translocation is neither completely sensitive nor specific in the diagnosis of MCL [19]. Around the time that MCL emerged as a distinct entity in 1992 [2], a veritable mountain of references, only some of which are represented here [19–22], described t(11; 14) in cases of atypical CLL as well as those lymphomas previously identified as intermediately differentiated lymphocytic lymphoma (IDLL) or centrocytic lymphoma. Although IDLL and centrocytic lymphoma are now classified as MCL, cases with t(11; 14) and atypical CLL morphology still remain somewhat controversial with regard to classification. Some authors [23, 24] have suggested that all cases of atypical CLL and leukemic MCL with t(11; 14) likely represent a common disorder. Indeed, cases of atypical CLL with t(11; 14) are not recognized as a distinct entity from MCL in the current WHO classification system [1].

Conventional cytogenetic analysis is not always sufficient for the diagnosis of *CCND1/IgH* gene rearrangements, and FISH has proven valuable in the identification of these otherwise cryptic events [23]. Secondary chromosomal abnormalities in MCL [7] may include +12, +9, del (9p21), del (6q21), del (13q14), and del (17p13), to name a few. The prognosis in cases of MCL with del (17p13) has been evaluated by several groups [9, 14, 15, 25], yielding mixed results. Recently, deletion of the *TP53* locus at 17p13 has been described in a case of non-nodal MCL with poor clinical outcome [15]. More evidence exists at the molecular level where mutation of the *TP53* gene has been linked to a poor prognosis in many studies [8–14].

Our case was remarkable for both cryptic rearrangement of *CCNDI/IgH* and cryptic deletion of 17p in a patient with CD5-negative non-nodal MCL. CLL was essentially ruled out by demonstration of the t(11; 14) gene rearrangement. Among the clinical forms of MCL, non-nodal disease has demonstrated a favorable prognosis when compared to the classical type [26]. In keeping with this trend, the present case had a low proliferation rate and lacked the significant atypia often seen in the more aggressive variants of disease. However, the additional chromosomal abnormalities in this case may have contributed to a poor initial therapeutic response. It is also possible, though this remains to be seen, that CD5-negative non-nodal MCL represents a subset of MCL with a more difficult and protracted clinical course. Indeed, the bulk of CD5-negative non-nodal MCL cases described in the literature are those briefly discussed in the backdrop of larger cohorts compiled for molecular profiling studies [26, 27]. As a result, much of the information regarding prognosis and clinical course of disease in these patients is still unknown. A recent study suggests that CD5-negative cases of MCL have significantly better progression-free survival (PFS) when compared to CD5-positive cases [28]. The authors found that this improved prognosis remained despite an enrichment of non-nodal cases in the CD5-negative group. Despite these results, further studies are necessary to fully characterize the interaction between CD5 negativity and non-nodal presentation with special emphasis on the effects of both findings occurring in concert as compared to either finding being present in isolation.

References

[1] S. H. Swerdlow, E. Campo, N. L. Harris et al., *WHO Classification of Tumours of Haematopoietic and Lymphoid Tissues*, IARC, Lyon, France, 2017.

[2] P. M. Banks, J. Chan, M. L. Cleary et al., "Mantle cell lymphoma A proposal for unification of morphologic, immunologic, and molecular data," *The American Journal of Surgical Pathology*, vol. 16, no. 7, pp. 637–640, 1992.

[3] N. D. Bell, J. A. C. King, C. Kusyk, B. P. Nelson, and K. M. Sendelbach, "CD5 negative diffuse mantle cell lymphoma with splenomegaly and bone marrow involvement," *Southern Medical Journal*, vol. 91, no. 6, pp. 584–587, 1998.

[4] J. Orchard, R. Garand, Z. Davis et al., "A subset of t(11;14) lymphoma with mantle cell features displays mutated IgVH genes and includes patients with good prognosis, non-nodal disease," *Blood*, vol. 101, no. 12, pp. 4975–4981, 2003.

[5] Y. Yatabe, S. Nakamura, M. Seto et al., "Clinicopathologic study of PRAD1/cyclin D1 overexpressing lymphoma with special reference to mantle cell lymphoma," *The American Journal of Surgical Pathology*, vol. 20, no. 9, pp. 1110–1122, 1996.

[6] S. Beà, M. Ribas, J. M. Hernández et al., "Increased number of chromosomal imbalances and high-level DNA amplifications in mantle cell lymphoma are associated with blastoid variants," *Blood*, vol. 93, no. 93, pp. 4365–4374, 1999.

[7] R. Bigoni, A. Cuneo, R. Milani et al., "Secondary chromosome changes in mantle cell lymphoma: cytogenetic and fluorescence in situ hybridization studies," *Leukemia & Lymphoma*, vol. 40, no. 5-6, pp. 581–590, 2001.

[8] T. Greiner, M. Moynihan, W. Chan et al., "p53 mutations in mantle cell lymphoma are associated with variant cytology and predict a poor prognosis," *Blood*, vol. 87, no. 10, pp. 4302–4310, 1996.

[9] A. M. Halldórsdóttir, A. Lundin, F. Murray et al., "Impact of TP53 mutation and 17p deletion in mantle cell lymphoma," *Leukemia*, vol. 25, no. 12, pp. 1904–1908, 2011.

[10] L. Hernandez, T. Fest, M. Cazorla et al., "p53 gene mutations and protein overexpression are associated with aggressive variants of mantle cell lymphomas," *Blood*, vol. 87, no. 8, pp. 3351–3359, 1996.

[11] D. Louie, K. Offit, R. Jaslow et al., "p53 overexpression as a marker of poor prognosis in mantle cell lymphomas with t(11; 14)(q13;q32)," *Blood*, vol. 86, no. 8, pp. 2892–2899, 1995.

[12] L. Nordström, S. Sernbo, P. Eden et al., "SOX11 and TP53 add prognostic information to MIPI in a homogenously treated cohort of mantle cell lymphoma-a Nordic Lymphoma group study," *British Journal of Haematology*, vol. 166, no. 1, pp. 98–108, 2014.

[13] J. Slotta-Huspenina, I. Koch, L. de Leval et al., "The impact of cyclin D1 mRNA isoforms, morphology and p53 in mantle cell lymphoma: p53 alterations and blastoid morphology are strong predictors of a high proliferation index," *Haematologica*, vol. 97, no. 9, pp. 1422–1430, 2012.

[14] L. Stefancikova, M. Moulis, P. Fabian et al., "Loss of the p53 tumor suppressor activity is associated with negative prognosis of mantle cell lymphoma," *International Journal of Oncology*, vol. 36, no. 36, pp. 699–706, 2010.

[15] J. Chapman-Fredricks, J. Sandoval-Sus, F. Vega, and I. S. Lossos, "Progressive leukemic non-nodal mantle cell lymphoma associated with deletions of TP53, ATM, and/or 13q14," *Annals of Diagnostic Pathology*, vol. 18, no. 4, pp. 214–219, 2014.

[16] S. L. Ondrejka, R. Lai, S. D. Smith, and E. D. Hsi, "Indolent mantle cell leukemia: a clinicopathological variant characterized by isolated lymphocytosis, interstitial bone marrow involvement, kappa light chain restriction, and good prognosis," *Haematologica*, vol. 96, no. 8, pp. 1121–1127, 2011.

[17] C. Royo, A. Navarro, G. Clot et al., "Non-nodal type of mantle

cell lymphoma is a specific biological and clinical subgroup of the disease," *Leukemia*, vol. 26, no. 8, pp. 1895–1898, 2012.
[18] A. K. Ho, S. Hill, S. N. Preobrazhensky, M. E. Miller, Z. Chen, and D. W. Bahler, "Small B-cell neoplasms with typical mantle cell lymphoma immunophenotypes often include chronic lymphocytic leukemias," *American Journal of Clinical Pathology*, vol. 131, no. 1, pp. 27–32, 2009.
[19] E. Vandenberghe, C. D. W. Peeters, I. Wlodarska et al., "Chromosome 11q rearrangements in B non Hodgkin's lymphoma," *British Journal of Haematology*, vol. 81, no. 2, pp. 212–217, 1992.
[20] A. Cuneo, M. Balboni, N. Piva et al., "Atypical chronic lymphocytic leukaemia with t(11;14)(q13;q32): karyotype evolution and prolymphocytic transformation," *British Journal of Haematology*, vol. 90, no. 2, pp. 409–416, 1995.
[21] D. Leroux, F. L. Marc'hadour, R. Gressin et al., "Non-Hodgkin's lymphomas with t(11;14)(q13;q32): a subset of mantle zone/intermediate lymphocytic lymphoma?" *British Journal of Haematology*, vol. 77, no. 3, pp. 346–353, 1991.
[22] M. Raffeld and E. Jaffe, "bcl-1, t(11;14), and mantle cell-derived lymphomas," *Blood*, vol. 78, no. 2, pp. 259–263, 1991.
[23] H. Avet-Loiseau, R. Garand, F. Gaillard et al., "Detection of t(11;14) using interphase molecular cytogenetics in mantle cell lymphoma and atypical chronic lymphocytic leukemia," *Genes, Chromosomes and Cancer*, vol. 23, no. 2, pp. 175–182, 1998.
[24] J. R. Neilson, C. D. Fegan, and D. W. Milligan, "Mantle cell leukaemia?" *British Journal of Haematology*, vol. 93, no. 2, pp. 494-495, 1996.
[25] M. Solenthaler, E. Matutes, V. Brito-Babapulle, R. Morilla, and D. Catovsky, "p53 and mdm2 in mantle cell lymphoma in leukemic phase," *Haematologica*, vol. 87, no. 87, pp. 1141–1150, 2002.
[26] A. Navarro, G. Clot, C. Royo et al., "Molecular subsets of mantle cell lymphoma defined by the IGHV mutational status and SOX11 expression have distinct biologic and clinical features," *Cancer Research*, vol. 72, no. 20, pp. 5307–5316, 2012.
[27] B. Espinet, A. Ferrer, B. Bellosillo et al., "Distinction between asymptomatic monoclonal B-cell lymphocytosis with cyclin D1 overexpression and mantle cell lymphoma: from molecular profiling to flow cytometry," *Clinical Cancer Research*, vol. 20, no. 4, pp. 1007–1019, 2014.
[28] Y. Miao, P. Lin, A. Saksena et al., "CD5-negative mantle cell lymphoma," *The American Journal of Surgical Pathology*, vol. 43, no. 8, pp. 1052–1060, 2019.

Haemophagocytic Lymphohistiocytosis in an Elderly Patient after Recent Cardiac Surgery

Eoghan Burke,[1] **Patricia Harkins,**[2] **and Jennifer Kieran**[2]

[1]*Royal College of Surgeons in Ireland, Dublin, Ireland*
[2]*St James's Hospital, Department of Medicine, Dublin, Ireland*

Correspondence should be addressed to Eoghan Burke; eoghanburke@rcsi.ie

Academic Editor: Gergely Feher

Introduction. The underlying pathophysiology of haemophagocytic lymphohistiocytosis (HLH) is characterised by excessive inflammation and tissue destruction secondary to abnormal immune activation. The term primary HLH refers to a genetic abnormality that predisposes to the condition whereas secondary refers to HLH being triggered by an underlying condition such as infection (often Epstein Barr Virus), autoimmune, or neoplastic disease. Its variable clinical presentation poses an obstacle to prompt diagnosis in the elderly patient. *Case.* A 70-year-old Caucasian man was admitted to hospital from a convalescence center with symptoms of fatigue, fever, decreased oral intake, and increasing shortness of breath on exertion. The patient was three weeks after coronary artery bypass grafting. Over the next two weeks, the patient continued to deteriorate both clinically and biochemically. The patient met criteria for haemophagocytic lymphohistiocytosis, likely driven by EBV infection. Bone marrow biopsy supported the diagnosis with evidence of active phagocytosis. The patient was commenced on high-dose dexamethasone and reviewed by haematology with further molecular testing confirming the diagnosis. *Discussion.* LH is becoming more common in older patients. We propose that new guidelines be developed to aid its prompt diagnosis in this age group.

1. Introduction

The underlying pathophysiology of haemophagocytic lymphohistiocytosis (HLH) is characterised by excessive inflammation and tissue destruction secondary to abnormal immune activation. This hyperimmune state is thought to be secondary to a failure of normal down-regulation of macrophage activity [1]. These macrophages release large volumes of proinflammatory cytokines which are thought to be responsible for the development of multiorgan failure in these patients [2]. Broadly speaking, it can be classified into primary and secondary. The term primary HLH refers to a genetic abnormality that predisposes to the condition whereas secondary refers to HLH being triggered by an underlying condition such as infection (often Epstein Barr Virus), autoimmune, or neoplastic disease [3]. Its variable clinical presentation poses an obstacle to prompt diagnosis in the elderly patient.

2. Case Report

A 70-year-old Caucasian man was admitted to hospital from a convalescence center with symptoms of fatigue, fever, decreased oral intake, and increasing shortness of breath on exertion. The patient was three weeks after coronary artery bypass grafting. His postoperative course included multiple blood transfusions secondary to intraoperative losses. The patient denied any chest pain, cough, nausea, diarrhoea, night sweats, or urinary symptoms concerning for post-op infection. His past medical history was remarkable for hepatic sarcoidosis, atrial fibrillation, hypertension, hyperlipidemia, and stage 3 chronic kidney disease.

On admission, clinical examination revealed a temperature of 39.6 degrees Celsius, heart rate was 80 beats per minute, blood pressure was 122/50 mmHg, respiratory rate was 16 breaths per minute, and he was saturating at 96% on room air. Heart sounds 1 and 2 were present and normal with no added sounds, and minimal crepitations in the left

Table 1: Laboratory data.

Indices	Day 1: emergency department	Day 5	Day 13	Others	Reference range adults
Haemoglobin (g/dl)	9.0		8.7		13.5 – 18.0
Mean corpuscular volume	82.8		79.4		83.0 – 99.0
Reticulocyte count (%)		1.1%			0.4 – 1.9
Nucleated red blood cell ($* 10^9$/L)		0.0	0.1		
White cell count ($* 10^9$/L)	4.1		2.7		4.0 – 11.0
Neutrophils ($* 10^9$/L)	3.1		1.5		2.0 – 7.5
Platelet count ($* 10^9$/L)	227		45		140 – 450
Sodium (mmol/L)	126		134		136 – 145
Potassium (mmol/L)	4.4		4.0		3.5 – 5.3
Urea (mmol/L)	9.4		8.8		2.5 – 7.8
Creatinine (μmol/L)	180		132		59 – 104
Total protein (g/L)	67		57		66 – 87
Serum albumin (g/L)	30		19		33 – 50
Alkaline phosphatase (IU/L)	353		1462		40 – 129
Gamma-glutamyl transferase (IU/L)	403		635		10 – 71
Bilirubin (μmol/L)	14		271		0 – 21
Alanine aminotransferase (IU/L)	148		336		0 – 41
Aspartate aminotransferase (IU/L)	134		1013		0 – 40
Lactic dehydrogenase (IU/L)	262				135 – 250
Corrected calcium (mmol/L)	2.10		2.13		2.15 – 2.50
Magnesium (mmol/L)	0.86		0.90		0.70 – 1.00
Phosphate (mmol/L)	1.12		1.00		0.81 – 1.45
C-reactive protein (mg/L)	80.46		16.49		0.00 – 5.00
Serum angiotension-converting enzyme (ACE) (IU/L)				106	<8 – 65
IgG (g/L)				16.35	6.26 – 14.96
IgM (g/L)				3.96	0.47 – 1.82
IgA (g/L)				14.52	0.62 – 2.90
Alpha 1 antitrypsin (g/L)				2.15	1.10 – 2.20
Ceruloplasmin (g/L)				0.35	0.22 – 0.66
Iron (μmol/L)				18	14 – 31
Unsaturated iron binding capacity (μmol/L)				10	20 – 66
Transferrin saturations (%)				64	30 – 40
Ferritin (ug/L)				35 164.8	23.0 – 393.0
Fibrinogen (g/L)				1.2	1.9 – 3.5
Haptoglobins (g/L)				<0.24	0.45 – 2.05
Triglycerides (mmol/L)				3.22	0.50 – 1.70
EBV DNA PCR				71 387	
EBV nuclear antigen IgG			Negative	Positive	
Viral capsid antigen IgM			Positive	Negative	
Viral capsid antigen IgG			Positive	Positive	

lung base were noted on auscultation. The abdomen was soft and nontender with no organomegaly. The patient was alert and oriented.

Laboratory results are displayed in Table 1. Chest X-ray revealed evidence of his recent sternotomy. A septic screen was performed with blood cultures and midstream urine sample taken for culture and sensitivity. The patient was commenced on IV piperacillin and tazobactam and admitted to the ward with the initial diagnosis of pneumonia.

Over the next two weeks, the patient continued to deteriorate both clinically and biochemically. CT thorax indicated small bilateral pleural effusions and a small pericardial effusion. Transthoracic and transoesophageal echo did not indicate any evidence of haemodynamic compromise caused by the pericardial effusion. He was reviewed by the cardiothoracic team who advised conservative management.

MSU and blood cultures did not grow any pathogen. The patient developed pancytopenia and worsening LFTs (Table 1).

The patient became frankly jaundiced with scleral icterus. His levels of consciousness began to fluctuate, and he was spiking temperatures, desaturating, and becoming increasingly hypotensive. Ultrasound of his liver did not indicate any intra- or extrabiliary tract obstruction, focal liver lesion, or sonographic evidence of acute cholecystitis. CT abdomen

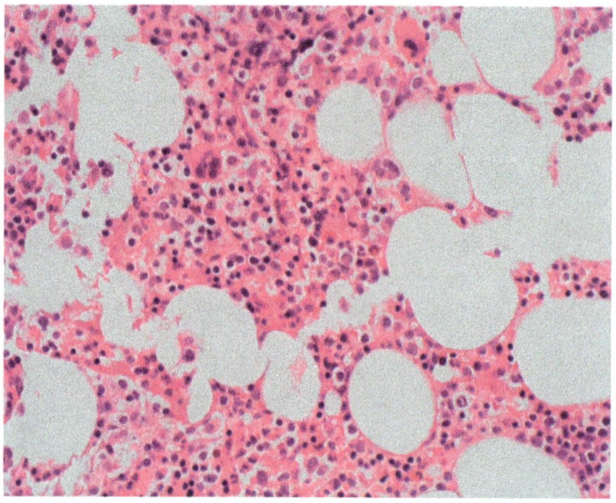

Figure 1: Haemotoxylin and eosin stained bone marrow trephine (x60) showing erythroid hyperplasia, normal megakaryocytes, and a subtle infiltrate of small lymphocytes and histiocytes.

Table 2: Diagnostic criteria for haemophagocytic lymphohistiocytosis.

Diagnostic criterion	Case	Criteria score
1. A molecular diagnosis consistent with HLH	Positive	1
2. Fulfillment of five out of the eight criteria below:		
Fever (>100.4°F, >38°C)	Present	1
Splenomegaly	Absent	0
Cytopenias affecting at least two of three lineages in the peripheral blood		1
Haemoglobin <9 g/100 ml	Present	
Platelets $<100 \times 10^9$/L	Present	
Neutrophils $<1 \times 10^9$/L	Absent	
Hypertriglyceridemia and/or hypofibrinogenemia		1
Fasting triglyceride levels >3 mmol/liter	Present	
Fibrinogen level <1.5 g/liter	Present	
Ferritin ≥500 ng/ml	Present	1
Haemophagocytosis in bone marrow, central nervous system, spleen, or lymph nodes	Present	1
Low or absent natural killer cell activity	Not tested	
Soluble CD25 (soluble IL-2 receptor) > 2400 U/ml	Not tested	
Total		**6/8**

HLH-HaemophagocyticLymphohistiocytosis Criteria 1 and/or 2 must be present to make a diagnosis of HLH.

indicated widespread lymphadenopathy which was likely reactive.

Serology for hepatitis B and C and HIV was negative. Serum plasma electrophoresis did not detect monoclonal bands. Alpha 1 antitrypsin and ceruloplasmin were within normal limits. Antinuclear, neutrophil-cytoplasmic, smooth muscle, mitochondrial, and liver-kidney antibodies were all negative. Iron overload studies indicated the following: iron within normal limits, a low total iron binding capacity, raised transferrin saturation, and ferritin of greater than 30,000 ug/L. Serum triglycerides were elevated at 3.22 mmol/L, and fibrinogen was noted to be low at 1.2 g/L. EBV DNA was detected using PCR and EBV. Nuclear antigen IgG became positive. There was no evidence of serological analysis being performed in this patient prior to surgery, nor was it evident in his medical chart from previous admissions.

The patient met criteria for haemophagocytic lymphohistiocytosis, likely driven by EBV infection. Bone marrow biopsy supported the diagnosis with evidence of active phagocytosis (Figure 1). The patient was commenced on high-dose dexamethasone and reviewed by haematology with further molecular testing confirming the diagnosis.

The patient made a full recovery and was subsequently discharged back to a convalescence center for further rehabilitation.

3. Discussion

HLH is a rare and devastating disorder of uncontrolled immune activation which is well described in paediatric populations but far less is known about an appropriate approach to diagnosis and treatment in older populations [4].

The incidence of HLH in the paediatric population is estimated at 1 to 225 per 300,000 live births [5]. The incidence in the adult population is unknown.

Adult patients with HLH will present with a myriad of clinical and laboratory abnormalities which often delays diagnosis. In an attempt to streamline early diagnosis, the Histiocyte Society has developed criteria for the diagnosis of HLH (see Table 2) [6].

It is important to understand, however, that these diagnostic criteria were developed to aid the diagnosis of HLH in the paediatric population and may be less effective in adults [7]. A serum ferritin level greater than 10,000 ng/ml, for example, is approximately 95% sensitive and specific for HLH in the paediatric population [8]; however, in the adult population, the differential for a similar serum ferritin level is much broader and includes more common pathologies such as renal and liver failure, sepsis, and haemochromatosis [9].

The mechanism of EBV infection in our patient is not clear. One potential mechanism is via blood transfusions the patient received intra- and postoperatively following his cardiac surgery. This has been well documented predominantly in the paediatric population [10].

The current treatment paradigms for HLH in the adult population were developed from studies in the paediatric population, namely, the HLH-94 study which was a large prospective paediatric study conducted in patients less than 16 years old [11].

In light of the increasing cases of HLH reported in adult populations, we propose that new guidelines be developed to aid its prompt diagnosis in this age group. Similarly, adult specific treatment guidelines must be developed in order to combat this frequently fatal pathology.

Consent

Informed written consent was obtained for this article. Guarantor: Dr. Eoghan Burke, eoghanburke@rcsi.ie.

References

[1] A. Filipovich, K. McClain, and A. Grom, "Histiocytic disorders: recent insights into pathophysiology and practical guidelines," *Biology of Blood and Marrow Transplantation*, vol. 16, no. 1, pp. S82–S89, 2010.

[2] K. Risma and M. B. Jordan, "Hemophagocytic lymphohistiocytosis," *Current Opinion in Pediatrics*, vol. 24, no. 1, pp. 9–15, 2012.

[3] E. Brisse, C. H. Wouters, and P. Matthys, "Advances in the pathogenesis of primary and secondary haemophagocytic lymphohistiocytosis: differences and similarities," *British Journal of Haematology*, vol. 174, no. 2, pp. 203–217, 2016.

[4] A. M. Schram and N. Berliner, "How I treat hemophagocytic lymphohistiocytosis in the adult patient," *Blood*, vol. 125, no. 19, 2015.

[5] J. I. Henter, G. Elinder, O. Söder, and A. Ost, "Incidence in Sweden and clinical features of familial hemophagocytic lymphohistiocytosis," *Acta Paediatrica Scandinavica*, vol. 80, no. 4, pp. 428–435, 1991.

[6] M. R. George, "Hemophagocytic lymphohistiocytosis: review of etiologies and management," *Journal of Blood Medicine*, vol. 5, pp. 69–86, 2014.

[7] N. Berliner, C. Kurra, and D. Chou, "Case 1-2016," *New England Journal of Medicine*, vol. 374, no. 2, pp. 165–173, 2016.

[8] C. E. Allen, X. Yu, C. A. Kozinetz, and K. L. McClain, "Highly elevated ferritin levels and the diagnosis of hemophagocytic lymphohistiocytosis," *Pediatric Blood & Cancer*, vol. 50, no. 6, pp. 1227–1235, 2008.

[9] A. M. Schram, F. Campigotto, A. Mullally et al., "Marked hyperferritinemia does not predict for HLH in the adult population," *Blood*, vol. 125, no. 10, pp. 1548–1552, 2015.

[10] P. R. EnokBonong, C. Buteau, G. Delage et al., "Transfusion-related epstein-barr virus (ebv) infection: a multicenter prospective cohort study among pediatric recipients of hematopoietic stem cell transplants (treasure study)," *Transfusion*, 2020.

[11] J.-I. Henter, A. Samuelsson-Horne, M. Arico et al., "Treatment of hemophagocytic lymphohistiocytosis with HLH-94 immunochemotherapy and bone marrow transplantation," *Blood*, vol. 100, no. 7, pp. 2367–2373, 2002.

Molecular Monitoring in Adult Philadelphia Chromosome-Positive Acute Lymphoblastic Leukemia with the Variant e13a3 *BCR-ABL1* Fusion

Mireille Crampe,[1] Laura Kearney,[1] David O'Brien,[2] C. Larry Bacon,[2] Derville O'Shea,[3] and Stephen E. Langabeer[1]

[1]*Cancer Molecular Diagnostics, St. James's Hospital, Dublin 8, Ireland*
[2]*Department of Haematology, St. James's Hospital, Dublin 8, Ireland*
[3]*Department of Haematology, Cork University Hospital, Cork, Ireland*

Correspondence should be addressed to Stephen E. Langabeer; slangabeer@stjames.ie

Academic Editor: Akimichi Ohsaka

Monitoring *BCR-ABL1* transcript levels in patients with Philadelphia chromosome-positive acute lymphoblastic leukemia (Ph+ ALL) is a widely adopted method to assess response to therapy. However, a small minority of Ph+ ALL patients express variant *BCR-ABL1* transcript types, usually due to splicing of alternative *BCR* or *ABL1* exons. Whether patients expressing these rare, variant *BCR-ABL1* transcripts have a distinct phenotype or response to therapy is not known due to the limited number of reported cases. Here, we report the presenting features of Ph+ ALL in a young adult with a variant e13a3 *BCR-ABL1* fusion. Molecular monitoring reflected the disease response from diagnosis through allogeneic stem cell transplantation which resulted in undetectable e13a3 *BCR-ABL1* transcripts. This case highlights the value of molecular monitoring in Ph+ ALL patients with variant *BCR-ABL1* transcripts and the requirement for standardization of such assays.

1. Introduction

Philadelphia chromosome-positive acute lymphoblastic leukemia (Ph+ ALL) in adults is an aggressive disease that responds poorly to conventional chemotherapy. Despite improvements in survival with the addition of tyrosine kinase inhibitors (TKI) to chemotherapy, hematopoietic allogeneic stem cell transplantation (ASCT) remains the only curative option in those eligible patients [1]. Molecular monitoring of *BCR-ABL1* transcripts is a valuable tool in assessing individual patient response to chemotherapy and ASCT [2–4]. The most common *BCR-ABL1* transcripts in Ph+ ALL are the e1a2, e13a2, and e14a2 fusions [5]; however, approximately 5% of adult patients express variant *BCR-ABL1* transcripts [6]. Of these variants, the e13a3 (b2a3) *BCR-ABL1* type is extremely rare with scant information regarding optimal therapeutic approach [7, 8]. Characterisation of these rare *BCR-ABL1* variants also affords the selection of appropriate primer/probe combinations for reverse-transcriptase quantitative PCR (RT-qPCR) assessment of residual disease. The presentation and clinical course of a patient with e13a3 *BCR-ABL1* Ph+ ALL is reported.

2. Case Report

A 23-year-old male presented with chest pain and dyspnoea, a hemoglobin count of 7.4 g/dL, platelet count of $<10\times10^9$/L, and white cell count of 11.6×10^9/L. Bone marrow (BM) biopsy and aspirate demonstrated a 95% infiltration of lymphoblasts (Figure 1). Immunophenotyping of the BM aspirate showed lymphoblasts were CD10-, CD19-, CD20-, CD34-, TdT-, and HLA-DR-positive. Cytogenetic analysis revealed a complex clone in 10 cells analysed by G-banding

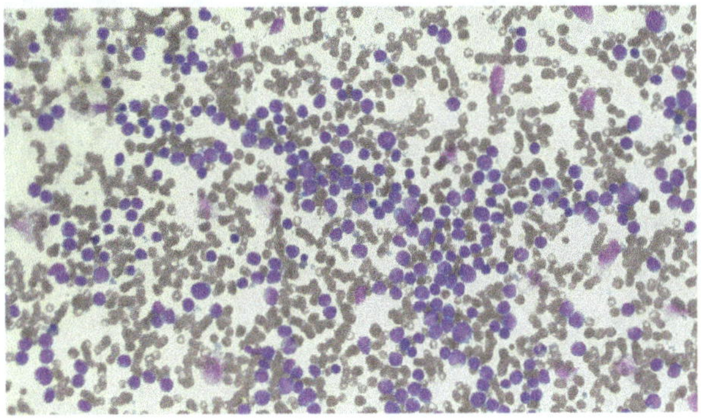

FIGURE 1: Bone marrow morphology at diagnosis showing infiltration by lymphoblasts.

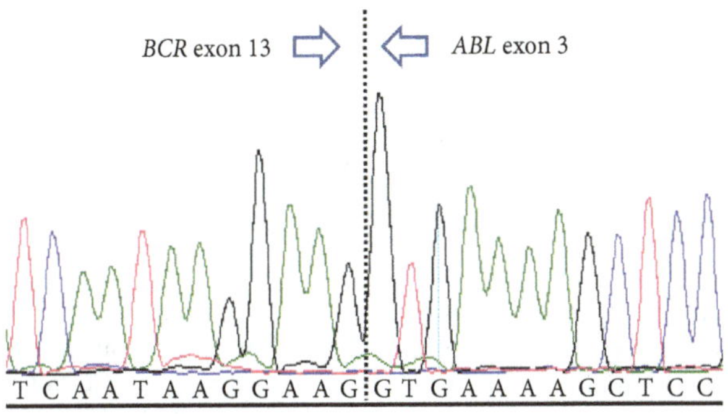

FIGURE 2: Sanger sequencing demonstrating presence of the e13a3 *BCR-ABL1* fusion gene.

containing various structural and numerical abnormalities including a derivative chromosome 22 from a translocation between the long arms of chromosomes 9 and 22. The composite karyotype was 44–48, *XY*, +*X*, *t*(1; 14)(p32; q32), −3, −6, add(6)(p21), add(7)(p21), add(8)(p21), −10, add(12)(p13), +16, add(19)(p13), der(22)*t*(9; 22)(q34; q11.2), +1~2mar, inc [cp10]. Interphase FISH analysis showed the presence of *BCR-ABL1* rearrangement in 64/100 cells analysed. Standardised RT-PCR and Sanger sequencing demonstrated e13a3 *BCR-ABL1* transcripts [9] (Figure 2). E13a3 *BCR-ABL1* transcripts lack *ABL1* exon a2, thus prohibiting the use of a standardised primer/probe combination for e13a2/e14a2 *BCR-ABL1* qPCR [10]. A modified *BCR-ABL1* qPCR assay was therefore adopted utilising *BCR* forward primer ENF501F2 [9] with *ABL1* reverse primer ENR1063 and *ABL1* probe ENP1043, the latter both complementary to *ABL1* exon a3 sequence [11]. The *BCR-ABL1* standard curve was constructed using serial dilutions of an e14a3 *BCR-ABL1* plasmid over a five log range (100% to 0.001% *BCR-ABL1* transcripts) with *ABL1* as the reference gene as previously described [12]. Best practice guidelines for *BCR-ABL1* qPCR and data interpretation were followed [13]. Presentation e13a3 *BCR-ABL1* transcripts were of a high level (*BCR-ABL1*/*ABL1* 75.7%) consistent with a diagnosis of pre-pre-B cell Ph+ ALL.

The patient commenced induction treatment with rituximab, dexamethasone, vincristine, and daunorubicin, with imatinib 400 mg oral daily started on day 15. After phase-one induction, the bone marrow aspirate demonstrated a complete morphological response with residual disease detected by immunophenotyping and RT-qPCR (*BCR-ABL1*/*ABL1* 8.11%). After phase-two induction, the bone marrow *BCR-ABL1*/*ABL1* level had fallen to 0.053%. Following high-dose methotrexate, the pre-ASCT *BCR-ABL1* level was 0.034%. The patient proceeded to ASCT from an unrelated donor after cyclophosphamide and total body irradiation conditioning and recommenced continued imatinib maintenance. *BCR-ABL1* transcripts were not detected in the peripheral blood at one, two, and three and a half months post-ASCT (Figure 3). Continued close molecular monitoring is planned.

3. Discussion

E13a3 *BCR-ABL1* transcripts lack *ABL1* exon a2 that encodes part of SH3 domain thought to contribute to leukemogenesis by inhibition of the kinase domain and by STAT5 activation [6]. In chronic myeloid leukemia patients, this transcript results in an indolent and TKI-responsive form of disease [14–16]; however, its prognostic significance in adult Ph+ ALL patients remains unknown due to the limited number of annotated cases. While the possibility exists of lymphoid blast crisis in chronic myeloid leukemia (CML), this transformation in e13a3 *BCR-ABL1* CML is rare [17]. In the absence of basophilia, thrombocytosis, and splenomegaly, this case likely represents *de novo* Ph+ ALL. Additional chromosomal abnormalities and complex karyotypes are frequently observed in Ph+ ALL, as witnessed in this case. There is some suggestion that in Ph+ ALL, additional cytogenetic abnormalities are associated with a shorter overall survival and might therefore be used for

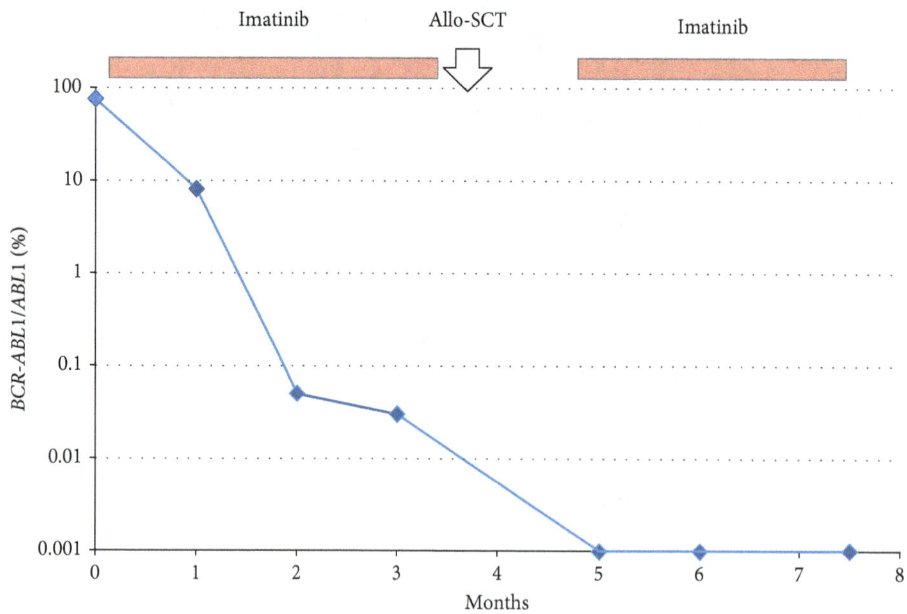

FIGURE 3: Molecular monitoring of e13a3 *BCR-ABL1* transcripts throughout clinical course. AlloSCT: allogeneic stem cell transplantation.

stratification purposes [18]. In the post-ASCT setting, monitoring *BCR-ABL1* transcript levels is an essential component of Ph+ ALL patient management [19] with effective standardisation of RT-qPCR assays for this and other variant *BCR-ABL1* fusion transcripts required [20].

Reporting of further cases would enable identification of any phenotypic characteristics of e13a3 *BCR-ABL1* Ph+ ALL and help establishing optimal treatment strategies for patients with this rare genotype.

References

[1] M. Yilmaz, H. Kantarjian, F. Ravandi-Kashani, N. J. Short, and E. Jabbour, "Philadelphia chromosome-positive acute lymphoblastic leukemia in adults: current treatments and future perspectives," *Clinical Advances in Hematology & Oncology*, vol. 16, no. 3, pp. 216–223, 2018.

[2] M. Yanada, I. Sugiura, J. Takeuchi et al., "Prospective monitoring of BCR-ABL1 transcript levels in patients with Philadelphia chromosome-positive acute lymphoblastic leukaemia undergoing imatinib-combined chemotherapy," *British Journal of Haematology*, vol. 143, no. 4, pp. 503–510, 2008.

[3] L. Zhang, R. T. Ramjit, C. E. Hill, M. Arellano, H. J. Khoury, and K. P. Mann, "Clinical significance of quantitative monitoring and mutational analysis of BCR-ABL1 transcript in Philadelphia chromosome positive B lymphoblastic leukemia," *Leukemia & Lymphoma*, vol. 57, no. 2, pp. 364-369, 2016.

[4] G. Cazzaniga, P. De Lorenzo, J. Alten et al., "Predictive value of minimal residual disease in Philadelphia-chromosome-positive acute lymphoblastic leukemia treated with imatinib in the European intergroup study of post-induction treatment of Philadelphia-chromosome-positive acute lymphoblastic leukemia, based on immunoglobulin/T-cell receptor and BCR/ABL1 methodologies," *Haematologica*, vol. 103, no. 1, pp. 107–115, 2018.

[5] S. E. Langabeer, "Variant BCR-ABL1 fusion genes in adult Philadelphia chromosome-positive B-cell acute lymphoblastic leukemia," *EXCLI Journal*, vol. 16, pp. 1144–1147, 2017.

[6] A. Tuszynski, S. Dhut, B. D. Young et al., "Detection and significance of bcr-abl mRNA transcripts and fusion proteins in Philadelphia-positive adult acute lymphoblastic leukemia," *Leukemia*, vol. 7, no. 10, pp. 1504–1508, 1993.

[7] T. Burmeister, S. Schwartz, A. Taubald et al., "Atypical BCR-ABL mRNA transcripts in adult acute lymphoblastic leukemia," *Haematologica*, vol. 92, no. 12, pp. 1699–1702, 2007.

[8] X. Zhang and J. Pan, "An e13a3 BCR-ABL1 fusion transcript in variant t(9;22;17)(q34;q11;q21)-positive adult acute lymphoblastic leukemia," *International Journal of Laboratory Hematology*, vol. 38, no. 3, pp. e52–e55, 2016.

[9] J. J. M van Dongen, E. A. Macintyre, J. A. Gabert et al., "Standardized RT-PCR analysis of fusion gene transcripts from chromosome aberrations in acute leukemia for detection of minimal residual disease," *Leukemia*, vol. 13, no. 12, pp. 1901–1928, 1999.

[10] J. Gabert, E. Beillard, V. H. J. van der Velden et al., "Standardization and quality control studies of 'real-time' quantitative reverse transcriptase polymerase chain reaction of fusion gene transcripts for residual disease detection in leukemia—a Europe against cancer program," *Leukemia*, vol. 17, no. 12, pp. 2318–2357, 2003.

[11] E. Beillard, N. Pallisgaard, V. H. J. van der Velden et al., "Evaluation of candidate control genes for diagnosis and residual disease detection in leukemic patients using 'real-time' quantitative reverse-transcriptase polymerase chain reaction (RQ-PCR)—a Europe against cancer program," *Leukemia*, vol. 17, no. 12, pp. 2474–2486, 2003.

[12] S. L. McCarron, S. E. Langabeer, K. Bolger et al., "Molecular response to imatinib in chronic myeloid leukemia with a variant e13a3 BCR-ABL1 fusion," *Medical Oncology*, vol. 32, no. 2, p. 452, 2015.

[13] L. Foroni, G. Wilson, G. Gerrard et al., "Guidelines for the measurement of BCR-ABL1 transcripts in chronic myeloid

leukaemia," *British Journal of Haematology*, vol. 153, no. 2, pp. 179–190, 2011.

[14] D. S. Snyder, R. McMahon, S. R. Cohen, and M. L. Slovak, "Chronic myeloid leukemia with an e13a3 BCR-ABL fusion: benign course responsive to imatinib with an RT-PCR advisory," *American Journal of Hematology*, vol. 75, no. 2, pp. 92–95, 2004.

[15] B. Pienkowska-Grela, R. Woroniecka, I. Solarska et al., "Complete cytogenetic and molecular response after imatinib treatment for chronic myeloid leukemia in a patient with atypical karyotype and BCR-ABL b2a3 transcript," *Cancer Genetics and Cytogenetics*, vol. 174, no. 2, pp. 111–115, 2007.

[16] B. Liu, W. Zhang, and H. Ma, "Complete cytogenetic response to Nilotinib in a chronic myeloid leukemia case with a rare e13a3(b2a3) BCR-ABL fusion transcript: a case report," *Molecular Medicine Reports*, vol. 13, no. 3, pp. 2635–2638, 2016.

[17] J. Ha, J.-W. Cheong, S. Shin, S.-T. Lee, and J. R. Choi, "Chronic myeloid leukemia with rare variant b2a3 (e13a3) BCR-ABL1 fusion," *Annals of Laboratory Medicine*, vol. 36, no. 3, pp. 287–289, 2016.

[18] C. A. Seol, Y.-U. Cho, S. Jang et al., "Prognostic significance of recurrent additional chromosomal abnormalities in adult patients with Philadelphia chromosome-positive acute lymphoblastic leukemia," *Cancer Genetics*, vol. 216-217, pp. 29–36, 2017.

[19] H. Pfeifer, B. Wassmann, W. Bethge et al., "Randomized comparison of prophylactic and minimal residual disease-triggered imatinib after allogeneic stem cell transplantation for BCR-ABL1-positive acute lymphoblastic leukemia," *Leukemia*, vol. 27, no. 6, pp. 1254–1262, 2013.

[20] S. E. Langabeer, "Standardized molecular monitoring for VariantBCR-ABL1Transcripts in chronic myeloid leukemia," *Archives of Pathology & Laboratory Medicine*, vol. 139, no. 8, p. 969, 2015.

NGS Analysis of Clonality and Minimal Residual Disease in a Patient with Concurrent Richter's Transformation and CLL/SLL

Shrihari S. Kadkol,[1] Joshua Bland,[1] Ashley Kavanaugh,[1] Hongyu Ni,[1] Vijeyaluxmi Nehru,[2] and David Peace[2]

[1]*Department of Pathology, University of Illinois, Chicago, Chicago, IL, USA*
[2]*Department of Medicine, University of Illinois at Chicago, Chicago, IL, USA*

Correspondence should be addressed to Shrihari S. Kadkol; skadkol@uic.edu

Academic Editor: Pier Paolo Piccaluga

B-cell lymphomas are neoplastic proliferations of clonal B lymphocytes. Clonality is generally determined by PCR amplification of VDJ rearrangements in the IgH heavy chain or VJ rearrangements in Igκ/Igλ light chain genes followed by capillary electrophoresis. More recently, next-generation sequencing (NGS) has been used to detect clonality in B-cell lymphomas because of the exponential amount of information that is obtained beyond just detecting a clonal population. The additional information obtained is useful for diagnostic confirmation, prognosis assessment, and response to therapy. In this study, we utilized NGS analysis to characterize two histologically distinct lymphomas (DLBCL and CLL/SLL) that were detected contemporaneously in an asymptomatic patient. NGS analysis showed that the same VDJ rearrangement was present in nodal (DLBCL) and marrow (CLL/SLL) biopsies confirming that the DLBCL resulted from Richter's transformation of a subclinical CLL/SLL. The V region of the rearrangement remained unmutated without somatic hypermutation. In silico analysis showed that the HCDR3 sequence was heterogeneous and not stereotypic. Minimal residual disease analysis by NGS showed that the tumor clone decreased by 2.84 logs in the bone marrow after R-CHOP therapy. However, a small number of tumor cells were still detected in the peripheral blood after R-CHOP therapy. Subsequent allogeneic transplantation was successful in eradicating the tumor clone and achieving deep molecular remission. We show that NGS analysis facilitated clinical management in our patient by helping to characterize the VDJ rearrangement in detail and by tracking minimal residual disease with high sensitivity and specificity.

1. Introduction

B-cell lymphomas are characterized by clonal expansion of B lymphocytes that contain specific VDJ or VJ rearrangements in IgH and Igκ/Igλ genes. There are approximately 50–60 functional *V*, 25 *D*, and 6 J segments on the IgH locus on chromosome 14 [1]. D-J followed by *V*-DJ joining results in the first level of heavy-chain diversity. This is followed by random nucleotide additions and/or deletions at the D-J and V-DJ junctions that result in the next level of diversity. Many of the rearrangements are unsuccessful and do not result in a functional IgH chain due to premature stop codons or frameshifts. If the rearrangement is unsuccessful on one allele, the B cell attempts rearrangement on the second IgH allele on chromosome 14. If one of the rearrangements in the IgH locus is successful, rearrangement proceeds to the light chains. In a successful VDJ rearrangement on the IgH gene, the 3′ end of *V* and *D* and 5′ end of the *J* segment code for the HCDR3 region of the heavy chain. As a result of nucleotide addition and deletion in the junctional regions, the HCDR3 region contributes maximally towards antibody diversity.

VDJ rearrangements can be detected by PCR amplification with primers that bind the V and *J* segments [2]. Subsequently, the amplicons are analyzed by capillary electrophoresis to determine clonality [3]. A rearrangement of a particular length that is overrepresented is suggestive of a clonal population. However, capillary electrophoresis resolves amplicons based on length alone. In contrast, VDJ amplicon sequencing by NGS has distinct advantages over just length separation and include the ability to determine the (i) identity of the *V*, *D*, and *J* segments, (ii) clonal relationship between histologically distinct lymphomas, (iii) somatic hypermutation (SHM) in the *V* region, (iv) B-cell receptor stereotypy based on HCDR3 length and composition, and (v) minimal residual disease (MRD) with high sensitivity. The ability to obtain multiple pieces of information with a single assay is particularly advantageous for optimizing clinical management in patients with B-cell lymphomas.

Recently, NGS has enabled the analysis of VDJ amplicons at an unprecedented level of depth with implications for diagnosis, prognosis, and therapy [4]. In this case report, we highlight the role of NGS analysis in confirming Richter's transformation of CLL/SLL to diffuse large B-cell lymphoma (DLBCL) in an asymptomatic patient. We demonstrate the power of NGS to characterize the clonal VDJ rearrangement in detail and to follow minimal residual disease (MRD) with exquisite sensitivity in peripheral blood and bone marrow with implications for prognosis and therapy.

2. Case Presentation

A 55-year-old woman presented with mild enlargement of a right posterior cervical node over a period of several months. She had an excellent performance status and denied any constitutional complaints. Excisional biopsy of the enlarged node demonstrated diffuse large B-cell lymphoma (Figure 1, LN, Supplementary File 2). H&E sections showed diffuse effacement of normal architecture by a lymphocytic infiltrate, consisting of sheets of large atypical cells in a background of small lymphocytes. The large atypical lymphocytes contained a small amount of cytoplasm, oval to round nuclei, vesicular chromatin, and one to three prominent nucleoli. The Ki-67 positivity was around 40%, a value much higher than generally observed in CLL/SLL and consistent with DLBCL [5]. Based on these findings, the histopathology in the lymph node was diagnosed as DLBCL. The immunophenotype suggested a possible origin from an underlying CLL/SLL consistent with Richter's transformation (CD20+, CD23+, CD5+, BCL2+, BCL6−, CD10−, and cyclin D1−). The patient's complete blood count and metabolic profile were normal with an absolute lymphocyte count of $3.6 \times 10^3/\mu l$ and serum LDH of 174 U/L (ULN 180). A CT-PET scan demonstrated bilateral FDG avid lymph nodes in the cervical, supraclavicular, and axillary regions. A staging bone marrow biopsy showed extensive involvement by small atypical lymphocytes with a kappa-restricted immunophenotype consistent with CLL/SLL (CD19+, CD20+, CD5+, CD23+, CD10−, and cyclin D1−). In contrast to the lymph node, there was no morphologic evidence of involvement by DLBCL in the bone marrow (Figure 1, BM). Cytogenetic analysis of the marrow aspirate showed a mosaic abnormal female karyotype with 40% of cells harboring a trisomy 12 abnormality.

2.1. Lymph Node and Bone Marrow Analysis by NGS (Supplementary File 1). First, we determined the clonal relationship between the DLBCL in the lymph node and CLL/SLL in the bone marrow by next-generation sequencing (NGS). DNA extracted from FFPE sections of the lymph node and fresh bone marrow aspirate was analyzed for clonality by the NGS Lymphotrack IgH FR1/FR2/FR3 assay according to the manufacturer's protocol (Invivoscribe Inc., Cat no. 7-121-0139, San Diego, CA). DNA was first amplified with FR1-J, FR2-J, and FR3-J primers. Subsequently, the amplicons were purified and sequenced on an Illumina Miseq machine. Prior to amplification, a LymphoQuant B-cell internal control DNA (Invivoscribe, LQ, Cat no. 7-121-0139, 50 cell equivalents/µl) was added to each DNA specimen as a process control. Meticulous attention was followed to avoid contamination at each step. IgH clonality analysis was performed by importing the fastq.gz files into Lymphotrack software v2.4.3 (Invivoscribe). Using the merged read summary, a clonal sequence was defined as a sequence with a read frequency of >2.5% and a frequency of >10X the background (generally the 3rd sequence in the merged read summary) [4].

V-J frequency graphs after Lymphotrack analysis showed that the lymph node and bone marrow specimens from the patient contained a clonal sequence in FR1, FR2, and FR3 reactions. A representative FR3-J analysis with clonal reads is shown in Figure 1. Alignment analysis showed that the clonal rearrangement contained an identical sequence in both specimens, indicating that the same clone of B cells was present in both locations (Figure 2). IMGT V-Quest and IgBLAST analysis showed that the rearrangement was V1-2* 02/*D*5-12* 01/J4* 02. As expected, the sequence derived from the LQ process control was detected in both specimens (V1-69* 01/*D*6-13* 01/J6* 03) suggesting that performance of the assay was acceptable throughout all stages of the workflow. The total number of reads, % clonal (C), and % LQ sequence are shown in Table 1. A lower number of NGS reads were present in FR1-J and FR2-J reactions from the lymph node. FR1-J and FR2-J amplify lengths close to 350 bp and 250 bp, and because DNA is generally fragmented in FFPE tissue, a lower number of reads are to be expected. Nevertheless, the number of reads was still adequate to definitively call clonality because (i) review of the H&E sections showed almost complete effacement of the architecture by DLBCL ruling out a paucity of B cells as a cause of a false clonal call and (ii) FastQC analysis of the fastq.gz files showed that majority of the sequences were between 105 and 155 bp (200,000) with fewer sequences around 250 bp (~100,000) reflecting the distribution of reads after Lymphotrack analysis. Furthermore, the per-base sequence quality was >Q30 in both paired reads until 250 bp indicating a high quality of the reads.

2.2. Detailed Characterization of the Clonal VDJ Rearrangement. The same V1-2* 02/*D*5-12* 01/J4* 02 rearrangement was present in both lymph node and bone marrow specimens (Figure 2) confirming that the DLBCL in the lymph node arose as a result of Richter's transformation of a subclinical CLL/SLL. No other clonal sequence was identified indicating that the clone originated from a B cell with a monoallelic rearrangement. IMGT V-Quest and

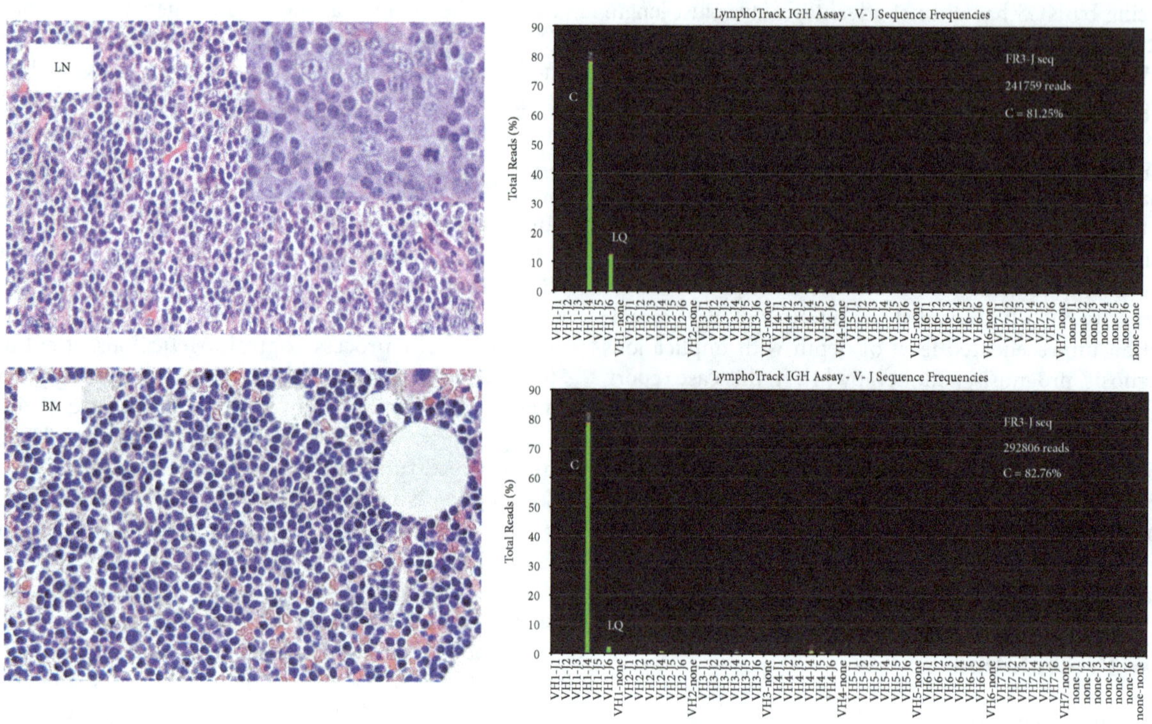

Figure 1: Tumor histology and V-J frequency graphs. On the left are H&E sections from the DLBCL in the lymph node and CLL/SLL in the bone marrow. Inset: high-power view of the DLBCL in the lymph node. On the right are the *V*-J frequency graphs from FR3-J primers showing the clonal and LQ reads. The *Y*-axis is the % of total reads, and *X*-axis is the specific *V*-J rearrangement. Clonal reads are present in both the lymph node and bone marrow. C: clonal, V1-2*02/*D*5-12*01/J4*02, LQ: LymphoQuant control, and V1-69*01/*D*6-13*01/J6*03.

```
V1-2*02/D5-12*01/J4*02

CLUSTAL O (1.2.4) multiple sequence alignment
Lymphnode     CTTCTGGATACACCTTCACCGGCTACTATATGCACTGGGTGCGACAGGCCCCTGGACAAG   60
Bonemarrow    CTTCTGGATACACCTTCACCGGCTACTATATGCACTGGGTGCGACAGGCCCCTGGACAAG   60
              ************************************************************

Lymphnode     GGCTTGAGTGGATGGGATGGATCAACCCTAACAGTGGTGGCACAAACTATGCACAGAAGT   120
Bonemarrow    GGCTTGAGTGGATGGGATGGATCAACCCTAACAGTGGTGGCACAAACTATGCACAGAAGT   120
              ************************************************************

Lymphnode     TTCAGGGCAGGGTCACCATGACCAGGGACACGTCCATCAGCACAGCCTACATGGAGCTGA   180
Bonemarrow    TTCAGGGCAGGGTCACCATGACCAGGGACACGTCCATCAGCACAGCCTACATGGAGCTGA   180
              ************************************************************

Lymphnode     GCAGGCTGAGATCTGACGACACGGCCGTGTATTACTGTGCGAGTGGATATAGTGGCTACG   240
Bonemarrow    GCAGGCTGAGATCTGACGACACGGCCGTGTATTACTGTGCGAGTGGATATAGTGGCTACG   240
              ************************************************************

Lymphnode     ACTCCCTTGACTACTGGGGCCAGGGAACCCT   271
Bonemarrow    ACTCCCTTGACTACTGGGGCCAGGGAACCCT   271
              *******************************

HCDR3 sequence

LN   GCGAGTGGATATAGTGGCTACGACTCCCTTGACTACTGG
BM   GCGAGTGGATATAGTGGCTACGACTCCCTTGACTACTGG
     V1-2        D5-12          N     J4

LN   A S G Y S G Y D S L D Y
BM   A S G Y S G Y D S L D Y
```

Figure 2: Alignment of the clonal sequence from lymph node and bone marrow. An identical clonal VDJ rearrangement is present in both specimens. The HCDR3 sequence is shown in red. The contribution of the *V*, *D*, and *J* segments to the HCDR3 sequence is shown (nucleotide, protein).

TABLE 1: Identification of a clonal population in the lymph node and bone marrow.

	Total reads	Clonal (%)	LQ (%)	PCB (%)
Lymph node				
FR1-J	29,955	41.81	40.96	0.92
FR2-J	83,646	47.94	26.23	0.25
FR3-J	241,759	81.25	12.56	0.43
Diagnostic bone marrow				
FR1-J	365,953	87.83	1.46	0.07
FR2-J	183,447	67.18	1.83	0.40
FR3-J	292,806	82.76	2.24	0.42

Total reads, % clonal, % LymphoQuant (LQ), and % polyclonal background (PCB) reads from FR1-J, FR2-J, and FR3-J primer sets are shown. The clonal VDJ rearrangement was V1-2*02/D5-12*01/J4*02. The LQ rearrangement was V1-69*01/D6-13*01/J6*03.

IgBLAST analysis showed that the rearrangement was productive. Alignment to the germline IGHV1-2* 02 sequence showed that the *V* region remained in an unmutated state suggesting an origin from a naïve B cell that had not yet experienced the germinal center reaction (Figure 3). The HCDR3 was 12 amino acids long: ASGYSGYDSLDY. The *V*-D junction did not show any additions or deletions. The D5-12*01 segment was mostly intact except for the deletion of the last four nucleotides (GTGGATATAGTGGCTA CGATTAC), but with an addition of five nucleotides (CTCCC) at the D-J junction.

2.3. Analysis of HCDR3 Stereotypy. It has been reported that the composition and length of the HCDR3 sequence may influence prognosis and risk of Richter's transformation [6–8]. Hence, we attempted to determine if the HCDR3 from the patient's sequence was stereotypic, because our patient seemed to have a rapid progression of CLL/SLL to DLBCL. Analysis of the FR1-J sequence by the web-based ARRest/AssignSubsets program (https://tools.bat.infspire.org/arrest/assignsubsets) showed that the patient's rearrangement was heterogeneous and did not fit into any of the 19 characterized subsets. Furthermore, the patient's HCDR3 protein sequence did not seem to align well by visual comparison with any of the reported 110 HCDR3 subsets [6,7]. As such, the patient's clonal HCDR3 sequence was considered to be heterogeneous.

2.4. Minimal Residual Disease Quantitation. Bone marrow and peripheral blood specimens were analyzed for minimal residual disease after the patient underwent 6 cycles of R-CHOP chemoimmunotherapy. A PET-CT scan at this time showed resolution of lymph node disease. Data were analyzed first by the Lymphotrack v2.4.3 software (Invivoscribe) and then by the LymphotrackMRD software v1.2.0 (Invivoscribe) to determine minimal residual disease. The clonal sequence that was unique to the tumor was tracked in follow-up specimens.

For each sample, the % clonal and % LQ sequence were calculated as follows:

(Exact match clonal sequence reads/total reads) × 100 = % clonal sequence

(LQ clonal sequence reads/total reads) × 100 = % LQ clonal sequence

MRD in cell equivalents/DNA input (ng) was calculated as follows:

MRD = (% clonal sequence/% LQ clonal sequence) × 100 cell equivalents

Figure 4 shows the VJ frequency graphs for the FR1-J reactions after R-CHOP therapy. Table 2 shows the MRD data. The diagnostic bone marrow contained a tumor clone content of 60,126 cell eq./1000 ng DNA (151,515 cells). After 6 cycles of R-CHOP therapy, the tumor clone decreased by 2.84 logs to 86 cell eq./1000 ng DNA. The clonal sequence was also detected in the peripheral blood at a level of 8 cell eq./1000 ng of DNA indicating that the tumor clone was also circulating in the peripheral blood, albeit at a very low level. Six months later, the patient underwent a successful matched unrelated donor peripheral stem cell transplant. Analysis of posttransplant peripheral blood at day 30 showed that the clonal sequence was still present at an extremely low level in both total DNA and CD19+ B-cell DNA (very few clonal reads). However, at day 60 after transplant, the clonal sequence was not detected in either total or CD19+ B-cell DNA indicating successful eradication of the tumor clone (Figure 5). Furthermore, both total DNA and CD19+ B-cell DNA from the day 30 and 60 peripheral blood specimens showed complete donor engraftment without any evidence of recipient DNA by STR analysis (analytical sensitivity of 3% chimerism). After R-CHOP, there was a sharp contraction of the B-cell repertoire that expanded successfully after transplantation. The patient remains in remission more than two years after transplant with an excellent performance status.

3. Discussion

Our patient presented with DLBCL in a cervical lymph node which proved to be Richter's transformation of a previously undiagnosed CLL/SLL. Richter's transformation of CLL/SLL is an uncommon occurrence with an annual incidence of 0.5–1.0% per year and a median latency of 1.8–1.9 years from the time of diagnosis of CLL/SLL [9, 10]. Prognosis is generally very poor with a median overall survival of approximately one year [11]. Concurrent diagnosis of DLBCL

```
CLUSTAL multiple sequence alignment by MUSCLE (3.8)
GL = Germline IgHV1-2*02

GL    TGAGAGCTCCGTTCCTCACCATGGACTGGACCTGGAGGATCCTCTTCTTGGTGGCAGCAG
LN    ------------------------------------------------------------
BM    ------------------------------------------------------------

GL    CCACAGGTAAGAGGCTCCCTAGTCCCAGTGATGAGAAAGAGATTGAGTCCAGTCCAGGGA
LN    ------------------------------------------------------------
BM    ------------------------------------------------------------

GL    GATCTCATCCACTTCTGTGTTCTCTCCACAGGAGCCCACTCCCAGGTGCAGCTGGTGCAG
LN    ------------------------------------------------------------
BM    ------------------------------------------------------------

GL    TCTGGGGCTGAGGTGAAGAAGCCTGGGGCCTCAGTGAAGGTCTCCTGCAAGGCTTCTGGA
LN    ----------------------------------------------------CTTCTGGA
BM    ----------------------------------------------------CTTCTGGA
                                                          ********

GL    TACACCTTCACCGGCTACTATATGCACTGGGTGCGACAGGCCCCTGGACAAGGGCTTGAG
LN    TACACCTTCACCGGCTACTATATGCACTGGGTGCGACAGGCCCCTGGACAAGGGCTTGAG
BM    TACACCTTCACCGGCTACTATATGCACTGGGTGCGACAGGCCCCTGGACAAGGGCTTGAG
      ************************************************************

GL    TGGATGGGATGGATCAACCCTAACAGTGGTGGCACAAACTATGCACAGAAGTTTCAGGGC
LN    TGGATGGGATGGATCAACCCTAACAGTGGTGGCACAAACTATGCACAGAAGTTTCAGGGC
BM    TGGATGGGATGGATCAACCCTAACAGTGGTGGCACAAACTATGCACAGAAGTTTCAGGGC
      ************************************************************

GL    AGGGTCACCATGACCAGGGACACGTCCATCAGCACAGCCTACATGGAGCTGAGCAGGCTG
LN    AGGGTCACCATGACCAGGGACACGTCCATCAGCACAGCCTACATGGAGCTGAGCAGGCTG
BM    AGGGTCACCATGACCAGGGACACGTCCATCAGCACAGCCTACATGGAGCTGAGCAGGCTG
      ************************************************************

GL    AGATCTGACGACACGGCCGTGTATTACTGTGCGAGAGACACAGTGTGAAAACCCACATCC
LN    AGATCTGACGACACGGCCGTGTATTACTGTGCGAG-------------------------
BM    AGATCTGACGACACGGCCGTGTATTACTGTGCGAG-------------------------
      ***********************************

GL    TGAGGGTGTCAGAAACCCAAGGGAGGAGGCAG
LN    --------------------------------
BM    --------------------------------
```

FIGURE 3: Alignment of the clonal VDJ sequence to germline V1-2*02 The clonal sequence (FR1-J) from the lymph node and bone marrow shows an unmutated *V* region when aligned to the germline *V* gene. GL: germline sequence, LN: lymph node, and BM: bone marrow.

and CLL/SLL, as in the present case, is rare but may be associated with improved survival compared to patients with sequential presentations. A retrospective study of patients with histologically proven Richter's transformation diagnosed between 1993 and 2018 at the Mayo clinic demonstrated that the median overall survival of patients with no prior treatment and concurrent diagnosis of CLL/SLL and Richter's transformation was 66.9 months compared to 29.4 months for patients with sequential presentations [11]. However, clonality analysis was successfully completed in less than 5% of patients in this study. Other investigators have shown that patients with CLL/SLL who develop

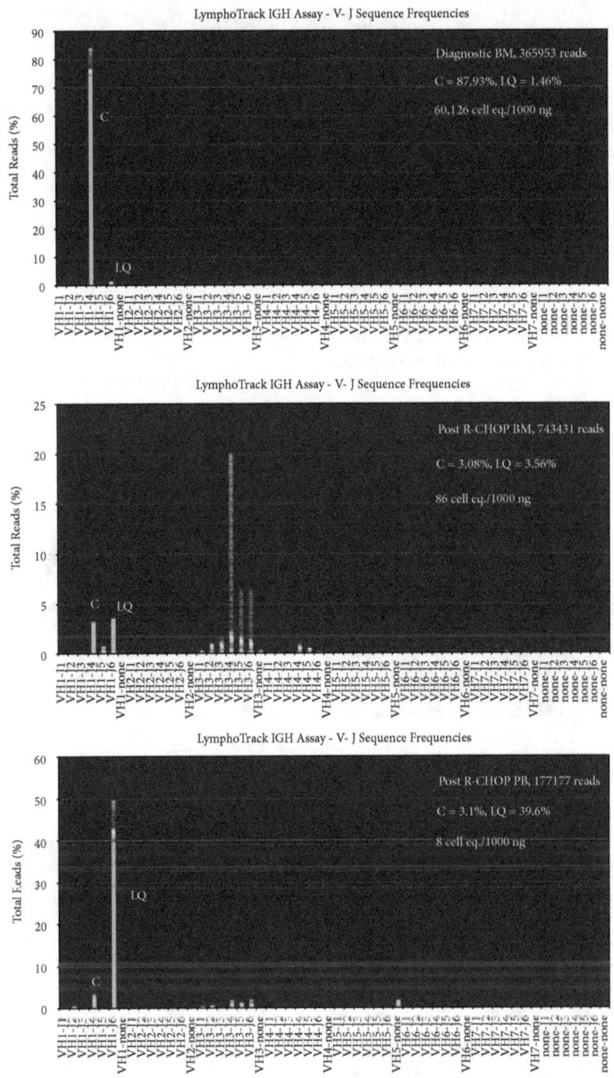

FIGURE 4: MRD after R-CHOP therapy. Clonal reads were detected at a low level in total DNA from bone marrow (BM) and peripheral blood (PB) and after R-CHOP therapy. The B-cell repertoire shows severe contraction in the peripheral blood after R-CHOP therapy. C: clonal and LQ: LymphoQuant.

TABLE 2: Minimal residual disease detection by NGS.

Specimen	Input DNA (ng)	Total reads	Reads				Clonal cell eq. per input DNA	Clonal cell eq. per 1000 ng	Tumor clone, interpretation
			Clonal	LQ	(%) clonal	(%) LQ			
Diagnostic BM	100	365953	321793	5352	87.93	1.46	6013	60126	Detected
After R-CHOP BM	1000	743431	22865	26454	3.08	3.56	86	86	Detected
After R-CHOP PB	1000	177177	5487	70158	3.10	39.60	8	8	Detected
Post Tx PB, TDNA, day 30	1000	220346	8	33874	0.0036	15.37	0.024	0.024	Detected
After Tx PB, CD19+ DNA, day 30	500	2049647	22	35956	0.001	1.754	0.061	0.122	Detected

TABLE 2: Continued.

Specimen	Input DNA (ng)	Total reads	Reads: Clonal	Reads: LQ	(%) clonal	(%) LQ	Clonal cell eq. per input DNA	Clonal cell eq. per 1000 ng	Tumor clone, interpretation
After Tx PB, TDNA, day 60	250	173948	0	4099	0	2.28	0	0	Not detected
After Tx PB, CD19+ DNA, day 60	250	301327	0	1652	0	0.55	0	0	Not detected

DNA input, total reads, % clonal or LQ reads, and clonal cell equivalents/1000 ng of DNA are shown. BM: bone marrow, PB: peripheral blood, TDNA: total DNA, CD19+: DNA from isolated CD19+ B cells, and Tx: allotransplant.

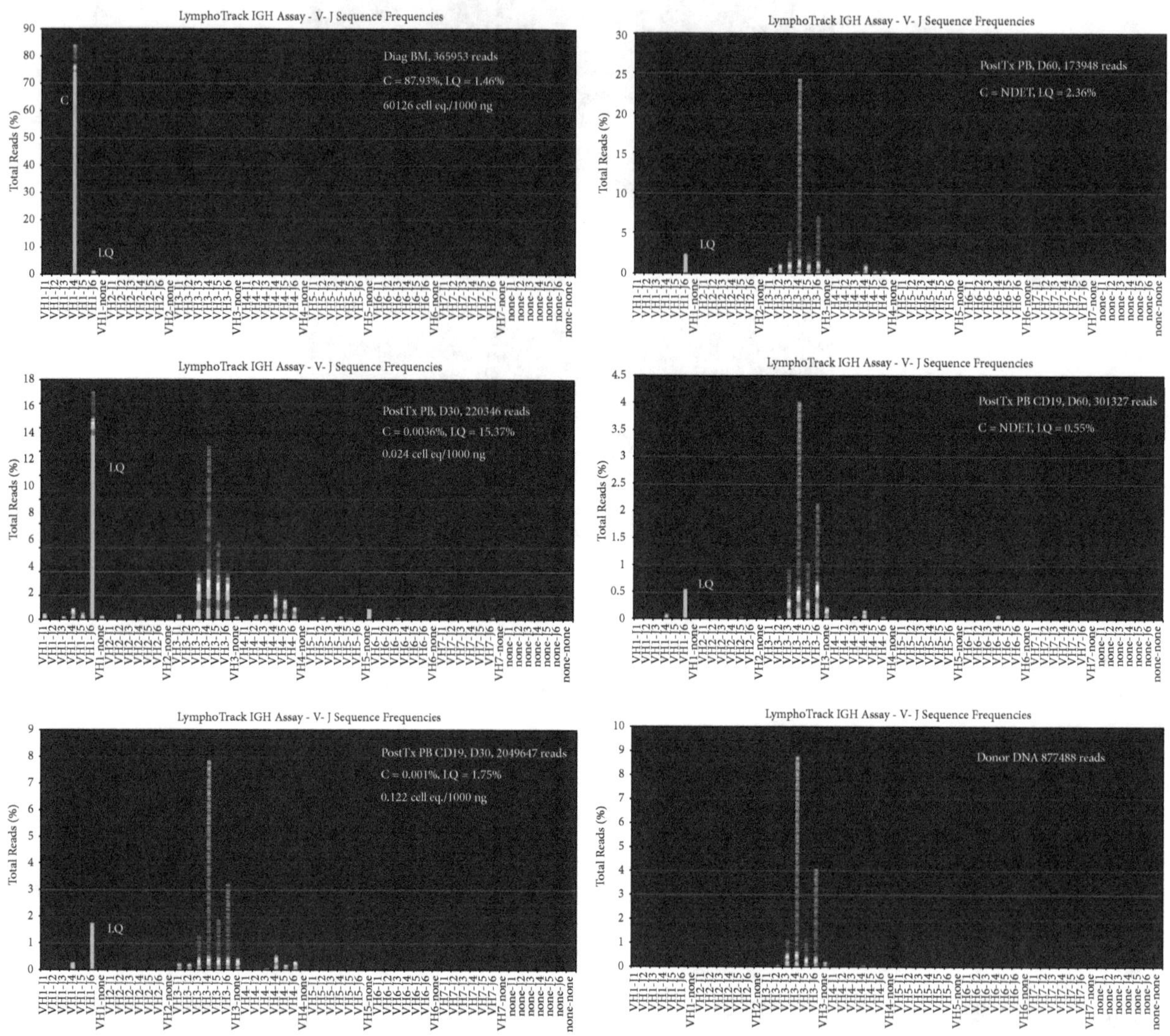

FIGURE 5: MRD after allogeneic transplant. Clonal reads were still present at day 30 after allotransplant in total DNA and CD19+ DNA but were extremely few in number to be visualized on the Y-axis. Clonal reads were not detected in total DNA and CD19+ B-cell DNA in peripheral blood (PB) at day 60 after transplant. The B-cell repertoire in the peripheral blood shows successful expansion and diversity at days 30 and 60 after transplant. C: clonal and LQ: LymphoQuant.

clonally related DLBCL have a much poorer prognosis than patients who develop clonally unrelated DLBCL [12, 13]. Rossi et al. reported that clonally related Richter's transformation was associated with a median survival of 14.2 months vs. 62.5 months for clonally unrelated Richter's transformation, underscoring the importance of definitively establishing clonal status in patients with suspected Richter's transformation [13].

Richter's transformation is well known for dramatic clinical presentations with rapid tumor growth, intense constitutional symptoms, abnormal blood counts, and metabolic aberrations, which were conspicuously lacking in our patient. The development of Richter's transformation in the context of unrecognized subclinical CLL/SLL is also unusual, although not without precedent [14]. It is likely that our patient's transformation to DLBCL was detected at a very early stage due to the obvious site of origin in a cervical node. It is also possible that idiosyncratic features of the patient's DLBCL or host factors such as attenuated immunity or blunted proinflammatory responses may have mitigated against the manifestation of constitutional symptoms and other abnormal parameters.

NGS analysis of the nodal and marrow specimens in our patient showed that, although histologically distinct, the two lymphomas shared an identical productive VDJ rearrangement. Alignment analysis showed that our patient's clonal sequence was unmutated when compared to germline V1-2 * 02 indicating lack of somatic hypermutation and an origin from a pregerminal center B cell that had not yet experienced the germinal center reaction. Furthermore, the patient's tumor also contained trisomy 12 by cytogenetic analysis. Unmutated V gene and trisomy 12 are associated with worse prognosis in CLL/SLL [15]. We next determined if the HCDR3 was stereotypic because BCR stereotypy has been reported to influence prognosis in CLL/SLL [16, 17]. Stereotypy is a feature whereby different patients with CLL have the same VDJ rearrangement with nearly identical HCDR3 sequences. Stereotypic BCRs have been identified in separate patients with CLL even though the random chance of this event occurring in different patients is almost impossible given the number of *V*, *D*, and *J* segments and the random additions and deletions of nucleotides that occur at the *V*-D and D-J junctions during VDJ rearrangement. Healthy persons also seem to carry stereotypic clones that can potentially transform into CLL/SLL [16]. In a study that included the analysis of 7596 IGH rearrangements in CLL/SLL, 18% of HCDR3 sequences were stereotypic [6]. Along with unmutated *V* genes, BCR stereotypy is associated with higher risk of Richter's transformation [15]. In particular, subsets #1, #2, and #8 stereotyped BCRs have the highest risk of transformation to large B-cell lymphoma, whereas subset #4 generally runs a more indolent course [7, 18]. Our patient's HCDR3 sequence was heterogeneous and did not fit into any of the described 19 stereotypic subsets. Because additional subsets are being defined, it is possible that our patient's HCDR3 may belong to a subset that is not yet well characterized at present. In the future, along with mutational status of the *V* gene, stereotypy might better refine prognosis in CLL/SLL patients.

We quantitated the minimal residual disease in our patient by NGS using the clonal VDJ sequence that was identified in the bone marrow specimen. In general, minimal residual disease in clonal B-cell proliferations can be detected by three methods, clone-specific PCR and detection by gel/capillary electrophoresis or real-time PCR, multiparameter flow cytometry, or NGS. For clone-specific PCR, the clonal VDJ rearrangement has to be Sanger sequenced initially. Once the sequence of the VDJ rearrangement is known, PCR primers specific to the clonal VDJ rearrangement must be designed and optimized. Because each patient's clone contains a different sequence, a PCR primer set specific to that clone must be designed for each patient. As such, this method is rather cumbersome and laborious and creates logistical problems with record keeping [19]. If the clonal sequence mutates in the primer-binding regions during follow-up, then false negative results may occur. Multiparameter flow cytometry is a sensitive method to track the malignant clone based on expression of CD markers on the surface of neoplastic B cells [20]. However, this technique requires expensive equipment and a significant level of expertise in interpreting results [19]. Therapy-induced changes in phenotypic expression in the neoplastic clone might lead to interpretation problems. Moreover, the sensitivity of detection may be less than that of PCR-based methods, especially if the assay is not fully optimized or if cellular integrity is compromised. NGS-based analysis of MRD is relatively straightforward in that the same assay that was used at diagnosis can be used during follow-up without the need to design clone specific primers. Compared to the other two methods mentioned above, the technique has superior analytical sensitivity and can detect at least 10^{-6} tumor cells if an adequate amount of DNA is analyzed. NGS also uses equipment that is available in most clinical laboratories and can shed light on the composition of the B-cell repertoire that is not possible with the previous two methods. Moreover, a significant advantage of our assay is that the software for bioinformatic analysis is included and as such, analysis of NGS data is relatively straightforward. The assay can be done in-house with access to the raw data as opposed to sending samples out for analysis to another lab and receiving only a report. Access to raw data allows assessment of quality metrics and detailed analysis of VDJ rearrangements including CDR3 sequences as detailed in this report.

A notable aspect of our NGS assay was the ability to quantitate the tumor clone in cell equivalents/input DNA using a LymphoQuant control that was added to the initial PCR step. The LymphoQuant control contains DNA from a specified amount of tumor cells mixed with polyclonal DNA. It also serves as a process control for the entire workflow. After R-CHOP therapy, the tumor clone decreased by 2.84 logs in the bone marrow when compared to the diagnostic specimen. Even though PET-CT scan showed resolution of lymph node disease, circulating tumor cells were still detected by NGS at a very low level in the peripheral blood after R-CHOP (8 clonal cell equivalents/1000 ng DNA) therapy with a potential for relapse at a later time. Interestingly, the clonal sequence was not detected in the bone marrow or peripheral blood after allogeneic transplantation at day 60 in both total DNA as well as in CD19+ B-cell DNA. These results suggest that R-CHOP alone was insufficient to eliminate the tumor clone and that allogeneic transplant was necessary for deep molecular remission. Our results show that the exquisite sensitivity and ability to track the clonal sequence make NGS the method of choice for MRD detection in lymphoma patients. MRD analysis may have utility in predicting response to therapy or risk of relapse and as such may help to optimize patient management by undertaking preemptive measures. Analyzing CD19+ B-cell DNA increases the sensitivity of detecting the B-cell tumor clone akin to lineage specific chimerism after transplant for leukemias and is required for optimal sensitivity. However, the clinically useful limits of MRD that are associated with prognosis or therapy response are unknown at the present time. More studies are needed to define the kinetics of NGS-based MRD detection in lymphoma, and it remains to be seen whether a deep molecular remission predicts long-term prognosis.

In summary, we show the utility of NGS-based clonality testing for in-depth analysis of B-cell lymphomas. First, we established the clonal relationship between the two lymphomas in our patient. Because NGS analysis provided us with the sequence and not just the length of the clonal VDJ rearrangement, we were able to determine that both lesions contained the same B-cell clone, despite having different histologies. As such, we confirmed that the DLBCL in the lymph node was due to Richter's transformation. At the same time, sequence analysis showed that the clone lacked SHM, a prognostic marker in CLL/SLL. NGS-based sequence analysis simultaneously allowed us to determine if the HCDR3 of the patient's clone belonged to a stereotypic subset. The ability to determine stereotypy is advantageous because different subsets are associated with variable prognosis. Our patient's HCDR3 however did not belong to any of the currently well-characterized subsets. As more subsets are characterized, it may be possible to use stereotypic analysis to refine prognosis. Finally, compared to flow cytometry or capillary electrophoresis, NGS analysis allowed us to monitor minimal residual disease in follow-up specimens with extremely high sensitivity and specificity. Our report illustrates that the exponential amount of information obtained by NGS can be harnessed not only to determine clonal relationships but also to refine prognosis and assess minimal residual disease with implications for prognosis and response to therapy.

Consent

Written consent was not obtained because no patient identifying data are included in the report. The University of Illinois at Chicago Institutional Review Board policy states that case reports pertaining to a single individual do not require IRB approval (https://research.uic.edu/human-subjects-irbs/policies/determination-whether-an-activity-represents-human-subjects-research-at-uic/).

Acknowledgments

The authors are very grateful to Dr. Fred Behm, Head, Department of Pathology, for his support. The authors also thank Carol Dodge, Manager, and the entire staff of the Molecular Pathology Laboratory for facilitating this work. This work was supported by the Department of Pathology at the University of Illinois at Chicago.

References

[1] W. S. DeWitt, P. Lindau, T. M. Snyder et al., "A public database of memory and naive B-cell receptor sequences," *PLoS One*, vol. 11, no. 8, Article ID e0160853, 2016.

[2] J. J. M. van Dongen, A. W. Langerak, M. Brüggemann et al., "Design and standardization of PCR primers and protocols for detection of clonal immunoglobulin and T-cell receptor gene recombinations in suspect lymphoproliferations: report of the BIOMED-2 Concerted Action BMH4-CT98-3936," *Leukemia*, vol. 17, no. 12, pp. 2257–2317, 2003.

[3] A. W. Langerak, P. J. T. A. Groenen, M. Brüggemann et al., "EuroClonality/BIOMED-2 guidelines for interpretation and reporting of Ig/TCR clonality testing in suspected lymphoproliferations," *Leukemia*, vol. 26, no. 10, pp. 2159–2171, 2012.

[4] M. E. Arcila, W. Yu, M. Syed et al., "Establishment of immunoglobulin heavy (IGH) chain clonality testing by next-generation sequencing for routine characterization of B-cell and plasma cell neoplasms," *Journal of Molecular Diagnostics*, vol. 21, no. 2, pp. 330–342, 2019.

[5] E. Gine, A. Martinez, N. Villamor et al., "Expanded and highly active proliferation centers identify a histological subtype of chronic lymphocytic leukemia ("accelerated" chronic lymphocytic leukemia) with aggressive clinical behavior," *Haematologica*, vol. 95, no. 9, pp. 1526–1533, 2010.

[6] A. Agathangelidis, N. Darzentas, A. Hadzidimitriou et al., "Stereotyped B-cell receptors in one-third of chronic lymphocytic leukemia: a molecular classification with implications for targeted therapies," *Blood*, vol. 119, no. 19, pp. 4467–4475, 2012.

[7] F. Murray, N. Darzentas, A. Hadzidimitriou et al., "Stereotyped patterns of somatic hypermutation in subsets of patients with chronic lymphocytic leukemia: implications for the role of antigen selection in leukemogenesis," *Blood*, vol. 111, no. 3, pp. 1524–1533, 2008.

[8] D. Rossi and G. Gaidano, "Biological and clinical significance of stereotyped B-cell receptors in chronic lymphocytic leukemia," *Haematologica*, vol. 95, no. 12, pp. 1992–1995, 2010.

[9] S. A. Parikh, K. G. Rabe, T. G. Call et al., "Diffuse large B-cell lymphoma (Richter syndrome) in patients with chronic lymphocytic leukaemia (CLL): a cohort study of newly diagnosed patients," *British Journal of Haematology*, vol. 162, no. 6, pp. 774–782, 2013.

[10] D. Rossi, E Berra, M Cerri et al., "Aberrant somatic hypermutation in transformation of follicular lymphoma and chronic lymphocytic leukemia to diffuse large B-cell lymphoma," *Haematologica*, vol. 91, pp. 1405–1409, 2006.

[11] Y. Wang, M. A. Tschautscher, K. G. Rabe et al., "Clinical characteristics and outcomes of Richter transformation: experience of 204 patients from a single center," *Haematologica*, vol. 105, no. 3, pp. 765–773, 2020.

[12] P. Abrisqueta, J. Delgado, M. Alcoceba et al., "Clinical outcome and prognostic factors of patients with Richter syndrome: real-world study of the Spanish Chronic Lymphocytic Leukemia Study Group (GELLC)," *British Journal of Haematology*, vol. 190, no. 6, pp. 854–863, 2020.

[13] D. Rossi, V. Spina, C. Deambrogi et al., "The genetics of Richter syndrome reveals disease heterogeneity and predicts survival after transformation," *Blood*, vol. 117, no. 12, pp. 3391–3401, 2011.

[14] S. Jelić, V. Jovanović, N. Milanović et al., "Richter syndrome with emphasis on large-cell non-Hodgkin lymphoma in

previously unrecognized subclinical chronic lymphocytic leukemia," *Neoplasma*, vol. 44, pp. 63–68, 1997.

[15] P. Boddu and A. Ferrajoli, "Prognostic factors in the era of targeted therapies in CLL," *Current Hematologic Malignancy Reports*, vol. 13, no. 2, pp. 78–90, 2018.

[16] D. Rossi, V. Spina, M. Cerri et al., "Stereotyped B-cell receptor is an independent risk factor of chronic lymphocytic leukemia transformation to Richter syndrome," *Clinical Cancer Research*, vol. 15, no. 13, pp. 4415–4422, 2009.

[17] E. ten Hacken, M. Gounari, P. Ghia, and J. A. Burger, "The importance of B cell receptor isotypes and stereotypes in chronic lymphocytic leukemia," *Leukemia*, vol. 33, no. 2, pp. 287–298, 2019.

[18] M. Marincevic, N. Cahill, R. Gunnarsson et al., "High-density screening reveals a different spectrum of genomic aberrations in chronic lymphocytic leukemia patients with 'stereotyped' IGHV3-21 and IGHV4-34 B-cell receptors," *Haematologica*, vol. 95, no. 9, pp. 1519–1525, 2010.

[19] D. Wu, R. O. Emerson, A. Sherwood et al., "Detection of minimal residual disease in B lymphoblastic leukemia by high-throughput sequencing of IGH," *Clinical Cancer Research*, vol. 20, no. 17, pp. 4540–4548, 2014.

[20] A. C. Rawstron, fnm au, C. Fazi et al., "A complementary role of multiparameter flow cytometry and high-throughput sequencing for minimal residual disease detection in chronic lymphocytic leukemia: an European Research Initiative on CLL study," *Leukemia*, vol. 30, no. 4, pp. 929–936, 2016.

Permissions

All chapters in this book were first published by Hindawi Publishing Corporation; hereby published with permission under the Creative Commons Attribution License or equivalent. Every chapter published in this book has been scrutinized by our experts. Their significance has been extensively debated. The topics covered herein carry significant findings which will fuel the growth of the discipline. They may even be implemented as practical applications or may be referred to as a beginning point for another development.

The contributors of this book come from diverse backgrounds, making this book a truly international effort. This book will bring forth new frontiers with its revolutionizing research information and detailed analysis of the nascent developments around the world.

We would like to thank all the contributing authors for lending their expertise to make the book truly unique. They have played a crucial role in the development of this book. Without their invaluable contributions this book wouldn't have been possible. They have made vital efforts to compile up to date information on the varied aspects of this subject to make this book a valuable addition to the collection of many professionals and students.

This book was conceptualized with the vision of imparting up-to-date information and advanced data in this field. To ensure the same, a matchless editorial board was set up. Every individual on the board went through rigorous rounds of assessment to prove their worth. After which they invested a large part of their time researching and compiling the most relevant data for our readers.

The editorial board has been involved in producing this book since its inception. They have spent rigorous hours researching and exploring the diverse topics which have resulted in the successful publishing of this book. They have passed on their knowledge of decades through this book. To expedite this challenging task, the publisher supported the team at every step. A small team of assistant editors was also appointed to further simplify the editing procedure and attain best results for the readers.

Apart from the editorial board, the designing team has also invested a significant amount of their time in understanding the subject and creating the most relevant covers. They scrutinized every image to scout for the most suitable representation of the subject and create an appropriate cover for the book.

The publishing team has been an ardent support to the editorial, designing and production team. Their endless efforts to recruit the best for this project, has resulted in the accomplishment of this book. They are a veteran in the field of academics and their pool of knowledge is as vast as their experience in printing. Their expertise and guidance has proved useful at every step. Their uncompromising quality standards have made this book an exceptional effort. Their encouragement from time to time has been an inspiration for everyone.

The publisher and the editorial board hope that this book will prove to be a valuable piece of knowledge for researchers, students, practitioners and scholars across the globe.

List of Contributors

Marika Okuni-Watanabe
Department of Hematology, Kobe City Medical Center West Hospital, 2-4, Ichiban-cho, Nagata-ku, Kobe City, Hyogo 653-0013, Japan

Keiji Kurata and Kimikazu Yakushijin
Department of Medical Oncology and Hematology, Kobe University Hospital, 7-5-2, Kusunoki-cho, Chuo-ku, Kobe City, Hyogo 650-0017, Japan

Sultan Aydın Köker
Department of Pediatric Hematology and Oncology, SB"U Van Education and Research Hospital, Van, Turkey

Alper Koker
Department of Pediatric Intensive Care, Hatay State Hospital, Antakya, Hatay, Turkey

Adem Yasin Köksoy, Ülkü Gül Şiraz and Emine Tekin
Department of Pediatrics, SBÜ Van Education and Research Hospital, Van, Turkey

Yasemin Kayadibi
Department of Radiology, SBÜ Van Education and Research Hospital, Van, Turkey

Fatima Zahra Rahali and Sanae Sayagh
Hematology Laboratory, University Hospital Centre Mohammed VI, Marrakesh, Morocco
Faculty of Medicine and Pharmacy, Marrakesh, Morocco

Fatima Taher and Houda Nassih
Faculty of Medicine and Pharmacy, Marrakesh, Morocco
Department of Pediatrics, University Hospital Centre Mohammed VI, Marrakesh, Morocco

David Palmer, Lauren Davis and Helena Sivaloganathan
Royal Sussex County Hospitals, University Hospitals Sussex, Brighton BN2 5BE, UK

Timothy Chevassut
Brighton and Sussex Medical School, University of Sussex, Brighton BN1 9PS, UK
Royal Sussex County Hospitals, University Hospitals Sussex, Brighton BN2 5BE, UK

Raisa Epistola and Tiffanie Do
Harbor-UCLA Medical Center, Department of Medicine, Torrance, CA, USA

Ritika Vankina, Daniel Wu, James Yeh and Jennifer M. Lee
Harbor-UCLA Medical Center, Department of Medicine, Division of Hematology & Medical Oncology, Torrance, CA, USA

Michael W. Fleischman
Harbor-UCLA Medical Center, Department of Medicine, Division of Gastroenterology, Torrance, CA, USA
University of California Los Angeles Division of Digestive Diseases, Los Angeles, CA, USA

Jeremy L. Ramdial, Ronan Swords, Mark Goodman and Robert A. Ali
Department of Hematology/Oncology, Sylvester Comprehensive Cancer Center, University of Miami Miller School of Medicine, Miami, FL, USA

Luis E. Aguirre
Department of Internal Medicine, University of Miami Miller School of Medicine, Miami, FL, USA

Rushad Machhi, Ashley M. Cunningham, Kenneth Hennrick, Karen A. Schaser, Eliot C. Williams and William Nicholas Rose
Department of Pathology and Laboratory Medicine, University of Wisconsin Hospital, 600 Highland Ave, D4/250, Madison 53792, WI, USA

Keiki Nagaharu
Department of Hematology and Oncology, Mie University Graduate School of Medicine, Edobashi 2-174, Tsu, Mie Prefecture 514-8507, Japan
Department of Hematology and Oncology, Suzuka General Hospital, Yamanohana 1275-53, Suzuka, Mie Prefecture 513-8630, Japan

Masahiro Masuya and Naoyuki Katayama
Department of Hematology and Oncology, Mie University Graduate School of Medicine, Edobashi 2-174, Tsu, Mie Prefecture 514-8507, Japan

Keiki Kawakami
Department of Hematology and Oncology, Suzuka General Hospital, Yamanohana 1275-53, Suzuka, Mie Prefecture 513-8630, Japan

Ibrahim Alharbi
Department of Pediatrics, Umm Al-Qura University, Makkah, Saudi Arabia
King Fahad Armed Forces Hospital, Jeddah, Saudi Arabia

Sarah Alqarni, Wed Khayyat and Amirah Almatrafi
Umm Al-Qura University, Makkah, Saudi Arabia

Mohsen Jari
Department of Pediatric Rheumatology, Imam Hossein Children's Hospital, Isfahan University of Medical Sciences, Isfahan, Iran

Samuele Ceruti, Andrea Glotta and Romano Mauri
Critical Care Department, Clinica Luganese Moncucco, Lugano, Switzerland

Harriet Adamson
CytoSorbents Europe GmbH, Berlin, Germany

Zsolt Molnar
CytoSorbents Europe GmbH, Berlin, Germany
Centre for Translational Medicine, Semmelweis University, Budapest, Hungary
Department of Anaesthesiology and Intensive Therapy, Poznan University of Medical Sciences, Poznan, Poland
Department of Anaesthesiology and Intensive Therapy, Semmelweis University, Budapest, Hungary

Neeraja Swaminathan, Jorge M. Vinicius and Jesse Serrins
Albert Einstein Medical Center, Philadelphia, PA 19141, USA

Xin Liao
Department of Hematology, Children's Hospital of Chongqing Medical University, Chongqing 400014, China

Yuxia Guo
Department of Hematology, Children's Hospital of Chongqing Medical University, Chongqing 400014, China
Ministry of Education Key Laboratory of Child Development and Disorders, Chongqing 400014, China
China International Science and Technology Cooperation Center for Child Development and Disorders, Chongqing 400014, China

Yali Shen
Department of Hematology, Children's Hospital of Chongqing Medical University, Chongqing 400014, China
China International Science and Technology Cooperation Center for Child Development and Disorders, Chongqing 400014, China
Chongqing Key Laboratory of Pediatrics, Chongqing 400014, China

Jianwen Xiao
Department of Hematology, Children's Hospital of Chongqing Medical University, Chongqing 400014, China
Ministry of Education Key Laboratory of Child Development and Disorders, Chongqing 400014, China
Chongqing Key Laboratory of Pediatrics, Chongqing 400014, China

Aristides Armas Villalba, Marya Haq and Jinen Thakkar
Internal Medicine Department, Kent County Hospital, Warren Alpert Medical School of Brown University, Providence, RI, USA

Cunxian Zhang
Associate Professor of Pathology and Laboratory Medicine, Brown University, Providence, RI, USA
Chief of Pathology, Kent County Hospital, Warwick, RI, USA

Mitali Sahni
Pediatrix Medical Group, Sunrise Children's Hospital, University of Nevada, Las Vegas, NV, USA

Pooja Patel and Akila Muthukumar
Department of Pediatrics, University of Texas Medical Branch, Galveston, TX, USA

Derya Demirtas and Hilmi Erdem Sumbul
Assistant Professor in Department of Internal Medicine, Adana Health Practice and Research Center, Health Sciences University, Adana, Turkey

Abdullah Orhan Demirtas
Assistant Professor in Department of Cardiology, Adana Health Practice and Research Center, Health Sciences University, Adana, Turkey

Ayse Selcan Koc
Assistant Professor in Department of Radiology, Adana Health Practice and Research Center, Health Sciences University, Adana, Turkey

Nada Agbariah and Alicia Rovó
Department of Hematology and Central Hematology Laboratory, Inselspital, Bern University Hospital, University of Bern, Bern, Switzerland

Javier Sanz
Department of Human Genetics, Inselspital University Hospital Bern, Bern, Switzerland

Kengo Hashimoto, Toru Nagao and Satoru Miyabe
Department of Oral and Maxillofacial Surgery, Aichi-Gakuin University School of Dentistry, Nagoya, Japan

Shin Koie and Terumi Saito
Department of Oral and Maxillofacial Surgery, Okazaki City Hospital, Okazaki, Japan

Alexander Pinhas, Oscar Otero-Marquez, Maria V. Castanos Toral and Justin V. Migacz
Department of Ophthalmology, New York Eye and Ear Infirmary of Mount Sinai, New York, NY, USA

Davis B. Zhou, Richard B. Rosen and Toco Y. P. Chui
Department of Ophthalmology, New York Eye and Ear Infirmary of Mount Sinai, New York, NY, USA
Department of Ophthalmology, Icahn School of Medicine at Mount Sinai, New York, NY, USA

Jeffrey Glassberg
Departments of Emergency Medicine,Hematology and Medical Oncology, Icahn School of Medicine at Mount Sinai, New York, NY, USA

Steve Biko Otieno, Alaa Altahan and Saradasri Karri
The University of Tennessee Health Science Center, Department of Hematology and Oncology, 19 S. Manassas, Memphis, TN 38103, USA
The Veterans Affairs Medical Center, 1030 Jefferson Ave, Memphis, TN 38104, USA
The West Cancer and Research Institute, 7945 Wolf River Blvd, Germantown, TN 38138, USA

Fnu Kaweeta
The University of Tennessee Health Science Center, Department of Hematology and Oncology, 19 S. Manassas, Memphis, TN 38103, USA

Fnu Alnoor
The Veterans Affairs Medical Center, 1030 Jefferson Ave, Memphis, TN 38104, USA
The University of Tennessee Health Science Center, Department of Pathology, 930 Madison Ave, Memphis, TN 38103, USA

Robert Johnson
The West Cancer and Research Institute, 7945 Wolf River Blvd, Germantown, TN 38138, USA

Benedetta Mariotti, Federico Meconi, Raffaele Palmieri, Eleonora De Bellis, Serena Lavorgna, Tiziana Ottone, Francesco Lo-Coco and Laura Cicconi
Department of Biomedicine and Prevention, University Tor Vergata, Rome, Italy

Vincenza Martini
UOC Ematologia, Ospedale "Fabrizio Spaziani", Frosinone, Italy

Albaraa T. Alfaraidi, Abdulaziz A. Alqarni, Mohammed T. Aqeel and Turki A. Albalawi
College of Medicine, King Saud Bin Abdulaziz University for Health Sciences, King Abdullah International
Medical Research Centre, King Abdulaziz Medical City, Ministry of the National Guard-Health Affairs, Jeddah, Saudi Arabia

Ahmed S. Hejazi
Department of Oncology, King Abdulaziz Medical City, Ministry of the National Guard-Health Affairs, Jeddah, Saudi Arabia

Alena Strýčková
National Centre of Hemostasis and Thrombosis, Department of Hematology and Blood Transfusion, Jessenius Faculty of Medicine in Martin, Comenius University in Bratislava, Martin, Slovakia
Department of Internal Medicine I, Jessenius Faculty of Medicine in Martin, Comenius University in Bratislava, Martin, Slovakia

Jakub Benko, Martin Jozef Péč, Tomáš Bolek , Matej Samoš and Marián Mokáň
Department of Internal Medicine I, Jessenius Faculty of Medicine in Martin, Comenius University in Bratislava, Martin, Slovakia

Monika Péčová, Jana Žolková, Monika Brunclíková and Ján Staško
National Centre of Hemostasis and Thrombosis, Department of Hematology and Blood Transfusion, Jessenius Faculty of Medicine in Martin, Comenius University in Bratislava, Martin, Slovakia

Noman Ahmed Jang Khan, Ashar Farooqi and Mohamed Alsharedi
Joan C. Edwards School of Medicine at Marshall University, Huntington, WV 25701, USA

Shoja Rahimian, Tushar Pawar, Ian Garrahy and Andrew Rettew
Department of Hematology & Oncology, Reading Hospital, West Reading, PA, USA

Rui Bergantim and José Eduardo Guimarães
Hematology Department, Centro Hospitalar São João, Porto, Portugal
i3S—Instituto de Investigação e Inovação em Sa´ude, Universidade do Porto, Porto, Portugal
Cancer Drug Resistance Group, IPATIMUP—Institute of Molecular Pathology and Immunology of the University of Porto, Porto, Portugal
Hematology & Oncology Unit, Department of Medicine, Faculty of Medicine of University of Porto, Porto, Portugal

Juliana Bastos
Hematology Department, Centro Hospitalar São João, Porto, Portugal
Hematology & Oncology Unit, Department of Medicine, Faculty of Medicine of University of Porto, Porto, Portugal

Maria José Soares
Hematology Department, Centro Hospitalar São João, Porto, Portugal
Cytogenetics Laboratory, Hematology Department, Centro Hospitalar São João, Porto, Portugal

Bruno Carvalho
Hematology & Oncology Unit, Department of Medicine, Faculty of Medicine of University of Porto, Porto, Portugal
Neurosurgery Department, Centro Hospitalar São João, Porto, Portugal

Pedro Soares
Radiotherapy Department, Centro Hospitalar São João, Porto, Portugal

Cristina Marques
Flow Cytometry Laboratory, Clinical Pathology Department, Centro Hospitalar São João, Porto, Portugal

Jennifer Costa
Pathologic Anatomy Department, Centro Hospitalar São João, Porto, Portugal

Fernanda Trigo
Hematology Department, Centro Hospitalar São João, Porto, Portugal

Kathie Wu
Geisinger Medical Center, 100 N Academy Ave, Danville 17822, PA, USA

Yvonne Dansoa and Priyanka Pathak
Geisinger Medical Center, 100 N Academy Ave, Danville 17822, PA, USA
Department of Hematology/Oncology, 100 N Academy Ave, Danville17822, PA, USA

Masato Yasumi, Takaya Endo and Takahiro Karasuno
Department of Hematology, Rinku General Medical Center, Izumisano, Japan

Hiroshi Sata
Division of Hematology, Department of Internal Medicine, Daini Osaka Police Hospital, Osaka, Japan

Venkata Rakesh Sethapati, Ra'ed Jabr, Leyla Shune, Wissam El Atrouni, Patrick R. Gonzales, Wei Cui, and Shivani Golem
University of Kansas Medical Center, Kansas City, KS, USA

Maria Kaparou, Zbigniew Rudzki, Hannah Giles, Vidhya Murthy, Swathy Srinath, Rebecca Lloyd, Maria Zahid Ahmed, Beena Salhan, Saleena Chauhan, Bhuvan Kishore, Richard Lovell, Claire Horgan, Shankara Paneesha, Evgenia Xenou, Anand Lokare, Joanne Ewing, Hansini Dassanayake, Emmanouil Nikolousis, and Alexandros Kanellopoulos
University Hospitals Birmingham NHS Foundation Trust, London, UK

Manuel Beltran
Division of General Internal Medicine, Mayo Clinic, Jacksonville, FL, USA

Sharad Khurana
Division of Hematology & Oncology, University of Arizona Cancer Center, Tucson, AZ, USA

Yennifer Gil
Department of Anesthesia and Preoperative Medicine, Mayo Clinic, Jacksonville, FL, USA

Jason T. Lewis
Department of Pathology, Mayo Clinic, Jacksonville, FL, USA

Rohit Kumar
Division of Medical Oncology and Hematology, University of Louisville, Louisville, KY, USA

James M. Foran
Department of Hematology & Oncology, Mayo Clinic, Jacksonville, FL, USA

Kane M. Laks, Cara Hirner and Barbara Gruner
Department of Pediatrics, University of Missouri School of Medicine, Columbia, MO, USA

Jared Coberly and Katsiaryna Laziuk
Department of Pathological Sciences, University of Missouri School of Medicine, Columbia, MO, USA

Bindu Kanathezhath Sathi
Department of Pediatrics, University of Missouri School of Medicine, Columbia, MO, USA
Pediatric Hematology Oncology, Valley Children's Hospital, Madera, CA, USA

Dan Han, Zhaodong Zhong and Rong Xie
Department of Hematology, Union Hospital, Tongji Medical College, Huazhong University of Science and Technology, Wuhan 430022, China

Yuqian Sun
Peking University Institute of Hematology, Peking University People's Hospital, Beijing Key Laboratory of Hematopoietic Stem Cell Transplantation, Beijing 100044, China

Xiaojian Zhu
Department of Hematology, Tongji Hospital, Tongji Medical College, Huazhong University of Science and Technology, Wuhan 430030, China

Runhui Zheng, Chunyan Wang, Pengfei Qin, Huo Tan and Xiaodan Luo
Department of Hematology, First Affiliated Hospital, Guangzhou Medical University, Guangzhou 510230, China

Xiaobo Chen
Guangzhou Institute of Respiratory Health, Guangzhou Medical University, Guangzhou 510120, China

Jui Choudhuri, Yanhua Wang and Yanan Fang
Department of Pathology, Montefiore Medical Center, Bronx, New York City 10467, NY, USA
Albert Einstein College of Medicine, Pelham PKWY South Bronx, New York City 10467, NY, USA

Leah Geiser Roberts
Liberty University College of Osteopathic Medicine (LUCOM), Lynchburg, VA, USA

Yan Zhang
Liberty University College of Osteopathic Medicine (LUCOM), Lynchburg, VA, USA
Jacobi Medical Center and NCB Hospital, Bronx, New York City 10467, NY, USA

Sepideh N. Asadbeigi and Chelsey D. Deel
Department of Pathology, University of Oklahoma Health Sciences Center, Oklahoma, USA

Alberto Santagostino, Laura Lombardi and Gerard Dine
Department of Clinical Hematology, Troyes General Hospital, 10000 Troyes, France

Pierre Hirsch
Sorbonne University, Inserm, Centre de Recherche Saint-Antoine, CRSA, AP-HP, Department of Laboratory Hematology Saint-Antoine Hospital, Paris, France

Srimanta Chandra Misra
Department of Clinical Hematology, Troyes General Hospital, 10000 Troyes, France
Department of Clinical Hematology, Saint Antoine Hospital, Paris, France

S. Nguyen
Department of Medicine, University of California San Diego, San Diego, CA, USA
Department of Medicine, University of California Riverside, Riverside, CA, USA

P. Teh
Department of Medicine, University of California Riverside, Riverside, CA, USA

J. Zhou and A. von Drygalski
Department of Medicine, University of California San Diego, San Diego, CA, USA
Department of Molecular Medicine, e Scripps Research Institute, La Jolla, CA, USA

E. Y. Chang
Radiology Service, VA San Diego Healthcare System, San Diego, CA, USA
Department of Radiology, University of California San Diego, San Diego, CA, USA

Robert K. McCall
Molecular Pathology Laboratory Network, Maryville, TN, USA

Changlee S. Pang
University of Colorado School of Medicine, Aurora, CO, USA

Mark J. Pettenati
Wake Forest Baptist Medical Center, Winston-Salem, NC, USA

Eoghan Burke
Royal College of Surgeons in Ireland, Dublin, Ireland

Patricia Harkins and Jennifer Kieran
St James's Hospital, Department of Medicine, Dublin, Ireland

Mireille Crampe, Laura Kearney and Stephen E. Langabeer
Cancer Molecular Diagnostics, St. James's Hospital, Dublin 8, Ireland

David O'Brien and C. Larry Bacon
Department of Haematology, St. James's Hospital, Dublin 8, Ireland

Derville O'Shea
Department of Haematology, Cork University Hospital, Cork, Ireland

Shrihari S. Kadkol, Joshua Bland, Ashley Kavanaugh and Hongyu Ni
Department of Pathology, University of Illinois, Chicago, Chicago, IL, USA

Vijeyaluxmi Nehru and David Peace
Department of Medicine, University of Illinois at Chicago, Chicago, IL, USA

Index